SPRINGER PUBLISHING

AF712593

GET THE MOST FROM YOUR BOOK

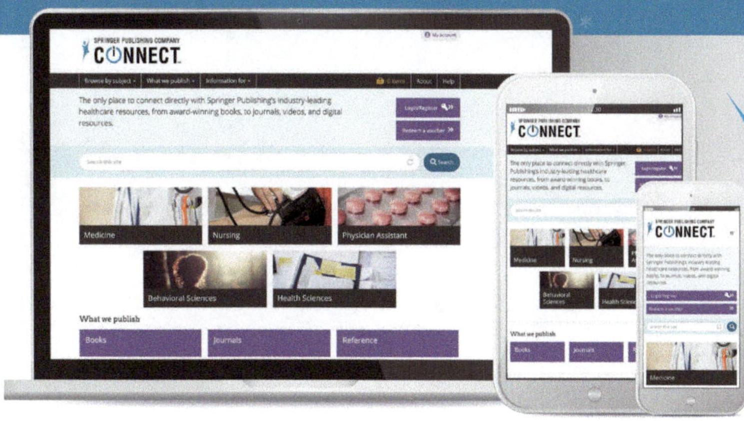

SPRINGER PUBLISHING
CONNECT™

VOUCHER CODE:

EDAH8DYN

Online Access

Your print purchase of *Managing Quality and Safety in Long-Term Care* includes **online access via Springer Publishing Connect™** to increase accessibility, portability, and searchability.

Insert the code at http://connect.springerpub.com/content/book/978-0-8261-4935-0 or scan the QR code and insert the voucher code today!

Having trouble? Contact our customer service department at ***cs@springerpub.com***

Instructor Resource Access for Adopters

Let us do some of the heavy lifting to create an engaging classroom experience with a variety of instructor resources included in most textbooks SUCH AS:

INSTRUCTOR MANUAL

POWERPOINTS

TEST BANK

Visit **https://connect.springerpub.com/** and look for the **"Show Supplementary"** button on your **book homepage** to see what is available to instructors! First time using Springer Publishing Connect?

Email **textbook@springerpub.com** to create an account and start unlocking valuable resources.

MANAGING QUALITY AND SAFETY IN LONG-TERM CARE

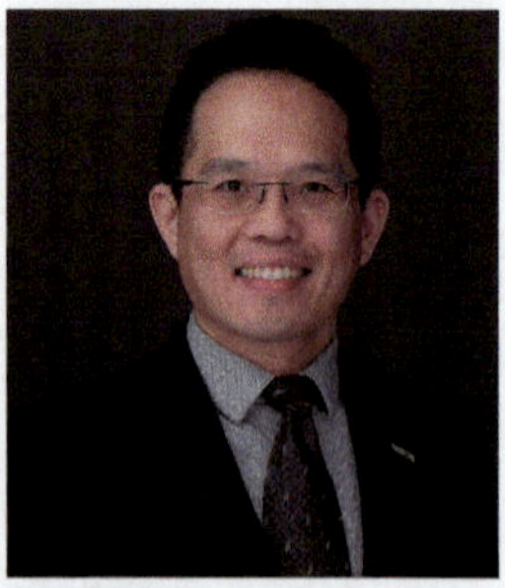

Darren Liu, DrPH, MS, FGSA, is a professor in the Department of Health Policy Management and Leadership at West Virginia University. He earned his master of science in biostatistics and doctor of public health degrees from the University of Pittsburgh. Dr. Liu has made significant contributions to the field through his authorship of two notable textbooks: *The Challenges of Health Disparities: Implications and Actions for Health Care Professionals* (2018) and *Isms in Health Care Human Resources: A Concise Guide to Workplace Diversity, Equity, and Inclusion* (2020). He has served on the board of directors for the Association of University Programs in Health Administration (AUPHA) and is a member of the Diversity and Inclusion Advisory Committee for the Association of Schools and Programs of Public Health (ASPPH). Additionally, Dr. Liu serves on the editorial boards of *Innovation in Aging* and *JMIR Aging*.

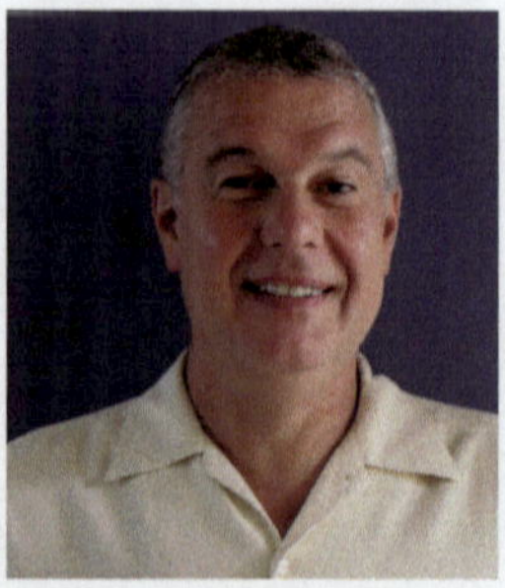

Nicholas G. Castle, PhD, MHA, FGSA, is a professor and chair of the Department of Health Policy Management and Leadership at West Virginia University, with a doctoral degree in health administration from Penn State University. A renowned expert in nursing home quality and safety, Dr. Castle has authored over 230 publications and served as the principal investigator on 14 grants. He also serves as the international editor for *The Gerontologist* and has received numerous accolades, including the American College of Health Care Administrators Long-Term Care Researcher of the Year Award (2001), the Public Health Service Award (2011), and the GSA Brody Thought Leader Award (2016). Additionally, Dr. Castle coleads a committee for the "Moving Forward Coalition," addressing recommendations from the 2022 National Academies of Sciences, Engineering, and Medicine report on nursing home care quality.

MANAGING QUALITY AND SAFETY IN LONG-TERM CARE

Darren Liu, DrPH, MS, FGSA

Nicholas G. Castle, PhD, MHA, FGSA

Editors

SPRINGER PUBLISHING

Springer Publishing Company, LLC
902 Carnegie Center/Suite 140, Princeton, NJ 08540
www.springerpub.com
connect.springerpub.com

Acquisitions Editor: David D'Addona
Production Editor: Susan White
Compositor: S4Carlisle Publishing Services

ISBN: 978-0-8261-4934-3
e-book ISBN: 978-0-8261-4935-0
DOI: 10.1891/9780826149350

SUPPLEMENTS:

SPRINGER PUBLISHING CONNECT™ | A robust set of instructor resources designed to supplement this text is located at http://connect.springerpub.com/content/book/978-0-8261-4935-0. Qualifying instructors may request access by emailing textbook@springerpub.com.

Instructor Materials:
LMS Common Cartridge—All Instructor Resources ISBN: 978-0-8261-5345-6
Instructor Manual ISBN: 978-0-8261-4936-7
Sample Syllabus ISBN: 978-0-8261-4939-8
Test Bank ISBN: 978-0-8261-4938-1
PowerPoint Slides ISBN: 978-0-8261-4937-4

24 25 26 27 / 5 4 3 2 1

Library of Congress Cataloging-in-Publication Data

Names: Liu, Darren (Professor of public health), editor. | Castle, Nicholas G., editor.
Title: Managing quality and safety in long-term care / Darren Liu, DrPH, MS, FGSA, Nicholas G. Castle, PhD, MHA, FGSA.
Identifiers: LCCN 2024039079 (print) | LCCN 2024039080 (ebook) | ISBN 9780826149343 (paperback) | ISBN 9780826149350 (ebook)
Subjects: LCSH: Long-term care facilities—Administration—Textbooks. | Long-term care facilities—Safety measures—Textbooks. | Long-term care facilities—Risk management—Textbooks.
Classification: LCC RA999.A35 M358 2024 (print) | LCC RA999.A35 (ebook) | DDC 362.16068—dc23/eng/20241107
LC record available at https://lccn.loc.gov/2024039079
LC ebook record available at https://lccn.loc.gov/2024039080

Printed in the United States of America by Gasch Printing.

This book is dedicated to:

All those who, including ourselves, have faced or will face the need for long-term services and supports, whether for themselves or their loved ones. Your resilience, courage, and dignity are an inspiration to us all. May this book offer valuable insights and inspire future generations to improve care and support for you and those who will follow.

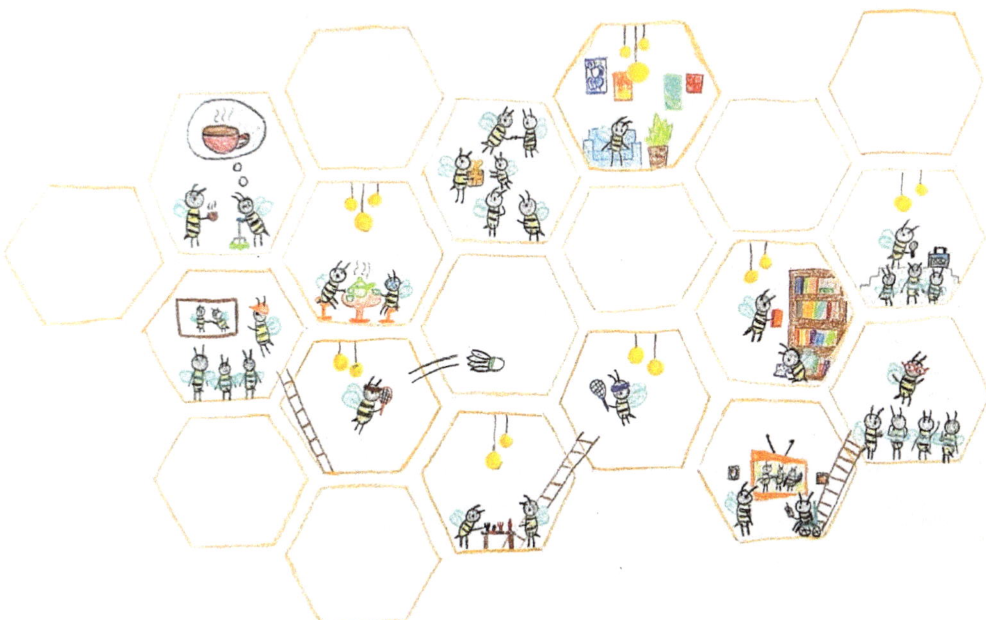

Source: Dora Liu. This artwork portrays the vibrant tapestry of human existence as we age.

Contents

Contributors

Katherine M. Abbott, PhD, MGS, FGSA, is the executive director of the Scripps Gerontology Center and a professor of gerontology at Miami University in Oxford, Ohio. Her research and teaching focus on preference-based, person-centered care, as well as the social networks and health of older adults receiving long-term services and supports. Dr. Abbott is also the co-founder of Preference Based Living, whose mission is to conduct studies that test innovative methods for honoring the preferences of individuals receiving care in diverse settings worldwide.

Kathleen Abrahamson, PhD, RN, CNE, FGSA, FAAN, is a professor at the University of Wisconsin Oshkosh College of Nursing in Oshkosh, Wisconsin.

Robert Applebaum, PhD, MSW, is the director of the Ohio Long-Term Care Research Project at the Scripps Gerontology Center and a professor emeritus in the Department of Sociology and Gerontology at Miami University in Oxford, Ohio.

Bailee Brekke, MGS, is a graduate research assistant at the Scripps Gerontology Center and a doctoral student in the Department of Sociology and Gerontology at Miami University in Oxford, Ohio.

Betty Burston, PhD, MA, is a professor-in-residence at the University of Nevada, Las Vegas. She began her college education at the age of 16 and became actively involved in the civil rights movement and the revolutionary action movement. Dr. Burston was awarded a Woodrow Wilson Fellowship and earned her PhD in economics from Cornell University and American University.

Nicholas G. Castle, PhD, MHA, FGSA, is a professor and chair of the Department of Health Policy, Management and Leadership at West Virginia University.

Heather Davila, PhD, MPA, is a research investigator at the Center for Access and Delivery Research & Evaluation (CADRE) at the Iowa City Veterans Health Administration and a research assistant professor at the University of Iowa Carver College of Medicine.

Natalie F. Douglas, PhD, CCC-SLP, is an associate professor of communicative disorders at the University of Louisiana at Lafayette. She actively collaborates with speech-language pathologists to develop and test interventions aimed at improving communication, life participation, and quality of life for people living with aphasia, traumatic brain injury, and dementia.

Suzanne Kunkel, PhD, is a senior research scholar and executive director emerita at the Scripps Gerontology Center, as well as a professor emerita in the Department of Sociology and Gerontology at Miami University in Oxford, Ohio.

Miranda C. Kunkel, PhD, LMSW, is a consultant at Collaborative Consulting and an adjunct assistant professor in the Department of Sociology and Gerontology at Miami University in Oxford, Ohio.

Sandi J. Lane, PhD, FACHE, LNHA, is an associate professor of public health sciences and the director of the Master of Healthcare Administration program at the University of North Carolina at Charlotte.

Michael Lin, PhD, MSPH, is a senior scientist at Telligen, a population health company in Des Moines, Iowa. He also serves as affiliate faculty at Metropolitan State University of Denver.

Darren Liu, DrPH, MS, FGSA, is a professor in the Department of Health Policy, Management & Leadership at West Virginia University.

Clare Luz, PhD, is an associate professor in the College of Osteopathic Medicine at Michigan State University (MSU) and the founding director of MSU's IMPART Alliance, which is dedicated to strengthening Michigan's direct care workforce.

Pamela Nadash, PhD, BPhil, is an associate professor of gerontology at the University of Massachusetts Boston and a fellow at the LeadingAge LTSS Center at UMass Boston. Her research focuses on health policy and aging, with an emphasis on policies that ensure access to supportive services.

Marcelo Coca Perraillon, PhD, is an associate professor at the University of Colorado Anschutz Medical Campus and codirector of the Population Health Shared Resources Core at the University of Colorado Comprehensive Cancer Center.

Lindsay J. Peterson, PhD, is a research assistant professor in the School of Aging Studies at the University of South Florida (USF), Tampa, and director of the Florida Policy Exchange Center on Aging at USF.

April Temple, PhD, is a professor of health services administration in the Department of Health Professions at James Madison University in Harrisonburg, Virginia.

Kimberly S. Van Haitsma, PhD, FGSA, is a professor in the Ross and Carol Nese College of Nursing at the Pennsylvania State University. She is also the director of the Program for Person-Centered Living Systems of Care, part of the Tresse Nese and Helen Diskevich Center of Geriatric Nursing Excellence. Additionally, she is an adjunct senior research scientist at the Polisher Research Institute at Abramson Senior Care. Dr. Van Haitsma is also the cofounder of Preference Based Living, whose mission is to conduct studies that test innovative methods for honoring the preferences of individuals receiving care in various settings worldwide.

David G. Wolf, PhD, MSJ, MSOL, is the academic program coordinator for the undergraduate and MBA graduate healthcare management programs at Lynn University in Boca Raton, Florida. He is a certified administrator in nursing home, assisted living, and subacute care, and serves as an academic board member of the American College of Health Care Administrators (ACHCA).

Huiwen Xu, PhD, is an associate professor in the Nell Hodgson Woodruff School of Nursing at Emory University in Atlanta, Georgia.

Preface

The U.S. demographic landscape of the past century, as depicted by population pyramids from 1900 to 2020, underscores the critical importance of healthcare management in aging populations. Over this period, profound shifts in population demographics have transformed the healthcare landscape, necessitating innovative approaches to address the unique challenges posed by an increasingly older adult population. From the broad-based pyramids of 1900, indicative of high birth rates and lower life expectancy, to the rectangular shapes of the mid-20th century, reflecting the demographic transition, and finally to the significant bulges in older age groups by 2020, the aging trend has become unmistakable (Blakeslee et al., 2023).

As population pyramids morphed into top-heavy structures, indicating longer life expectancies and dwindling birth rates, healthcare systems underwent a profound transformation. The focus pivoted from primarily addressing maternal and child health and infectious diseases to managing the chronic conditions prevalent among older adults. This demographic shift, from traditionally young societies to ones experiencing a *silver tsunami* of aging populations, has necessitated a reimagining of healthcare delivery globally (Jakovljevic et al., 2021). Consequently, there has been a surge in demand for geriatric care, specialized services, and long-term care (LTC) facilities, prompting the need for comprehensive and integrated care tailored to address the challenges associated with aging.

However, as the demand for older adult care in the United States surged, pressing issues such as shortages in staffing, particularly within direct care workforces, came to the forefront. To effectively address these challenges, healthcare systems must adopt innovative solutions. This entails leveraging technology to enhance care delivery and implementing workforce development initiatives. Additionally, strategies such as task shifting and incentivizing flexible work arrangements are crucial steps toward ensuring the sustainability and effectiveness of healthcare management in aging populations.

In 2023, one of the book's editors, Castle, had the privilege of coleading one of the seven national committees for the *Moving Forward Coalition* (Moving Forward, n.d.). Their mission was driven by the objectives outlined in a 2022 report by the National Academies of Sciences, Engineering, and Medicine (2022), with a specific focus on enhancing the quality of care in nursing homes. Their endeavors encompassed various initiatives, including the enhancement of the LTC workforce. However, as they delved deeper, it became evident that there was a significant gap in preparing the next generation of caregivers through higher education. It was this recognition that propelled us to develop the text you are now reading.

Central to our endeavor is a commitment to prioritizing critical aspects such as quality and safety. We acknowledge their indispensable roles in shaping the well-being and overall contentment of consumers within the realm of LTC. With growing concern over the declining interest among younger generations in topics related to the aging population, we developed this text in collaboration with a team of scholars and practitioners with the aim of guiding interprofessional students in reevaluating the significance of LTC in the United States.

This book comprises four parts, each dedicated to illuminating critical facets of LTC quality and safety. Part I, "Fundamentals of Long-Term Care Quality and Safety," provides a foundational exploration of the broad spectrum of LTC. Part II, "Quality and Safety Practice in Long-Term Care," delves into practical strategies for ensuring excellence in care delivery. Part III, "Strategies for Continuous Improvement of Quality and Safety," addresses complexities in enhancing care outcomes, while Part IV, "Shaping the Future," explores the evolving landscape of the LTC workforce and forecasts upcoming trends and challenges.

Of utmost significance is this book's relevance, particularly in the context of President Biden's executive order (The White House, 2023) aimed at enhancing access to high-quality LTC services. Through its pages, our objective is to kindle students' interest in reconsidering the LTC system as a career goal with a fresh perspective focused on *innovation, addressing health disparities,* and *embracing diversity*. Readers are also introduced to the principles and methodologies of *implementation sciences,* serving as a guide for successfully integrating evidence-based practices into everyday care delivery. We invite you to delve into the pages of this book, where evidence meets practice, and innovation meets real-world impact.

Through the conversations in the final chapter, our intention is to illuminate the perspectives and questions of future leaders in LTC, inspiring them to envision a future where *aging is met with confidence and dignity*. As you navigate through each chapter of this book, you will uncover the fundamental importance of quality and safety in the landscape of LTC, both nationally and globally. These principles serve as the cornerstone of our exploration, guiding us toward a future where individuals can thrive as they age, supported by a culture of excellence and compassion.

While this book uses examples primarily from the U.S. context, readers in the international community should be able to recognize the relevance of these principles to their local cultural contexts. The fundamental concepts of ensuring quality and safety in LTC, along with strategies for addressing challenges such as staffing shortages as well as healthcare disparities, transcend geographical boundaries. By understanding and adapting these principles to their own cultural and institutional settings, readers worldwide can apply the insights gleaned from this book to enhance the provision of care for aging populations in their respective regions.

As the field of LTC continues its evolution, it is essential to acknowledge that this book cannot cover every topic. We extend our sincere gratitude to each chapter author who, amid their demanding teaching schedules and ongoing research endeavors, graciously contributed their firsthand research insights and market acumen to enrich higher education through this volume. We also want to express our appreciation to those who generously devoted their time to review the drafts and provide valuable feedback, enhancing the overall quality and relevance of this publication. Together, let us embark on a journey toward excellence in LTC management.

Darren Liu
Nicholas G. Castle

REFERENCES

Blakeslee, L., Rabe, M., Caplan, Z., & Roberts, A. (2023, May 25). *Age profiles of smaller geographies don't always mirror the national trend*. U.S. Census Bureau. https://www.census.gov/library/stories/2023/05/aging-united-states-population-fewer-children-in-2020.html

Jakovljevic, M., Westerman, R., Sharma, T., & Lamnisos, D. (2021). Aging and global health. In R. Haring, I. Kickbusch, D. Ganten, & M. Moeti (Eds.), *Handbook of global health* (pp. 73–102). Springer Nature.

Moving Forward. (n.d.). *Home page*. Retrieved November 5, 2024, from https://movingforwardcoalition.org

National Academies of Sciences, Engineering, and Medicine. (2022). *The national imperative to improve nursing home quality: Honoring our commitment to residents, families, and staff*. National Academies Press. https://doi.org/10.17226/26526

The White House. (2023, April 18). *Executive order on increasing access to high-quality care and supporting caregivers*. https://www.whitehouse.gov/briefing-room/presidential-actions/2023/04/18/executive-order-on-increasing-access-to-high-quality-care-and-supporting-caregivers

Acknowledgments

We are grateful to our students for their careful proofreading of the drafts, which helped us correct many errors and improve the manuscript.

We especially wish to acknowledge the following individuals for their invaluable assistance bringing this book to fruition:

Steven M. Albert, PhD, MS, FGSA, FAAN
Professor, Behavioral and Community Health Sciences, School of Public Health, University of Pittsburgh, PA

Matt Dameron, LNHA
Executive Director, Summit Square Retirement Community, VA

Debra Dobbs, PhD, FGSA
Professor, School of Aging Studies, University of South Florida, FL

Katherine Kennedy, PhD, MSG, LNHA
Health Science Specialist, VA Providence Healthcare System, RI

Jennifer Kenyon
Subject Matter Expert, BCT Partners, LLC

Tsuann Kuo, PhD, MHA, FGSA
Associate Professor, Department of Medical Sociology and Social Work, College of Medicine, Chung Shan Medical University, Taichung, Taiwan

Edward Alan Miller, PhD, MPA, FGSA
Professor and Chair, Department of Gerontology, University of Massachusetts Boston, MA

Rajean P. Moone, PhD
Faculty Director—Long Term Care Administration, University of Minnesota, MN

Riikka Salonen, MA
Managing Director of Health Equity, BCT Partners, LLC

France Weaver, PhD, MS
Associate Professor and Director, Master of Health Administration, Department of Health Policy, Management, and Leadership, West Virginia University, WV

Takashi Yamashita, PhD, MA, MPH, FGSA
Professor of Sociology & Gerontology, Department of Sociology, Anthropology, and Public Health, University of Maryland, Baltimore County, MD

Instructor Resources

SPRINGER PUBLISHING CONNECT™

A robust set of instructor resources designed to supplement this text is located at http://connect.springerpub.com/content/book/978-0-8261-4935-0. Qualifying instructors may request access by emailing textbook@springerpub.com.

- **LMS Common Cartridge—All Instructor Resources**
- **Instructor Manual**
- **Sample Syllabus** with a course description, course objectives, course requirements, course schedules, and more
- **Test Bank** with 150 multiple-choice questions (including answers and full rationales)
- **Instructor Chapter PowerPoints** summarizing chapter content

SPRINGER PUBLISHING

Visit https://connect.springerpub.com/ and look for the "**Show Supplementary**" button on the book homepage.

PART I

FUNDAMENTALS OF LONG-TERM CARE QUALITY AND SAFETY

CHAPTER 1

INTRODUCTION TO LONG-TERM CARE, QUALITY, AND SAFETY

Nicholas G. Castle and Darren Liu

Learning Objectives

After completing this chapter, each learner will be able to:

- Understand the definition and scope of long-term care (LTC) and long-term services and supports (LTSS).
- Comprehend the difference between activities of daily living (ADLs) and instrumental activities of daily living (IADLs).
- Understand the role of informal caregivers and their challenges in providing care.
- Gain an understanding of the different care approaches, including aging-in-place and continuing care retirement communities (CCRCs), and how they can benefit individuals and families.
- Gain insights into the types of LTC services available, including memory care and hospice care, to facilitate informed decision-making.

INTRODUCTION

Long-term care (LTC) has assumed increasing significance in the U.S. healthcare system. As an overarching introduction for this text, we first expand upon this increased significance. Moreover, in some areas LTC has also provided below par quality of care. This is further described, along with why quality and safety can and do matter in LTC. Also, to further understand quality and safety in LTC we introduce the services and providers used in LTC, and the intertwined lexicon of terms commonly used. Finally, we address how these providers and services comprise the long-term continuum.

LTC is generally viewed as care and services provided to individuals over long periods of time. Few specific time periods are given; rather, LTC is most often defined by the services and settings it encompasses (described in the text that follows). These services and settings are used by many groups, including the disabled and seniors. For example, 70% of adults 65 and over will require some type of LTC during the remainder of their lives. In 2018, approximately 1.32 million individuals resided in U.S. nursing homes, with an additional 900,000 in residential communities, highlighting the substantial demand for institutional LTC (Sengupta et al., 2022). Moreover, 3 million individuals received care from community-based services, indicating additional demand for noninstitutional LTC services. Various factors, including an aging population, advancements in healthcare leading to longer life expectancy, fewer available family caregivers due to smaller family sizes, and increased female employment, contribute to the escalating demand for LTC.

While essential, LTC is complex and expensive, with many aspects subject to stringent regulation, particularly in nursing homes. The COVID-19 pandemic brought attention to longstanding issues of inadequate nursing home quality, prompting calls for reform (Shippee et al., 2020). The 2022 report from the National Academies of Sciences, Engineering, and Medicine (NASEM) highlighted numerous deficiencies in nursing home care and proposed urgent reforms across key objectives, aiming for comprehensive, person-centered care; fair compensation for the workforce; transparent finances; and quality assurance (NASEM, 2022).

In response to the challenges outlined in the NASEM report, the Biden–Harris administration initiated significant reforms, targeting minimum staffing standards, oversight improvements, and transparent ownership in nursing homes. Subsequent efforts in October 2022 introduced stricter oversight, penalties for underperforming facilities, and increased funding to support the nursing home workforce. An executive order signed in 2023 (Executive Order No. 14095, 2023) acknowledged the critical need for accessible and high-quality LTC, recognizing the financial strain on families and the labor-intensive nature of quality care, particularly impacting women of color in the caregiving workforce. As nursing homes care for vulnerable populations, comprehensive reform is imperative, especially considering the aging population, healthcare advancements, and systemic weaknesses revealed by the pandemic, emphasizing the urgent need for reform across all LTC settings.

THE IMPORTANCE OF QUALITY AND SAFETY IN LONG-TERM CARE

Quality and safety matter in many respects. Quality and safety in LTC have ethical, outcome, provider, and regulatory imperatives. Ethically, consumers entrust their well-being to LTC providers, expecting not only adequate care but also an environment that upholds their dignity, security, and overall quality of life. In the realm of health outcomes, quality and safety directly impact consumers' physical, mental, and emotional well-being. High-quality care ensures timely medical attention, assistance with daily activities, and emotional support, contributing to improved overall health outcomes and quality of life for residents. For instance, proper medication management and skilled nursing care mitigate the risk of complications, preserving seniors' dignity while enhancing their overall well-being (Crotty et al., 2004).

The benefits of high-quality LTC for seniors extend beyond the obvious, encompassing less visible yet equally significant advantages. Notably, high-quality care fosters greater job satisfaction among caregivers, reducing turnover rates and potentially attracting more qualified individuals to the profession. Providers offering superior care often attract more business, including higher-paying business, thus positively impacting their financial bottom-line. Furthermore, regulatory compliance is essential for LTC providers, as failure to meet federal and state standards can result in severe penalties, sanctions, or even the revocation of licenses. Regulatory bodies such as the Centers for Medicare & Medicaid Services (CMS) establish guidelines governing staffing ratios, safety protocols, and quality benchmarks, underscoring the critical importance of adherence to these standards for sustained operations and certification.

QUALITY AND SAFETY MEASUREMENT

Quality and safety measurement in LTC involves a multifaceted approach, encompassing various assessments and protocols to ensure optimal resident well-being and satisfaction. Quality indicators, ranging from patient and family satisfaction surveys to external assessments such as state inspections, serve as crucial accountability tools, allowing providers to evaluate their performance against established benchmarks and standards. This comprehensive evaluation enables the identification of areas for improvement and ensures alignment with accepted levels of care.

Conversely, safety measures within LTC facilities are geared toward proactively preventing accidents, injuries, or incidents that could jeopardize residents' health and safety (Castle & Ferguson, 2010; Mor, 2006). These measures include protocols for fall prevention, infection control, medication management, and emergency preparedness, among others. Adherence to safety protocols not only mitigates risks but also fosters a sense of security among residents, significantly enhancing their overall quality of life. Incident reporting systems play a pivotal role by encouraging workers to report safety concerns anonymously (Wagner et al., 2006), facilitating the identification and resolution of potential risks and systemic issues (Serre et al., 2022).

Maintaining high standards of quality and safety in LTC requires more than meeting prescribed criteria; it necessitates cultivating a culture of excellence. This culture is characterized by a commitment to delivering compassionate, person-centered care that transcends regulatory frameworks and permeates daily practices and interactions within the facility (Abusalem et al., 2021). Such an environment ensures that residents feel valued, respected, and secure, fulfilling the fundamental purpose of LTC. Additionally, this approach underscores the importance of continuous improvement, making it an essential skill for LTC leadership to cultivate.

UNDERSTANDING LONG-TERM CARE AND LONG-TERM SERVICES AND SUPPORTS

The LTC encompasses a diverse range of services aimed at meeting the health, personal care, and social needs of individuals requiring ongoing assistance due to chronic illness, disabilities, or aging-related issues. These services support individuals who cannot manage their care independently and cover activities known as activities of daily living (ADL) and instrumental activities of daily living (IADL). Table 1.1 provides a comparison between ADLs and IADLs, outlining their definitions, scopes, examples, and impacts on independence and assistance needs.

The terms *long-term care* (LTC) and *long-term services and supports* (LTSS) are often used interchangeably, yet they possess subtle differences in origin and scope. LTC initially referred to a range of services addressing both medical and nonmedical needs of individuals with chronic illnesses and disabilities, often involving assistance with ADLs and encompassing medical care, personal assistance, and social support. On the other hand, LTSS takes a broader approach, acknowledging that healthcare alone may not adequately address the multifaceted needs essential to an individual's well-being. While LTSS encompasses healthcare services, it also includes an array of nonmedical support systems, social services, community-based assistance, and even transportation or counseling. These components are pivotal in fostering independence and delivering comprehensive care. Table 1.2 delineates the distinguishing features between LTC and LTSS.

TABLE 1.1 Comparison: ADLs Versus IADLs

ASPECT	ADLs	IADLs
Definition	Fundamental self-care tasks	Skills related to managing one's environment
Scope	Personal care and hygiene	Managing household, community, and social tasks
Examples	Bathing, dressing, eating	Meal preparation, managing finances, transportation
Dependency level	Essential for personal well-being and survival	Important for community engagement and autonomy
Impact on independence	Critical for basic functioning	Contributes to autonomy and social participation
Assistance needs	Often requires more direct assistance	May involve guidance or support rather than direct assistance
Assessment in care planning	Key focus in assessing care needs	Assesses broader functional independence

ADLs, activities of daily living; IADLs, instrumental activities of daily living.

TABLE 1.2 Differences Between LTC and LTSS

ASPECT	LTC	LTSS
Focus	Primarily healthcare-centered care	Comprehensive, includes healthcare and nonmedical support
Scope	Emphasizes medical care, ADL assistance	Broader, encompasses medical, social, and community support
Services provided	Medical care, ADLs (bathing, dressing, etc.)	Healthcare, social services, transportation, counseling, community support
Setting	Often institutional (nursing homes, ALFs)	Inclusive of institutional and community-based care
Duration of care	Can include both short-term care and LTC	Primarily focuses on LTC needs
Regulatory focus	Compliance with healthcare-related regulations	Integrates healthcare regulations with social services
Holistic approach	Emphasizes essential healthcare and custodial care	Prioritizes holistic well-being and independence
Example programs/ initiatives	Medicare-certified nursing homes, rehab centers	Aging-in-place initiatives, Medicaid HCBS waivers

ADLs, activities of daily living; ALF, assisted-living facility; HCBS, home- and community-based services; LTC, long-term care; LTSS, long-term services and supports.

While LTC and LTSS overlap in usage, understanding their nuances is crucial for navigating the diverse care options available in the United States. Depending on the context or focus of discussion, one term may be preferred over the other. However, both concepts aim to provide a continuum of care tailored to meet the unique needs of individuals requiring extended assistance, whether in institutional settings or within their communities. This understanding lays the foundation for exploring the continuum of care further.

UNDERSTANDING LONG-TERM CAREGIVERS: FORMAL VERSUS INFORMAL

LTC is vital for individuals requiring extended assistance due to chronic illness, disabilities, or age-related challenges. It is provided by caregivers who are either formal or informal. These caregivers form a diverse network dedicated to enhancing the quality of life for those in need. Table 1.3 offers an overview comparing the key components of formal caregivers versus informal caregivers.

Formal caregivers are professionally trained individuals employed in various healthcare facilities or agencies, including nursing homes, assisted living facilities, hospice centers, and hospitals. They offer skilled medical care, assist with ADLs, provide therapy, and ensure social support for their patients. Typically formal caregivers hold certifications or degrees in healthcare and receive salaries or wages for their services, which are regulated by healthcare governing bodies. Their availability is aligned with the schedules of their facilities or agencies, granting them access to professional resources, ongoing training, and support networks. By maintaining a professional caregiver–patient relationship, formal caregivers offer consistent and structured support to ensure continuity of care. This consistency serves as a quality indicator; in settings such as nursing homes, metrics are often used to measure the presence of the same caregiver caring for a resident, a practice known as consistent resident assignment (Castle, 2011).

Nursing staff in LTC, including RNs, LPNs, licensed vocational nurses (LVNs), and certified nursing assistants (CNAs) or aides, play crucial roles in healthcare delivery. These nursing staff

TABLE 1.3 Formal Versus Informal Caregivers: The Comparison

ASPECT	FORMAL CAREGIVERS	INFORMAL CAREGIVERS
Care setting	Employed in healthcare facilities (nursing homes, hospitals) or agencies	Provide care in various settings (homes, community)
Training and qualifications	Professional training and certifications (e.g., nursing degrees, licenses)	Typically lack formal healthcare training
Scope of responsibilities	Provide skilled medical care, ADL assistance, therapy, and social support	Offer emotional support, assist with ADLs, advocate for care
Employment	Employed by healthcare facilities or agencies	Not employed specifically as caregivers
Payment	Paid salaries or hourly wages	Unpaid or may receive some financial support
Regulation and oversight	Regulated by healthcare governing bodies and certifications	Less formal regulation and oversight
Availability	Available on schedules within care facilities	Available based on personal availability and commitment
Professional support and resources	Access to healthcare resources, training, and support networks	Limited access to formal training or resources
Relationship with recipients of care	Professional and structured caregiver–patient relationship	Often familial or close relationships, personal connections
Continuity of care	Consistent and structured caregiving support	Dependent on personal availability and circumstances

ADL, activities of daily living.

perform a variety of healthcare functions typically linked to their training. However, some counterintuitive relationships are evident; for example, the vast majority of care in nursing homes is delivered by CNAs (caregivers with the least training). The characteristics of these nursing staff can have a profound influence on quality. Factors such as staff satisfaction, staff training, staffing levels, turnover, and retention are all linked to quality. Not surprisingly, in many settings the characteristics of nursing staff are key quality metrics. However, many of these metrics are under the jurisdiction of administration (e.g., satisfaction, staff training, staffing levels, turnover, and retention). This also makes LTC administration extremely influential.

In addition to the clinical or nursing staff, the landscape of LTC providers is enriched by an ensemble of other vital formal (nonclinical) caregivers. These professionals, including therapists, dietitians, social workers, and activities coordinators, form an intricate support network aimed at enhancing residents' overall quality of life. While not directly involved in medical care, these caregivers play an equally significant role in facilitating emotional well-being, social engagement, and personalized assistance. Their collective efforts contribute to creating an environment that transcends just medical treatment, emphasizing the importance of many forms of care in ensuring residents' happiness, comfort, and sense of belonging within their LTC community.

In contrast, *informal caregivers* usually refer to individuals who are typically not employed specifically as caregivers and may receive limited or no compensation. Their roles extend beyond the conventional framework of formal caregiving and often involve family members, friends, or neighbors who undertake various responsibilities to aid individuals in need. These informal caregivers are diverse and can range from high-school students helping care for their grandparents to 85-year-old seniors caring for their 90-year-old spouses. They play multifaceted roles, offering emotional support, assisting with IADLs and ADLs, providing companionship, and advocating for the well-being of their loved ones. Their support ranges from helping with household chores, providing transportation to medical appointments, and administering medications to offering companionship and moral support. Subject to less formal regulation and oversight, their availability relies on personal commitment and availability. These informal caregivers are in fact the most numerous LTC caregivers, with figures in the millions.

Informal caregivers, although not professionally trained in healthcare, exhibit unwavering dedication and commitment, driven by personal relationships and a desire to ensure the comfort and well-being of their loved ones. Their roles can be demanding, often requiring significant time, effort, and emotional investment. This can come at a cost. A substantial body of research has shown informal caregivers can be predisposed to physical and emotional strain, affecting their own well-being.

Acknowledging and supporting these caregivers through respite care, access to resources, and emotional support becomes imperative to sustain both the caregivers' and care recipients' quality of life. It is also worth noting that informal caregivers often lack access to formal training or resources and provide care based on familial or personal connections, resulting in a caregiving continuity largely determined by their personal circumstances and availability.

THE CONTINUUM OF LONG-TERM CARE

The previous text highlights that, in general, LTC is a process. For most individuals, this process involves a spectrum of services tailored to meet diverse and evolving needs. From initial diagnosis or injury through rehabilitation, recovery, and ongoing supportive care, this continuum theoretically ensures a seamless journey for those in need. But for many the journey is not as seamless as we would like, and real quality problems exist. The transitions in care involved are not always timely and vital information is not always readily available.

Part of the LTC process often involves acute care, such as hospitalization or ED visits, preceding LTC. Collaborative efforts between acute care and postacute care settings, detailed in a discharge plan, can foster continuity of care, reduce errors, and maintain consistent treatment across diverse care settings, ensuring quality care and achievable recovery goals.

Navigating LTC planning requires a nuanced understanding of individual needs and preferences. The continuum of care comprises various models, each tailored to address specific requirements and circumstances. Table 1.4 provides an overview of different care models, highlighting their descriptions, key emphases, and key features. These models cater to diverse needs and preferences, emphasizing aspects such as independence, specialized care, social engagement, and support levels within different settings.

For example, the aging-in-place model advocates for individuals remaining in their familiar homes while receiving essential care and services (Forsyth & Molinsky, 2021). While the book may not explore every aspect of each care model extensively, it highlights the critical importance of maintaining high standards of care and safety, particularly in contexts such as aging-in-place, which prioritize personal autonomy and familiarity. Assisted living offers moderate support, while nursing homes provide varying levels of care, including comprehensive medical care and rehabilitation. Memory care units offer specialized support for individuals dealing with memory-related conditions, emphasizing comfort and tailored care. Hospice facilities, providing end-of-life care, focus on comfort and palliative care; this service is often covered by Medicare, with a strong emphasis on family involvement.

Continuing care retirement communities (CCRCs) stand as multifaceted ecosystems within the LTC spectrum. Offering diverse care levels within one campus, these communities cater to varying needs—from independent living to skilled nursing care. By encapsulating various levels of care within a unified environment, CCRCs provide a seamless transition for individuals requiring escalating levels of support as their needs evolve.

TABLE 1.4 Comparison of Long-Term Care Models

CARE MODEL	DESCRIPTION	EMPHASIS	KEY FEATURES
Aging-in-place	Allows individuals to stay in their homes while receiving necessary care and support.	Independence, familiarity	Home modifications, community-based services, personalized care plans; cost-effective long-term
Assisted living	Offers moderate support and personal care services within a community setting.	Supportive environment, social engagement	Assistance with daily activities, social activities and events, varying levels of care
Nursing homes/ skilled nursing	Provides comprehensive medical care, rehabilitation, and various levels of assistance.	Medical care, specialized support	Skilled nursing care, rehabilitation services, safety protocols, varied levels of medical support; can be expensive based on level of care
Memory care units	Tailored care for individuals dealing with memory-related conditions, focusing on specialized support and comfort.	Specialized care, enhanced safety	Structured programs, safety features, specialized care for cognitive challenges
Hospice care	Focuses on comfort and palliative care, offering specialized medical support, often covered by Medicare.	Palliative care, family involvement	End-of-life care, comfort-focused, family involvement
Continuing care retirement communities	Provides various levels of care within a single community, allowing for seamless transitions as care needs evolve.	Continuum of care, diverse care options	Independent living to skilled nursing, multiple levels of care available within one campus; entry fees, monthly fees, healthcare costs

Source: Alzheimer's Association. (n.d.). *Hospice care.* Retrieved May 12, 2024, from https://www.alz.org/help-support/caregiving/care-options/hospice-care; Alzheimer's Association. (n.d.). *Long-term care.* Retrieved May 12, 2024, from https://www.alz.org/help-support/caregiving/care-options/long-term-care; Kane, R. A. (2001). Long-term care and a good quality of life: Bringing them closer together. *The Gerontologist, 41*(3), 293–304. https://doi.org/10.1093/geront/41.3.293; Wiles, J. L., Leibing, A., Guberman, N., Reeve, J., & Allen, R. E. S. (2012). The meaning of "aging in place" to older people. *The Gerontologist, 52*(3), 357–366. https://doi.org/10.1093/geront/gnr098

In addition to traditional care settings, home- and community-based services (HCBS) have emerged as important alternatives. HCBS encompass various services—from personal care to skilled nursing care—fostering independence while delivering vital assistance, enabling individuals to remain in their homes or community settings. Integrating HCBS into the LTC discourse broadens the spectrum of possibilities, highlighting individualized care plans and community resource integration to bolster support.

Each model within the LTC continuum brings its unique focus, ensuring comprehensive addressing of individuals' needs, whether through independence, specialized medical care, social engagement, or tailored support services. Aligning the chosen model with an individual's needs and preferences harnesses the versatility offered by this continuum, ultimately enhancing the quality of care and quality of life for those in need. Case Study 1.1 demonstrates a scenario where a coordinated transition through different care settings optimizes patient outcomes and family involvement, underscoring the importance of seamless care coordination and interdisciplinary collaboration.

Case Study 1.1 Smith Family's Journey Through Stroke Recovery

The Smith family consists of Mr. and Mrs. Smith, both in their late 70s, and their daughter, Sarah, who lives in another state. Mr. Smith recently had a stroke, requiring immediate hospitalization for acute care.

Acute care phase: Mr. Smith was admitted to the hospital where he received acute medical treatment and stabilization. During his stay, the hospital team initiated discussions about the next phase of care.

Transition to subacute care: Following his initial treatment, Mr. Smith was transferred to a subacute care facility specializing in stroke rehabilitation. Here, he received intensive therapy, including physical, occupational, and speech therapies to regain his motor skills and speech.

Postacute care at home: After several weeks of progress, Mr. Smith's condition improved significantly. The care team, in collaboration with Mrs. Smith and their daughter Sarah, developed a discharge plan. They arranged for home health services to continue Mr. Smith's rehabilitation and provide ongoing support at home.

Continued support and follow-up: Once at home, Mr. Smith received regular visits from home health professionals. The care plan included medication management, therapy sessions, and assistance with daily activities. Sarah ensured that her parents had access to community resources for additional support.

Long-term planning: As Mr. Smith continued to progress, the focus shifted to long-term strategies for maintaining his health. The care team provided guidance on lifestyle modifications, home safety measures, and regular check-ins to monitor his well-being.

Case Study Discussion Questions

1. What are the key considerations in coordinating care transitions for a patient like Mr. Smith moving through various care settings? How can effective communication among the care team, patient, and family members be ensured during these transitions?
2. In what ways does the involvement of family members, particularly Sarah, impact Mr. Smith's care journey? Discuss the significance of family support in the postacute and long-term phases of care, considering its role in both emotional well-being and practical care management.
3. Reflecting on the continuum of care provided to Mr. Smith, what systemic improvements or strategies could enhance the integration and effectiveness of care across acute, subacute, home, and LTC settings? How might technology or interdisciplinary collaboration play a role in optimizing this continuum for stroke rehabilitation and ongoing support?

When considering care choices, evaluating the quality and safety of care spans across crucial dimensions. It involves assessing the level of care provided, the reputation of the facility, the available medical services, opportunities for social engagement, and the financial implications. This comprehensive assessment forms the foundation for informed decision-making.

Initiating planning well in advance is instrumental in ensuring that decisions about care are well-considered. This preparatory phase allows individuals to take into account their health conditions, personal preferences, and financial considerations. By addressing these aspects proactively, individuals and their families can navigate care choices more effectively. However, in many cases illness (say a fall) can be unexpected, and individuals and their families are put in situations wherein they have to make quick LTC choices.

In this decision-making process, the involvement of family members, legal advisors, and financial planners is invaluable. Their collective expertise contributes to creating a comprehensive care plan that not only addresses healthcare needs but also encompasses financial and legal aspects. This inclusive approach ensures that care decisions are made with a full understanding of the individual's needs and circumstances. Case Study 1.2 depicts this decision-making process.

Case Study 1.2 Navigating Care Choices Through Care Compare

Background

Mr. and Mrs. Johnson, both in their early 80s, found themselves in a challenging situation as Mr. Johnson's health deteriorated, requiring specialized care due to Parkinson disease. Their daughter, Emily, residing in the same city, took on the responsibility of researching and coordinating her father's care. Aware of the complexities involved, Emily turned to online resources for guidance, landing on the Care Compare website (www.medicare.gov/care-compare).

Initial Phase: Research and Decision-Making

Emily delved into the Care Compare website, navigating its user-friendly interface and selected "nursing homes" as the type of provider to explore various nursing homes in their area. She prioritized factors such as quality ratings, staffing levels, health inspections, and the facility's report card. With these insights, she compiled a list of potential nursing homes that aligned with her father's specific care needs and preferences.

Engaging With Family and Health Professionals

Armed with information from the Care Compare website, Emily initiated discussions with her family and Mr. Johnson's healthcare team. She shared her findings, emphasizing the importance of involving them in the decision-making process. Together, they reviewed the details, discussing each facility's strengths and weaknesses, considering how they aligned with Mr. Johnson's requirements.

Collaborative Decision-Making

The family and healthcare professionals engaged in open dialogues, weighing the pros and cons of each facility based on their search results of the Care Compare data. This collaborative effort ensured that everyone had a voice in the decision-making process. They narrowed down the options, considering factors such as specialized Parkinson care programs, proximity to family, and the facility's track record in managing similar cases.

Outcome and Action

After thorough discussions and deliberation, the family, with input from the healthcare professionals, finalized a nursing home that met Mr. Johnson's needs and aligned with their collective preferences. Emily actively participated in communicating their decision to the chosen facility, ensuring a seamless transition for her father's care.

Ongoing Support and Review

As Mr. Johnson settled into the new nursing home, Emily continued to refer to the Care Compare website for ongoing monitoring and evaluation. She regularly engaged with the facility staff, communicating any concerns or queries while utilizing the platform's resources to ensure her father received the best possible care. Through the utilization of the Care Compare website as a pivotal tool for research and decision-making, the Johnson family navigated the challenging landscape of finding suitable care for Mr. Johnson. Their collaborative approach, involving both family members and healthcare professionals, led to a well-informed choice that prioritized Mr. Johnson's comfort and well-being.

Case Study Discussion Questions

1. How might Emily's use of the Care Compare website have influenced the decision-making process differently if she hadn't engaged the healthcare team and family members in the discussion? What critical perspectives or insights might have been missed in this scenario?

(continued)

Case Study 1.2 Navigating Care Choices Through Care Compare (*continued*)

2. Considering the prioritization of factors such as quality ratings, staffing levels, and specialized care programs, how might these elements vary in importance for different families or individuals seeking nursing home care? Are there situations where certain factors might take precedence over others?
3. Reflecting on the Johnson family's approach to ongoing support and review after Mr. Johnson settled into the nursing home, what proactive strategies could families employ to continually assess and ensure the quality of care in such facilities beyond the initial decision-making phase? How might technology or other resources aid in this ongoing evaluation process?

CONTEMPORARY STRATEGIES IN LONG-TERM CARE ADMINISTRATION

LTC administration encompasses the management of services and facilities providing extended care to individuals with chronic illnesses or disabilities. It is not just about overseeing operations; it embodies a commitment to preserving life's sanctity and ensuring well-being. Successful administrators in this field possess a multifaceted skill set, combining empathy, strategic thinking, and adept management abilities (Association of University and Programs of Health Administration [AUPHA], 2022). They prioritize compassionate and person-centered care, recognizing the individuality and diverse needs of each resident. Effectively managing resources, including skilled staff, medical supplies, and facility maintenance, is integral to their role. These administrators navigate complex regulatory frameworks, ensuring compliance while fostering environments that prioritize residents' safety, dignity, and quality of life. They are champions of transparency and accountability, instituting robust oversight mechanisms to continuously improve care standards and mitigate risks. Moreover, they foster collaborative and supportive environments that empower their caregiving teams, acknowledging their pivotal role in delivering exceptional care. A successful LTC administrator is an advocate, a leader, and a steward of compassionate, high-quality care, dedicated to enhancing the lives of those entrusted to their facilities.

Quality and safety are the pillars of LTC, ingrained in every facet of care. Initially, the focus was on regulations and standardized protocols to streamline processes and reduce errors. However, contemporary strategies like implementation sciences, person-centered care, cultural competence, and addressing health disparities have gained prominence. This shift signifies a personalized approach, honoring residents' uniqueness and cultural nuances while aiming for fairness and equity. The fusion of modern and traditional methods forms a robust framework that caters to individual needs while fostering inclusivity and diversity. Additionally, strong community ties are vital. Engaging with the local community provides essential support during crises, ensuring access to resources and expertise. It is a proactive measure to fortify community resilience and protect residents in times of adversity (Koliou et al., 2020). For example, participation in community-wide emergency drills, access to specialized training, and establishing reciprocal agreements for resource sharing during crises are vital facets of this engagement.

In this evolving healthcare landscape, administrators and leaders are responsible for innovation to maintain the highest care standards. Effective leadership cultivates a robust safety culture, encouraging open reporting and setting clear safety standards (Bonner et al., 2008; Thomas et al., 2012). Collaboration between practitioners and researchers is crucial. Together, they analyze root causes impacting care outcomes and develop evidence-based solutions. Implementation science aids in applying novel concepts to enhance outcomes for older adults (Bobitt & Jarrott, 2023).

At the core of contemporary strategies are person-centered care (Behrens et al., 2019), cultural competence (Diederich et al., 2022), and addressing health disparities (Liu et al., 2018). Tailoring care to individual preferences, respecting diverse backgrounds, and recognizing and alleviating disparities among caregivers are essential for equitable care. Striving for fairness in resident experiences and addressing caregivers' diverse needs fosters an environment where everyone receives the necessary resources and support for optimal well-being and quality care (Fabius et al., 2020; Park, 2021).

CURRENT CHALLENGES AND FUTURE DIRECTIONS

In the sphere of LTC, significant hurdles stand in the way; particularly concerning are the costs of services. LTC services often come with large expenses that can financially strain both individuals and families. This situation frequently leads to challenges in obtaining essential care, as funding sources are limited, leaving many without adequate support. With the aging population on the rise, finding solutions to these financial challenges becomes more pressing, calling for new and sustainable financial models to ensure everyone can access quality care. However, given the high costs of services and increased demand for payors such as Medicare and Medicaid, finding sustainable financial models remains a challenge.

Furthermore, within LTC settings, persistent health disparities deepen inequalities in healthcare access and outcomes among different groups. Certain communities face disparities in care quality, resulting in differing health outcomes. Tackling these disparities requires comprehensive strategies that involve tailored interventions, culturally sensitive care approaches, and specific plans to bridge gaps in access and outcomes. It is crucial to recognize and mitigate these disparities by promoting equitable care practices that cater to the unique needs of every individual.

Strategies for bolstering the quality and safety of LTC services take center stage for the future. The changing landscape emphasizes a shift toward individual-focused care, cultural understanding, and the integration of innovative technologies. Implementing practices grounded in evidence, nurturing a culture that prioritizes safety, and strengthening care coordination are key to improving overall quality. Additionally, investing in workforce training and development, alongside robust regulatory frameworks, is pivotal in raising standards and ensuring consistent, high-quality care across various care settings.

SUMMARY

Looking ahead, the future of LTC demands a comprehensive approach to address financial barriers, address health disparities, and fervently pursue strategies to enhance care quality and safety. It requires collaborative efforts among policymakers, healthcare providers, communities, and stakeholders to pave the way for a more equitable, accessible, and higher-quality LTC system. As we embark on this exploration of LTSS, each of the following chapters will delve into the various facets that shape this landscape, unraveling the interconnected threads of healthcare.

END-OF-CHAPTER RESOURCES

DISCUSSION QUESTIONS

1. What factors did Emily consider while choosing a nursing home for her father?
2. What is the importance of collaborative decision-making in choosing suitable LTC services?
3. How can LTC services promote quality and safety through customized interventions and cultural approaches?

4. How can informal caregivers take better care of aging adults while also supporting their personal autonomy and decision-making?
5. How does aging-in-place differ from other home-based care models, such as hospice or home healthcare?
6. What are some of the key features of CCRCs?

SPRINGER PUBLISHING CONNECT™ | A robust set of instructor resources designed to supplement this text is located at http://connect.springerpub.com/content/book/978-0-8261-4935-0. Qualifying instructors may request access by emailing textbook@springerpub.com.

REFERENCES

Abusalem, S., Polivka, B., Coty, M. B., Crawford, T. N., Furman, C. D., & Alaradi, M. (2021). The relationship between culture of safety and rate of adverse events in long-term care facilities. *Journal of Patient Safety, 17*(4), 299–304. https://doi.org/10.1097/PTS.0000000000000587

Association of University and Programs of Health Administration. (2022). *2022–2023 body of knowledge and curriculum guidance*. https://www.aupha.org/publications/bokcg

Behrens, L. L., McGhan, G., Abbott, K. M., Fick, D. M., Kolanowski, A. M., Liu, Y., Buck, H. G., Roes, M., Heid, A. R., Spector, A., & Van Haitsma, K. (2019). Mapping core concepts of person-centered care in long-term services and supports. *Journal of Gerontological Nursing, 45*(2), 7–13. https://doi.org/10.3928/00989134-20190111-02

Bobitt, J., & Jarrott, S. E. (2023). Strengthening aging research through dissemination and implementation science methods. *The Gerontologist, 63*(3), 401–404. https://doi.org/10.1093/geront/gnac189

Bonner, A. F., Castle, N. G., Perera, S., & Handler, S. M. (2008). Patient safety culture: A review of the nursing home literature and recommendations for practice. *The Annals of Long-Term Care, 16*(3), 18. https://www.ncbi.nlm.nih.gov/pmc/articles/PMC3119574

Castle, N. G. (2011). The influence of consistent assignment on nursing home deficiency citations. *The Gerontologist, 51*(6), 750–760. https://doi.org/10.1093/geront/gnr068

Castle, N. G., & Ferguson, J. C. (2010). What is nursing home quality and how is it measured? *The Gerontologist, 50*(4), 426–442. https://doi.org/10.1093/geront/gnq052

Crotty, M., Rowett, D., Spurling, L., Giles, L. C., & Phillips, P. A. (2004). Does the addition of a pharmacist transition coordinator improve evidence-based medication management and health outcomes in older adults moving from the hospital to a long-term care facility? Results of a randomized, controlled trial. *The American Journal of Geriatric Pharmacotherapy, 2*(4), 257–264. https://doi.org/10.1016/j.amjopharm.2005.01.001

Diederich, F., König, H. H., & Brettschneider, C. (2022). Cultural differences in the intended use of long-term care services in the United States: The role of family ties. *The Journals of Gerontology: Series B, 77*(1), 201–211. https://doi.org/10.1093/geronb/gbab035

Exec. Order No. 14095, 88 FR 24669 (July 21, 2023). https://www.govinfo.gov/content/pkg/DCPD-202300309/pdf/DCPD-202300309.pdf

Fabius, C. D., Wolff, J. L., & Kasper, J. D. (2020). Race differences in characteristics and experiences of Black and White caregivers of older Americans. *The Gerontologist, 60*(7), 1244–1253. https://doi.org/10.1093/geront/gnaa042

Forsyth, A., & Molinsky, J. (2021). What is aging in place? Confusions and contradictions. *Housing Policy Debate, 31*(2), 181–196. https://doi.org/10.1080/10511482.2020.1793795

Koliou, M., van de Lindt, J. W., McAllister, T. P., Ellingwood, B. R., Dillard, M., & Cutler, H. (2020). State of the research in community resilience: Progress and challenges. *Sustainable and Resilient Infrastructure, 5*(3), 131–151. https://doi.org/10.1080/23789689.2017.1418547

Liu, D., Burston, B., Stewart, S. C., & Mulligan, H. H. (2018). *The challenges of health disparities: Implications and actions for health care professionals*. Jones & Bartlett Learning.

Mor, V. (2006). Defining and measuring quality outcomes in long-term care. *Journal of the American Medical Directors Association*, *7*(8), 532–540. https://doi.org/10.1016/j.jamda.2006.08.001

National Academies of Sciences, Engineering, and Medicine. (2022). *The national imperative to improve nursing home quality: Honoring our commitment to residents, families, and staff*. National Academies Press. https://doi.org/10.17226/26526

Park, S. S. (2021). Caregivers' mental health and somatic symptoms during COVID-19. *The Journals of Gerontology: Series B*, *76*(4), e235–e240. https://doi.org/10.1093/geronb/gbaa121

Sengupta, M., Lendon, J. P., Caffrey, C., Melekin, A., & Singh, P. (2022). Post-acute and long-term care providers and services users in the United States, 2017–2018. *Vital & Health Statistics*, (47), 1–93. https://doi.org/10.15620/cdc:115346

Serre, N., Espin, S., Indar, A., Bookey-Bassett, S., & LeGrow, K. (2022). Long-term care nurses' experiences with patient safety incident management: A qualitative study. *Journal of Nursing Care Quality*, *37*(2), 188–194. https://doi.org/10.1097/NCQ.0000000000000583

Shippee, T. P., Akosionu, O., Ng, W., Woodhouse, M., Duan, Y., Thao, M. S., & Bowblis, J. R. (2020). COVID-19 pandemic: Exacerbating racial/ethnic disparities in long-term services and supports. *Journal of Aging & Social Policy*, *32*(4–5), 323–333. https://doi.org/10.1080/08959420.2020.1772004

Thomas, K. S., Hyer, K., Castle, N. G., Branch, L. G., Andel, R., & Weech-Maldonado, R. (2012). Patient safety culture and the association with safe resident care in nursing homes. *The Gerontologist*, *52*(6), 802–811. https://doi.org/10.1093/geront/gns007

Wagner, L. M., Capezuti, E., & Ouslander, J. G. (2006). Reporting near-miss events in nursing homes. *Nursing Outlook*, *54*(2), 85–93. https://doi.org/10.1016/j.outlook.2006.01.003

CHAPTER 2

NO PLACE LIKE HOME: AN OVERVIEW OF HOME- AND COMMUNITY-BASED SERVICES IN THE UNITED STATES

Robert Applebaum, Suzanne Kunkel, and Bailee Brekke

Learning Objectives

After completing this chapter, each learner will be able to:

- Understand what long-term services and supports (LTSS) are and how they are delivered in the United States
- Explain the shift from institutional care to home- and community-based services (HCBS)
- Identify major legislative changes that led to the development of HCBS as an option for individuals with high need for long-term services
- Recognize the importance of quality and reliability of support in HCBS
- Explain the benefits of HCBS over institutional care for people with severe disabilities.

INTRODUCTION

For many of us, our morning routines of showering, dressing, preparing breakfast, and commuting to work or school are simply the tasks of our daily lives. However, to those who require assistance with these actions, getting the right support, in the right place, and in the right manner is vital for maintaining a high quality of life. These individuals, who require aid with these day-to-day tasks, are classified as needing long-term services and supports (LTSS).

In the United States, LTSS can be provided in an array of settings. Historically, before the advent of public funding for LTSS, support was predominantly provided at home, often by family members. However, with the establishment of national health programs such as Medicaid and Medicare in 1965, there was a shift toward institutional settings for long-term care (LTC), accompanied by formal regulations, monitoring, and fiscal accountability. It became commonplace to assume that individuals with high need for long-term services and financial constraints required nursing home care. However, this assumption began to be questioned by older adults, their families, gerontologists, and policy makers alike.

Major legislative changes in 1981 ushered in a new era, making home- and community-based services (HCBS) a viable option for individuals with severe disabilities. Today, the majority of people in need of assistance, even those with severe disability, receive support within their communities rather than in a nursing home. Dorothy's iconic line from *The Wizard of Oz*, "There's no place like home" (Baum, 1900), provides a powerful message for those needing long-term services. In this chapter we describe the HCBS that are now available across the nation.

EVOLUTION AND EXPANSION OF HOME- AND COMMUNITY-BASED SERVICES

The landscape of LTC in the United States underwent significant shifts, rooted in the incentives outlined in the 1965 Medicaid program and a prevailing societal belief favoring institutional care for older individuals with severe disability. During the 1970s, nursing home utilization surged, driven by these incentives and perceptions (Hawes & Phillips, 1986). At that time, Medicaid would cover nursing home care but not community-based services, reflecting a bias toward institutional care. However, in 1981, recognizing the potential benefits of home-based care, pivotal federal legislation allowed states to seek *waivers* from the Centers for Medicare & Medicaid Services (CMS) to use Medicaid for noninstitutional long-term services (Medicaid and CHIP Payment and Access Commission [MACPAC], n.d.). This marked the beginning of widespread support for HCBS across all states.

Today, HCBS under Medicaid serves more individuals with severe disabilities than nursing homes. For example, in 1988, HCBS comprised only 10% of Medicaid LTSS expenditures, but by 2018, this figure had soared to 56% (Murray et al., 2021). These waiver programs cater to various target populations, with the two largest groups being older adults (80 programs) and individuals with intellectual and developmental disabilities (119 programs).

OVERVIEW OF HOME- AND COMMUNITY-BASED SERVICES

HCBS encompasses a wide rage of services designed to support individuals with their daily living activities. These include personal care, homemaker services, home-delivered meals, transportation, adult day services, emergency response systems, home modification, home medical equipment, and companionship (CMS, 2023). While many households rely on family or friends for such assistance, formal service providers become necessary as care needs increase. These providers can be a mix of private and nonprofit organizations, with most home care workers employed by agencies. Notably, some consumers opt to hire workers directly, bypassing traditional agency-based providers. This model, known as consumer self-direction, is gaining traction as individuals take control of their care through hiring and supervising their own workers. Additionally, it is worth mentioning that assisted living, a residential care option, falls within the home- and community-based category, as individuals residing in these settings are considered part of the community.

PROVIDERS OF HOME- AND COMMUNITY-BASED SERVICES

The expansion of HCBS funding has led to a proliferation of providers, with over 20,000 agencies offering services to older individuals in the community. These providers vary in specialization, from offering single services such as transportation to providing comprehensive care like home delivered meals or personal care and homemaking under one roof. There are two types of providers for hands-on personal care: skilled home health agencies, which deliver nursing services for acute care illness, and home care agencies, which provide ongoing personal care services.

In the early days of HCBS, nonprofit organizations dominated the provider landscape. Many of these had philanthropic roots and were established to meet the needs of a growing older population. However, with increased funding allocated to HCBS, the provider community has undergone a transformation. Presently, a substantial portion of providers operate as for-profit businesses, and, in some instances, as multistate corporate chains. For instance, in the past, skilled home health agencies receiving Medicare funds were mandated to be nonprofits until a regulatory amendment in 1980. Today, over half of the nation's home health and home care agencies operate as for-profit entities.

Family and Friend Care

The role of family and friend as caregiver is paramount, including a diverse range of relationships such as spouses, adult children, siblings, grandchildren, friends, and neighbors. Their contributions, from assisting with daily tasks to providing emotional support, constitute a significant aspect of care provision nationwide. Notably, this caregiving responsibility often falls disproportionately on women, particularly spouses and adult daughters, leading to challenges in balancing work and caregiving responsibilities with dual-worker households (Brody, 2003). While some states offer extended family leave options for caregiving, the level of support for caregiving in the United States lags behind many countries globally.

Despite the expansion of formal HCBS, family and friends remain essential caregivers for individuals with disabilities. More than 80% of the care for these individuals is provided by family and friends (Feinberg et al., 2011). These unpaid care providers represent a significant economic contribution, with approximately 38 million family caregivers contributing an estimated $600 billion in value (Reinhard et al., 2023).

Recognizing the significance of caregiver support, various national initiatives have been implemented to address their needs. For instance, the inclusion of the National Family Caregiver Support Program in the Older Americans Act (OAA) in 2000 marked a pivotal step in providing direct federal support to caregivers (Administration for Community Living [ACL], 2023). The program is designed to provide information to caregivers about available services, to assist caregivers in gaining access to services, to provide individual counseling and training to caregivers, and to support respite care. This was the first program that allocated federal funds to directly support caregivers.

A recent initiative enacted in 2021, the **R**ecognize, **A**ssist, **I**nclude, **S**upport, and **E**ngage (RAISE) Act, includes 26 recommendations for how the federal government, states, tribes, territories, and communities—in partnership with the private sector—can better support caregivers (ACL, 2024). The importance of supporting family and friend caregivers has been recognized, but the demographic changes associated with increased longevity and lower fertility rates means that our nation still needs to make better progress in efforts to support informal caregivers.

Consumer Self-Direction

The concept of consumer self-direction challenges ageist and ableist assumptions that older adults, or those with disabilities, are incapable of making decisions regarding their care. These assumptions, rooted in prejudicial stereotypes, undermine individuals' autonomy and dignity. Regardless of age or level of disability, most of us desire control over our lives, including the type and quality of assistance we receive.

In a self-direction model, care recipients take charge of their care needs. They have the authority to hire, fire, train, schedule, and supervise the workers who are assisting them with daily tasks (CMS, n.d.). Of course, individuals with adequate private resources do this all the time, but such opportunities have been limited to individuals receiving services supported by public funds. Some state Medicaid HCBS, such as California's In-Home Supportive Services (IHSS) program, extend self-direction opportunities to a significant number of consumers (California Department of Social Services [CDSS], n.d.). However, in most states, agency-based providers remain the primary source of services.

Despite the norm of relying on agencies, studies such as the National Cash and Counseling Demonstration have shown overwhelmingly positive outcomes associated with self-direction (Carlson et al., 2007). Through randomized experimental designs, such studies have demonstrated that individuals directing their own care experience higher satisfaction levels and are more likely to remain independent within their community, rather than transitioning to institutional settings. These findings have led to the replication of self-direction programs in numerous states, with the vast majority now offering self-direction opportunities through their Medicaid waiver programs. We delve into these developments in the following sections.

FUNDING SOURCES AND FINANCIAL MODELS FOR HOME- AND COMMUNITY-BASED SERVICES

In addition to the growth in HCBS under Medicaid, there has been an expansion of consumers paying privately for an array of HCBS. About 35% to 40% of older people with severe disability report buying some services through the private market. This means that entry into the HCBS system comes from two directions. HCBS for some individuals is provided by public programs and for others it is a private pay endeavor, where individuals pay out of pocket to buy the needed assistance.

The bulk of public financing for HCBS primarily comes from two programs, one federal/state and one solely federal. Public sector funding most often comes from the Medicaid program, through the use of Medicaid waivers or through another component of Medicaid called the personal care option. The joint federal/state Medicaid program, which is designed to serve low-income Americans of all ages, allocates a substantial amount of funds to HCBS for older individuals with severe disability; a recent report estimated that Medicaid HCBS allocations exceeded $60 billion in 2020 (Murray et al., 2021). However, to receive these services an individual must be classified as needing nursing home care and be very low income. The use of Medicaid to finance HCBS requires states to apply for a waiver from the federal government, and the use of Medicaid funds varies dramatically across the nation. Some states have very large HCBS programs, while others continue to spend the majority of their Medicaid funds on nursing home care.

Another public program is the OAA. Initially passed in 1965, the program allocates funds to states and Native American tribes for an array of social services. The OAA is designed to support individuals aged 60 and over with a variety of services to help them remain healthy and independent in the community. These services include congregating meals, health promotion and disease management, legal services and elder abuse mitigation, home modification, support for volunteer activities, and senior employment. The entire act adds up to about $3 billion, compared to almost $2 trillion spent on Medicare and Medicaid (Colello & Napili, 2024). A 1973 reauthorization to the OAA established a network of Area Agencies on Aging (AAAs), and these organizations have the responsibility to assist older people in finding the needed community services. AAAs often use their funding allocation to contract with community-based providers to deliver needed community-based services. The AAAs are the core of the formally designated Aging Network. The agencies that make up the Aging Network are often at the center of HCBS systems, providing access and coordination of services.

The Role of Care Management

The expansion of Medicaid HCBS, and additional funding from the OAA and other federal initiatives, marked a growing availability of home care services (Office of Community Services [OCS], 2023). In addition, state and local governments and philanthropic organizations became more involved in offering services to older people. The needs of the growing older population were now being recognized at federal, state and local levels. This was certainly an important milestone. However, because options were being developed and delivered by an array of agencies, from very different funding sources, coordination and information sharing across programs was problematic. Older consumers and their families reported having very limited information about potential services and the differing eligibility criteria required to even access such services. In response to this problem, the concept of care management in HCBS was developed.

Care managers in HCBS are now widely used. Care managers assist consumers and their families in navigating the array of programs and services offered by different organizations. The role of care managers is an attempt to rationalize an uncoordinated system. Care managers are often trained as social workers or nurses, but some are trained in gerontology, counseling, and rehabilitation services. In addition, the care manager is trained to know about the array of programs and services that are available in a specific community and the eligibility criterion for each program. The care manager, working with the care recipient and family or friend supporters, assesses the day-to-day needs of the individual. The support provided by family and friends provides a starting point for the development of a formal plan of care to support the care recipient. The care manager then develops a specific plan of care, determines eligibility, and arranges the necessary services. Once services are arranged, the care manager is involved in monitoring both the care recipient's ongoing condition and the quality of the services being provided. Periodic reassessments, usually in the individual's home, and continued contacts via the telephone are part of the care manager's monitoring efforts.

For individuals eligible for the Medicaid HCBS waiver program, it is likely that the care manager, who works for the waiver program itself, will be able to arrange services funded directly though the program. Care managers could also be working for state and local entities, and they may have to identify services that are funded from several different program sources, such as the OAA, the local United Way, and state-supported programs. Care management has become a core component of the HCBS system. Virtually all of the state Medicaid waiver programs across the nation include a care management component. Additionally, most of the state and local programs that provide HCBS also include care managers in program design. In response to widespread fragmentation across health and long-term services, care management has become an integral part of the overall system.

ISSUES AND OPPORTUNITIES FACING THE HOME- AND COMMUNITY-BASED SERVICES SYSTEM

State Variation in Home- and Community-Based Services

The long-standing debate in the United States about the role of states versus the role of federal government is visible in many current discussions such as healthcare, gun control, and education. Within LTSS, this tension is present, since the federal/state Medicaid program is the largest public funder. However, while the federal government has regulatory oversight and approval responsibilities, the administration and day-to-day regulation of long-term services is largely left to the individual states. The result of this structure is considerable variation in the design of long-term services systems for older people and individuals with physical disabilities. As an example, in the states of California (83.2%), Washington (76.2%), Vermont (73.2%), and Minnesota (72.1%), leaders in developing HCBS, a high proportion of Medicaid long-term services expenditures are allocated to noninstitutional care (AARP, n.d.-a). States with lower HCBS expenditures are New Hampshire (13.5%), Alabama (14.6%), and Kentucky (18.4%); these states spend less than one-fifth of their Medicaid LTSS funds on HCBS (AARP, n.d.-a).

In addition to the variation in overall HCBS expenditures, there are widespread differences across the state on a number of factors, such as using public dollars to allow consumers to self-direct for HCBS. California leads the nation with almost 17% of home care consumers self-directing (AARP, n.d.-b). On the other hand, Ohio, Arizona, and Indiana report that fewer than 2% of their consumers participate in HCBS Medicaid self-direction (AARP, n.d.-b). Another state difference is that some states, such as Massachusetts and Oregon, have state-funded programs to support HCBS, while other states rely on the federal/state Medicaid program for the bulk of their HCBS funding. Fifteen states around the nation actually have HCBS programs that are funded at the local level, typically through property taxes (Koumoutzis et al., 2021). All of these differences result in states having very different HCBS systems that impact access and eligibility, the type and amount of services available, and program structure and quality.

Quality and Supply of Workforce

Without question one of the biggest challenges facing the entire long-term services workforce is attracting and retaining high-quality direct care workers (DCWs) who provide the hands-on care to individuals with disability. These personal care workers typically receive low wages (Paraprofessional Healthcare Institute [PHI], 2022) and face physical and emotional work demands (Stevens, 2022). The challenges associated with the home care workforce have been a concern since the late 1980s and have been the subject of a number of studies and interventions since then. The COVID-19 pandemic brought the issue to the forefront, as many individuals with disability who were eligible to receive in-home services were simply unable to get those services due to a lack of workers (Cimarolli et al., 2022).

Ultimately, retaining DCWs has been a challenge for the entire system of LTSS. However, the worker shortage not only undermines the ability to provide care; the shortage also calls into question the ability to provide good quality care. The provision of LTC services transitioned from traditional provider-driven care models to a focus on a person-centered care (PCC) approach that prioritizes individuals' preferences, values, beliefs, experiences, and needs (Jones, 2011; Yee et al., 2021). PCC has been proven to improve cognitive and psychologic functioning, care satisfaction, and quality of life of older adults receiving care (Bhattacharyya et al., 2022; Yee et al., 2021).

The pandemic has heightened efforts to address the DCW crisis. Federal funding from the American Rescue Plan Act (ARPA) was allocated to states to address the unique needs of older adults. Many states chose to allocate funding to DCWs in unique ways, including increased training, wage-pass throughs, and matching services registries. While wages and benefits are certainly a necessary element in addressing the problem, they don't appear to be the sole contender in alleviating this crisis. As an example, a study of certified nursing assistants in skilled nursing facilities found supervisory turnover significantly reduced DCW retention (Kennedy et al., 2021). Recruiting and retaining DCWs is a long-standing challenge, one that will require a multifaceted approach. Increased wages, a prioritization of work culture, and increased community recognition of the work will be needed to improve DCW retention and the overall provision of care for older adults moving forward (Karmacharya et al., 2023).

Growing Pressure on Family and Friend Caregivers

The fact that more older people with disability are receiving services in the community than in nursing homes represents an important step forward in ensuring that consumers are better able today to choose their care setting. A review of utilization data shows that three-quarters of older individuals experiencing disability do not live in nursing homes (Applebaum et al., 2024). As noted earlier, we spend more public dollars on HCBS than on nursing home care, which reflects this shift to services being provided at home.

Caregiving pressures come from multiple sources. First, older people are being sent home from the hospital sooner because of changes in the Medicare hospital reimbursement system; the average length of stay for older people has dropped by more than 5 days since 1980 (Administration on Aging, 2011). Leaving the hospital sooner may be a good thing for patients, but it does mean that family and friend caregivers are now being called in to assist with more complicated health-focused tasks than ever before. Second, the shift to more HCBS means that individuals with more severe levels of disability, both physical and cognitive, are being cared for at home. The complexity of the care needed by the recipient, such as those with dementia, places more demands both physically and psychologically on the caregiver. While caregivers embrace their role, complex health and long-term needs make the role more complicated than ever. Spousal caregivers, who are sometimes often facing their own health challenges, bear tremendous caregiving responsibilities often without respite. The caregiving provided by adult children, often daughters, includes these same formidable challenges, with work and children adding to the complexity of the role. Caregivers also often talk about satisfaction and rewards of their role.

Ensuring Quality of Home- and Community-Based Services

Increased investment of public dollars and the growth of HCBS have been accompanied by concerns about the quality of care being provided, mirroring criticisms of nursing home care. A vulnerable population being cared for by individuals with low pay and limited training has been an enduring concern regarding nursing home care. Data on nursing home quality have shown a decline as the industry has become increasingly dominated by for-profit and corporate ownership (Harrington et al., 2012). HCBS, and particularly in-home services, face many of the same challenges, complicated by the fact that care is provided in one's home, with less public visibility than a residential care setting. But one of the advantages that help improve the quality of in-home care is the presence of family members who are part of the ecosystem of care. Having additional individuals in the home to observe and advocate results in higher quality care (Johnson et al., 2023).

As Medicaid has increased its investment in HCBS, the federal government and states have developed quality assurance and improvement approaches. At the federal level, each state operating a waiver that allows people to receive services at home is required to have a quality assurance and improvement plan that is approved by the CMS. The states must specify the types and amount of monitoring data to be collected, the approach to collect data, and a plan for how data will be used. The states are responsible for developing the quality plan and to work with local entities to implement such a plan. In general, the quality plan involves direct data collection from care recipients, provider audits, a review of service plans and billing, and a review of client tracking data. As an example, agencies collect satisfaction data from consumers about the services they are receiving. Agencies also compare the services authorized by care managers to the number of hours that were actually provided and billed for through provider audits. Agencies also track client progress from initial application for services to when they received the needed assistance. While challenges remain, there has been considerable progress in developing approaches to ensuring the quality of HCBS.

Accessible and Affordable Housing

One of the most formidable challenges faced by older people with a disability is the lack of adequate housing. Housing challenges include affordability, accessibility, and the availability of needed support services.

In many communities there is a shortage of *affordable* housing. This problem has grown as a result of the pandemic, and a recent study reported that more than 11 million older Americans were housing cost burdened, meaning that more than 30% of their income was allocated to housing (Joint Center for Housing Studies of Harvard University, 2023). Historically, the challenge has been particularly acute for individuals with low incomes, women, minorities, and those living alone (Pynoos & Nishita, 2006).

Despite the desire of many older individuals to age in place, not all housing is *accessible* or adaptable to physical and health changes. Having accessibility to a physically supportive environment is also important in allowing older adults the opportunity to age in place (Pynoos & Nishita, 2006). In many communities, the housing stock has existed for decades and often homes and apartments do not offer adequate access for individuals who may not be able to negotiate stairs. This could include apartments with no elevators or private homes where bedrooms and/or bathrooms are on the second floor. Another component of accessibility involves the community itself. For example, studies have recognized the importance of access to everyday needs, such as grocery stores, pharmacies, doctors, social and religious activities, and health and LTC providers (Golant, 2019). Individuals with disability have a very difficult time finding options. In a Scripps study examining barriers to individuals being able to leave the nursing home setting, the number one reason why individuals could not return to the community was inadequate housing (Applebaum et al., 2011).

Even housing designed for older residents may not include the *necessary services* (Pynoos & Nishita, 2006). In an effort to address these barriers, home modifications have been a more recent addition to the HCBS package to promote successful aging (Sheth & Cogle, 2023). Home modifications include installing grab bars in the bathroom, building wheelchair ramps, and replacing uneven carpets in an effort to increase the livability of an individual's home. Ultimately, considerations will need to be made in the future to ensure that older adults are aging in the *right* place to ensure their overall health and well-being (Golant, 2015).

Lastly, with the growing population there has been a recent increase in the number of unhoused older adults. Recent work found that those aged 65 and older are the fastest growing population who are unhoused. One-third of those who are chronically unhoused are aged 55 and older (Office of Policy Development and Research, 2023). Various factors, including fixed incomes, physical and cognitive conditions, and lacking LTSS and healthcare coverage, increase the likelihood of being unhoused. A recent critique of housing policy indicated that government support for affordable housing has not kept pace with the current population and the unique needs of older adults (Pynoos, 2018).

THE ROLE OF TECHNOLOGY

We have all experienced the profound effects of technology on our daily lives. Whether it is through personal computers, cell phones, or artificial intelligence, the world that we live and work in today is vastly different from what it was even a decade ago. A critical question is what future technological changes will mean for HCBS. One of the most potentially impactful changes involves robotics. Facing an unprecedented growth in their aging population, government and private industry in Japan has invested billions of dollars in robotics.

While still in the very early stages of feasibility assessment and technological development, the idea of a personal care robot that will assist a person with tasks of daily living now seems quite likely. Robotic assistance already exists to help a person with making breakfast or to transfer from their bed to a chair. The self-driving car, while maybe not ready for prime time, has already become a reality. The idea for such a technological change 20 years ago would have seemed like something from science fiction. Of course, there are many ethical and preference questions about how robotics technology can and will be used. If it is part of a network of support for individuals with disability, it could enhance independence and have a profound impact on one's quality of life. If, however, it is a substitute for human interaction and becomes the primary source of support for a person who is somewhat isolated it could lead to negative outcomes.

There are other technological innovations that have been and will continue to be used. Driven by changing needs and options related to the COVID-19 pandemic, telehealth is increasingly utilized for certain kinds of healthcare interventions. These communication mechanisms have also been useful for family caregivers who can now have enhanced interactions with their loved ones who may be living alone and receiving in-home services. Other changes in practice include sophisticated medication management systems, improved cell phone and computer access for individuals with disability, emergency systems such as LifeLine, and development of monitoring systems such as bed, door, and water sensors in the home. The growth in the number of older individuals with disability receiving services in their own home will catalyze further product development in this area. Technology will be an important component of the future HCBS system across the nation and globally.

GROWTH IN MEDICAID HOME- AND COMMUNITY-BASED SERVICES AND MANAGED CARE

One of the hallmarks of America's economic system is that industry will follow the opportunity for financial growth. The amount of funds now going into the health and long-term services system for older people has skyrocketed. Because such a high proportion of the funding comes from the public sector programs, Medicare and Medicaid, a number of companies have developed managed care products for this market. Today more than half of Medicare beneficiaries in the nation are enrolled in Medicare Advantage plans, which is the managed care option (Freed et al., 2024). On the Medicaid side, 41 states have some type of managed LTSS program in place (Hinton & Raphael, 2024). Both the states and the federal government have been concerned about the consistent increase in Medicare and Medicaid expenditures and have seen managed care products as a mechanism to control costs and possibly increase quality.

While it is difficult to know how the shift to more managed care products and participants will impact HCBS over the long run, we have seen some important changes thus far. As an example, individuals who require nursing home rehabilitation care under Medicare are now recording shorter stays in nursing homes, as the Medicare Advantage plans do not provide the automatic 20 days of coverage, as is the case for fee-for-service Medicare enrollees. This means individuals are going home faster, with higher care needs that need to be met by informal caregivers or through formal services. On the managed Medicaid LTSS programs, concerns have been expressed about the amount and scope of HCBS. While data are limited, a review of the experience from some demonstrations that have attempted to integrate Medicaid and Medicare services indicate this concern. A related critique has been that the large Medicaid LTSS plans have been less encouraging of the consumer self-direction.

As noted, definitive data on how managed care will impact quality and costs of health and long-term services, and in particular its effects on HCBS, are unknown. What does seem to be clear is that the growth of managed care products in the health and long-term services arena will continue. State governments are especially interested in stability and cost control and feel like the managed care products will address those concerns. The growth of the older population, the continuing rise in healthcare costs, and the emphasis on cost control will result in the continued reliance on managed care products in the future.

SUMMARY

This chapter has highlighted the tremendous expansion of HCBS across the nation, reflecting success in honoring people's preferences to receive care at home. With both private and public sector providers of HCBS on the rise, more and more older individuals with severe disability will have the opportunity to receive care in their own homes, in their communities. The steady decline in nursing home occupancy over the past three decades signals a continuing shift in the system toward alternative care options such as assisted living and in-home care, a tread expected to persist. The HCBS system will likely undergo considerable change over the next 20 years. While technological advancements, such as robotics, hold promise for revolutionizing home care delivery, it is essential to recognize that compassionate and skilled caregivers will remain the cornerstone of in-home care. However, challenges persist within the workforce, including low pay and inadequate benefits, particularly in the in-home personal care industry serving older individuals with disability (Janssen et al., 2023). With continued costs pressures on organizations in this industry, exacerbated by the expansion of managed care, the prospect of increased funding for the home care and assisted living workforce remains uncertain. There are no easy answers to the workforce challenges of today and tomorrow. Addressing these workforce challenges demands a comprehensive, system-wide strategy that recognizes their reality and establishes tangible plans for mitigation. HCBS will continue to be a critical component of the care system for older individuals with disabilities, underscoring the importance of striving for a system capable of delivering the high-quality care that everyone desires for their loved ones and themselves.

END-OF-CHAPTER RESOURCES

DISCUSSION QUESTIONS

1. HCBS have brought significant changes to the LTSS landscape in the United States. Discuss the benefits of receiving care in a home and community setting versus an institutional setting.
2. The COVID-19 pandemic has exposed vulnerabilities in LTSS communities, particularly nursing homes. How do you think this vulnerability in institutional care will affect the future of LTSS in the United States?

3. The direct care workforce in the United States plays a crucial role in providing HCBS. Discuss some of the challenges that this workforce faces and potential solutions to address these challenges.
4. HCBS is funded through a patchwork of funding streams, including Medicaid, Medicare, OAA, and state-funded programs. What are the pros and cons of this fragmented approach to funding LTSS?
5. Policy changes and initiatives have attempted to make it easier for individuals to live independently at home and in the community. What are some of the gaps and limitations of these initiatives? What else can be done to support individuals with disabilities to live independently at home or in the community?

SPRINGER PUBLISHING CONNECT™ | A robust set of instructor resources designed to supplement this text is located at http://connect.springerpub.com/content/book/978-0-8201-4935 0. Qualifying instructors may request access by emailing textbook@springerpub.com.

REFERENCES

AARP. (n.d.-a). *Medicaid LTSS balance: Spending.* Retrieved August 13, 2024, from https://ltsschoices.aarp.org/scorecard-report/2023/dimensions-and-indicators/medicaid-ltss-balance-spending

AARP. (n.d.-b). *Self-directed program enrollment.* Retrieved August 13, 2024, from https://ltsschoices.aarp.org/scorecard-report/2023/dimensions-and-indicators/self-directed-program-enrollment

Administration for Community Living. (2023, February 15). *National Family Caregiver Support Program.* https://acl.gov/programs/support-caregivers/national-family-caregiver-support-program

Administration for Community Living. (2024, July 12). *Recognize, Assist, Include, Support, & Engage (RAISE) Family Caregivers Act Advisory Council.* https://acl.gov/programs/support-caregivers/raise-family-caregiving-advisory-council

Administration on Aging. (2011). *A profile for older Americans: 2011.* U.S. Department of Health & Human Services. https://acl.gov/sites/default/files/aging%20and%20disability%20in%20america/2011profile.pdf

Applebaum, R., Bardo, A., Kunkel, S., & Carpio, E. (2011, June). *Right place, right time, right care: An evaluation of Ohio's nursing home diversion and transition.* Scripps Gerontology Center, Miami University. https://sc.lib.miamioh.edu/bitstream/handle/2374.MIA/4449/Right_Place_Right_Time_Right_Carev1.pdf

Applebaum, R., Bowblis, J. R., Nelson, M., Dikhtyar, O., McClure, M., & Bakht, N., N. (2024, March). *A profile of nursing homes in Ohio.* Scripps Gerontology Center, Miami University. https://sc.lib.miamioh.edu/bitstream/handle/2374.MIA/6958/A-Profile-of-Nursing-Homes-in-Ohio.pdf

Baum, L. F. (1900). *The Wizard of Oz.* George M. Hill Company.

Bhattacharyya, K. K., Craft Morgan, J., & Burgess, E. O. (2022). Person-centered care in nursing homes: Potential of complementary and alternative approaches and their challenges. *Journal of Applied Gerontology, 41*(3), 817–825. https://doi.org/10.1177/07334648211023661

Brody, E. M. (2003). *Women in the middle: Their parent-care years.* Springer Publishing Company.

California Department of Social Services. (n.d.). *In-Home Supportive Services (IHSS) program.* Retrieved April 3, 2024, from https://www.cdss.ca.gov/in-home-supportive-services

Carlson, B. L., Foster, L., Dale, S., & Brown, R. (2007). Effects of cash and counseling on personal care and well-being. *Health Services Research, 42*(1 Pt 2), 467–487. https://doi.org/10.1111/j.1475-6773.2006.00673.x

Centers for Medicare & Medicaid Services. (n.d.). *Self-directed services.* Retrieved April 3, 2024, from https://www.medicaid.gov/medicaid/long-term-services-supports/self-directed-services/index.html

Centers for Medicare & Medicaid Services. (2023, September 6). *Home- and community-based services.* https://www.cms.gov/training-education/partner-outreach-resources/american-indian-alaska-native/ltss-ta-center/information/ltss-models/home-and-community-based-services

Cimarolli, V. R., Bryant, N. S., Falzarano, F., & Stone, R. (2022). Job resignation in nursing homes during the COVID-19 pandemic: The role of quality of employer communication. *Journal of Applied Gerontology, 41*(1), 12–21. https://doi.org/10.1177/07334648211040509

Colello, K. J., & Napili, A. (2024, May 6). *Older Americans Act: Overview and funding* [CRS R43414]. Congressional Research Service. https://crsreports.congress.gov/product/pdf/R/R43414

Feinberg, L., Reinhard, S. C., Houser, A., & Choula, R. (2011). *Valuing the invaluable: 2011 update: The growing contributions and costs of family caregiving.* AARP Public Policy Institute. https://www.researchgate.net/publication/260403580_Valuing_the_Invaluable_2011_Update_The_Growing_Contributions_and_Costs_of_Family_Caregiving

Freed, M., Fuglesten Biniek, J., Damico, A., & Neuman, T. (2024). *Medicare Advantage in 2024: Enrollment update and key trends.* Kaiser Family Foundation. https://www.kff.org/medicare/issue-brief/medicare-advantage-in-2024-enrollment-update-and-key-trends

Golant, S. M. (2015). *Aging in the right place* (p. 406). Health Professions Press.

Golant, S. M. (2019). Connectivity as an indicator of older people's housing quality. In K. B. Anacker, M. T. Nguyen, & D. P. Varady (Eds.), *The Routledge handbook of housing policy and planning* (pp. 231–242). Routledge.

Harrington, C., Olney, B., Carrillo, H., & Kang, T. (2012). Nurse staffing and deficiencies in the largest for-profit nursing home chains and chains owned by private equity companies. *Health Services Research, 47*(1Pt.1), 106–128. https://doi.org/10.1111/j.1475-6773.2011.01311.x

Hawes, C., & Phillips, C. D. (1986). The changing structure of the nursing home industry and the impact of ownership on quality, cost and access. In B. H. Gray (Ed.), *For-profit enterprise in health care* (pp. 492–541). National Academies Press.

Hinton, E., & Raphael, J. (2024, May 1). *10 things to know about Medicaid managed care.* Kaiser Family Foundation. https://www.kff.org/medicaid/issue-brief/10-things-to-know-about-medicaid-managed-care

Johnson, B. H., Lee, M., & Mossburg, S. E. (2023, June 14). *Patient and family roles in safety.* Agency for Healthcare Research and Quality. https://psnet.ahrq.gov/perspective/patient-and-family-roles-safety

Joint Center for Housing Studies of Harvard University. (2023). *Housing America's older adults.* https://www.jchs.harvard.edu/housing-americas-older-adults-2023

Jones, C. S. (2011). Person-centered care. *Journal of Gerontological Nursing, 37*(6), 18–23. https://doi.org/10.3928/00989134-20110302-04

Karmacharya, I., Janssen, L. M., & Brekke, B. (2023). "Let Them Know That They're Appreciated": The importance of work culture on direct care worker retention. *Journal of Gerontological Nursing, 49*(8), 7–13. https://doi.org/10.3928/00989134-20230706-03

Kennedy, K. A., Applebaum, R., Bowblis, J. R., & Straker, J. K. (2021). Organizational factors associated with retention of direct care workers: A comparison of nursing homes and assisted living facilities. *The Gerontologist, 61*(4), 530–539. https://doi.org/10.1093/geront/gnaa130

Koumoutzis, A., Stemen, S. E., Maharjan, R., Heston-Mullins, J., Mayberry, P. S., & Applebaum, R. (2021). Local initiatives to fund services for older Americans: Community recognition of the importance of social care. *Journal of Applied Gerontology, 40*(9), 980–984. https://doi.org/10.1177/0733464820944325

Medicaid and CHIP Payment and Access Commission. (n.d.). *Waivers.* Retrieved April 3, 2024, from https://www.macpac.gov/medicaid-101/waivers

Murray, C., Tourtellotte, A., Lipson, D., & Wysocki, A. (2021). *Medicaid long-term services and supports annual expenditures report: Federal fiscal years 2017 and 2018.* Centers for Medicare & Medicaid Services. https://www.medicaid.gov/medicaid/long-term-services-supports/downloads/ltssexpenditures-2017-2018.pdf

Office of Community Services. (2023). *Social Services Block Grant Program (SSBG).* https://www.acf.hhs.gov/ocs/programs/ssbg

Office of Policy Development and Research. (2023, December 5). *Homelessness and housing insecurity among older adults.* PD&R Edge. https://www.huduser.gov/portal/pdredge/pdr-edge-featd-article-120523.html

Paraprofessional Healthcare Institute. (2022, September 6). *Direct care workers in the United States: Key facts (PHI Report 2020).* Paraprofessional Healthcare Institute, The John A. Hartford Foundation. https://www.phinational.org/resource/direct-care-workers-in-the-united-states-key-facts-3

Pynoos, J. (2018). The future of housing for the elderly: Four strategies that can make a difference. *Public Policy & Aging Report*, *28*(1), 35–38. https://doi.org/10.1093/ppar/pry006

Pynoos, J., & Nishita, C. M. (2006). The elderly and a right to housing. In R. G. Bratt, M. E. Stone, & C. Hartman (Eds.), *A right to housing: Foundation for a new social agenda* (p. 279–295). Temple University Press.

Reinhard, S. C., Caldera, S., Houser, A., & Choula, R. B. (2023). *Valuing the invaluable: 2023 update: Strengthening supports for family caregivers.* AARP Public Policy Institute. https://www.aarp.org/content/dam/aarp/ppi/2023/3/valuing-the-invaluable-2023-update.doi.10.26419-2Fppi.00082.006.pdf

Sheth, S., & Cogle, C. R. (2023). Home modifications for older adults: A systematic review. *Journal of Applied Gerontology*, *42*(5), 1151–1164. https://doi.org/10.1177/07334648231151669

Stevens, K. A. (2022). *An assessment of the personal care workforce shortage in the Ohio Area Agency on Aging PSA 2 program area and recommendations to address.* http://info4seniors.org/wp-content/uploads/2022/10/PCA-WORKFORCE-SHORTAGE_FINAL-REPORT_KAStevens-1.pdf

Yee, J., Ribeiro Souza, M. C. M., Horta, N. de C., & Kartoz, C. (2021). Person-centered care for older adults living in long-term care facilities: A systematic literature review. *Journal of Public Health Issues and Practices*, *5*(2). https://doi.org/10.33790/jphip1100184

CHAPTER 3

NURSING HOMES

Heather Davila and Kathleen Abrahamson

Learning Objectives

After completing this chapter, each learner will be able to:

- Describe Donabedian's "structure-process-outcome" framework and how it applies to nursing home quality.
- Describe important components of quality and safety in nursing homes.
- Describe key milestones in the history of quality and safety in nursing homes.
- Discuss differences between quality assurance and quality improvement approaches to nursing home quality.
- Understand general approaches to improving quality and safety in nursing homes.
- Discuss challenges and opportunities for improving nursing home quality and safety.

INTRODUCTION

Nearly 1.2 million adults received care in one of the approximately 15,000 skilled nursing facilities (SNFs, commonly referred to as nursing homes) in the United States in 2022 (Chidambaram & Burns, 2024). Although postacute and long-term care is increasingly delivered in home- and community-based settings (HCBS), including residential settings such as assisted living facilities, nursing homes remain an important source of care for many Americans and represent a major bucket of long-term care spending. Care in nursing homes is multifaceted, involving clinical services (e.g., nursing, rehabilitation/therapy, social work), functional assistance (e.g., mobility, toileting, bathing), meals and nutrition, psychosocial and behavioral support, activities, and housing. Nursing home quality likewise involves multiple components, including the assessment of the processes and outcomes of clinical and supportive assistance (quality of care), resident quality of life (e.g., dietary quality, services such as laundry, comfort level of the facility), and resident safety (e.g., infection prevention measures and emergency preparedness plans).

Defining, assessing, and improving nursing home quality is made more complicated by the fact that nursing homes provide postacute short-stay services that are primarily rehabilitative in nature as well as long-term care services, which have fundamentally different goals. For postacute care, services are typically covered by Medicare, a federal program for those aged 65 or over, or private insurance. The primary goal of postacute services, often after a hospitalization, is discharge to a community setting or similar discharge goal with the return of maximum functional ability. This differs from the reimbursement for most long-term, residential care in nursing homes, for which about 60% nationally is covered by Medicaid (Chidambaram & Burns, 2024), a program administered by individual states and funded jointly by states and the federal government to serve persons with few individual assets to pay for care services. The primary goal of long-term services is to maintain the maximum level of functional independence while achieving the highest possible quality of life.

Over time, changes to Medicare have led to shorter hospital stays and a dramatic increase in the amount of postacute care provided by nursing homes. The care goals of short-stay, postacute residents differ from those of residents who receive nursing home care for longer periods, such as months or even years. For those receiving long-term care in nursing homes, the nursing home is not just a source of care but also home: the setting of daily life activities, relationships, activities, meals, and social interactions. Many nursing homes must therefore meet regulatory requirements that address the needs of both long and short-stay residents, as well as both Medicare and Medicaid reimbursement requirements, which adds to the challenge and complexity of measuring quality outcomes and meeting quality metrics in the nursing home setting. This complexity is also reflected in the Centers for Medicare & Medicaid Services (CMS) public online reporting system for nursing homes, Care Compare (formerly Nursing Home Compare), which reports separate long-stay and short-stay quality indicators. Because Medicare payment rates are higher than those provided by Medicaid, there can be an incentive for nursing home providers to focus primarily on performing well—achieving "high quality"—in their postacute operations. Thus, the growing dominance of postacute care in nursing homes could have unintended consequences for long-term nursing home residents, whose needs weigh more heavily in the quality of life and functional care domains than those of postacute residents, whose needs are focused on acute rehabilitation and discharge. Factors that influence quality of daily life, such as control over one's regular routines, interpersonal relationships, enjoyable activities, and meals, take on added importance for long-term residents of nursing homes. For long-term residents, one's overall quality of life may be the ultimate measure of care quality.

Nearly six decades ago, physician Avedis Donabedian proposed that healthcare quality be evaluated in terms of three domains: the structures, process, and outcomes of care (Donabedian, 1966). Donabedian's "structure, process, outcome" model remains the most common approach to understanding and assessing healthcare quality today. According to Donabedian, the structural factors surrounding care (e.g., facility size, number and types of staff, features of the physical environment) influence the processes of care delivery (e.g., clinical assessments of residents, communication between staff related to resident care), which in turn impact care outcomes (the ultimate goals of care). Donabedian's model provides a useful framework for understanding nursing home quality and how approaches to assessing and improving quality have changed over time (Castle & Ferguson, 2010; Figure 3.1 displays Donabedian's model with examples representing each of the model's three domains).

Building upon Donabedian's work in their seminal report addressing needed changes to the U.S. healthcare system, the Institute of Medicine (IOM) defined *quality* as "the degree to which health services for individuals and populations increase the likelihood of desired health outcomes and are consistent with current professional knowledge" (2001, p. 232). The IOM outlined six major aims for healthcare—that it be "safe, effective, patient-centered, timely, efficient, and

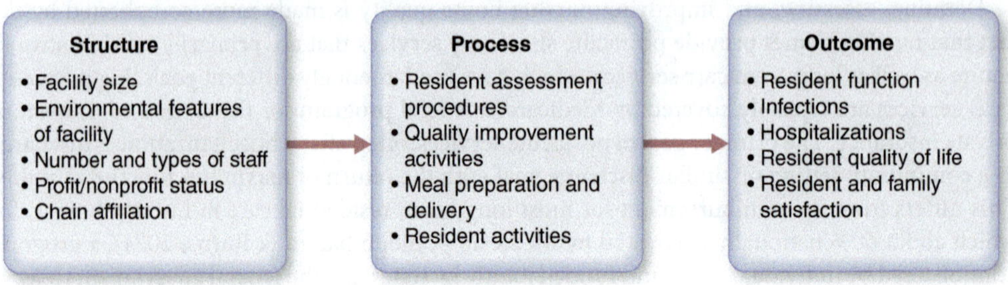
Structure
• Facility size
• Environmental features of facility
• Number and types of staff
• Profit/nonprofit status
• Chain affiliation
Process
• Resident assessment procedures
• Quality improvement activities
• Meal preparation and delivery
• Resident activities
Outcome
• Resident function
• Infections
• Hospitalizations
• Resident quality of life
• Resident and family satisfaction

FIGURE 3.1. Examples of structure, process, and outcome aspects of quality in nursing homes (Donabedian's model).

Source: Data from Donabedian, A. (1966). Evaluating the quality of medical care. *The Milbank Memorial Fund Quarterly*, *44*(3), 166–206. https://doi.org/10.2307/3348969

equitable" (2001, p. 6). These aims remain relevant to examining the quality of care provided across the U.S. healthcare system today, including in nursing homes.

The quality of care in nursing homes is an important public policy issue because the majority of nursing home care is paid for by government agencies using taxpayer dollars. Further, nursing home care is provided to some of the most vulnerable citizens. Government agencies, both state and federal, have assumed the fundamental responsibility for establishing quality standards in nursing homes, monitoring nursing home quality to protect both persons and resources, and assuring compliance and accountability (including penalties) among nursing home providers. Government agencies also report nursing home performance on quality measures to the public for additional accountability and assistance with informed consumer decision-making. Thus, performance on quality measures and regulatory compliance with quality metrics are important aspects of administration of services in the nursing home setting.

THE EVOLUTION OF NURSING HOME QUALITY

Current approaches to assessing the quality and safety of care in nursing homes have been heavily shaped by legislation that directs how nursing homes are regulated and financed. From the regulatory standpoint, in general, state governments are responsible for certifying that nursing homes comply with state and federal requirements for operation. The relationship between regulatory oversight and quality is fundamental to nursing home operations given the highly regulated nature of the nursing home industry relative to other healthcare delivery settings. Regulatory oversight is primarily achieved through health inspections, which are typically conducted annually and consist of in-person visits by inspectors who are commonly called surveyors. Health inspection surveys address a wide range of domains, including resident rights, threats to resident safety, incident reporting, care documentation, and observation of care provision, among others. Results of health inspection surveys are used to create part of the equation that results in the quality rating, or "five-star rating," that is reported to the public by the CMS. Inspection results also carry the potential for punitive consequences such as fines or loss of licensure if regulatory standards are not achieved, including clinical quality standards. In addition to state inspections, for nursing homes that participate in Medicare or Medicaid, which includes most nursing homes, the federal government bears ultimate responsibility for ensuring these facilities comply with federal standards and works with state agencies to assure documentation of standards. See Chapter 4 for more detailed information about the role of state and federal agencies in nursing home regulatory processes.

As touched upon earlier, the government's role in defining and overseeing nursing home quality is a result of several factors, including rising costs of nursing home care borne largely by states and the federal government, historical evidence of abuse and neglect of nursing home residents, and growing emphasis over recent decades on a value-based approach to care delivery and reimbursement that emphasizes achieving the highest quality outcomes at the most efficient cost. The value-based reimbursement approach has increased the emphasis on accurate definition and measurement of quality because it often attaches financial incentives to achieving quality outcomes.

In the past, the government primarily used structural measures to assess nursing home quality, such as safety plans, features of the facility, and adherence to staffing requirements. Structural measures address the resources needed to provide care and remain an important part of the quality measurement equation. Over time, however, there has been a shift to use of more process and outcome measures in assessments of nursing home quality (Castle & Ferguson, 2010). Process measures address what is done, or how care is provided. Outcome measures address the end result of the use of structural resources to carry out care processes, and ideally are a reflection of adequate and appropriate care. A challenge, however, is that outcomes may be influenced by other factors such as individual disease progression and baseline clinical status that are not within the nursing home's control. For example, a resident who enters the nursing home with immobility, dehydration, and a nutritional deficit may develop skin breakdown despite the nursing home having adequate staffing and utilizing evidence-based nursing processes of care. By utilizing multiple types of quality measures (structure, process, outcome), regulators and the public get a clearer picture of what is being done in the facility to increase the potential for the best possible outcomes for individual residents despite risk factors. Current quality measures for nursing homes used by the CMS include a mix of structure, process, and outcome measures. Structural measures include factors such as staffing levels and provision of safe physical spaces. Examples of currently used process measures include the percentage of residents receiving flu shots or taking antipsychotic medications. Examples of currently used outcome measures include the percentage of residents with urinary tract infections or number of residents rehospitalized after being admitted to the nursing home. The development and use of nursing home quality measures will be discussed in more depth later in this chapter.

The remainder of this chapter outlines major developments in the evolution of nursing homes and strategies to assess and improve nursing home quality. (Also see Figure 3.2.) It ends with a brief discussion of some of the important challenges, opportunities, and future directions for the quality of nursing homes and other residential long-term care settings.

Early Nursing Homes

Facilities that we now refer to as nursing homes (SNFs) developed in response to rapidly changing social and economic conditions taking place during the middle of the 20th century. As industrialization changed how families were structured, caregiving responsibilities normally fulfilled within families increasingly went unmet. Initially care for older adults and others in need of supportive services, such as younger persons with disabilities, was the role of religious or charity organizations. However, medical science was developing rapidly in conjunction with the professionalization of nursing and physician education and services, sometimes referred to as an increased "medicalization" to the approach of caring for persons in need. With expanding need for social programs to address the growing numbers of older adults and people with disabilities who had inadequate financial resources and access to supportive care, the government and medical professionals began the development of the long-term care system, which applied a medical/institutional approach to the care of persons in need.

At the height of the Great Depression, the enactment of the Social Security Act in 1935 provided qualifying individuals with funds to pay for modest costs associated with housing and supportive care. However, the Social Security Act prohibited the funds from going to residents of "public institutions," which at the time included almshouses (charitable congregate housing) and "poor farms" (Watson, 2009). Small, independently run nursing homes emerged in response. In 1950, amendments to the Social Security Act expanded program eligibility, increasing the number of Americans who received Social Security benefits. The amendments also reversed the previous policy by allowing Social Security payments to "residents of public institutions," as well as payments directly to nursing homes. Social Security Act amendments also stipulated that states establish standards for nursing homes, but stopped short of dictating what those standards should entail. Eventually, many of the small informal nursing homes that had emerged after the passage of the 1935 Social Security Act were driven out of business as larger firms took over.

The Institutionalization of Long-Term Care

The enactment of the Medicare and Medicaid programs in 1965 represented another major turning point in cementing the government's role in the oversight of nursing homes and the quality of care they provide. The legislation began requiring public programs to provide health insurance coverage to certain groups of Americans, principally adults aged 65 and over, persons with disabilities, and those with low incomes. Institutional long-term care, including care in nursing homes, became eligible for Medicaid coverage for qualifying individuals. Medicaid, however, would not cover the cost of long-term care in HCBS until many years later. Policymakers did

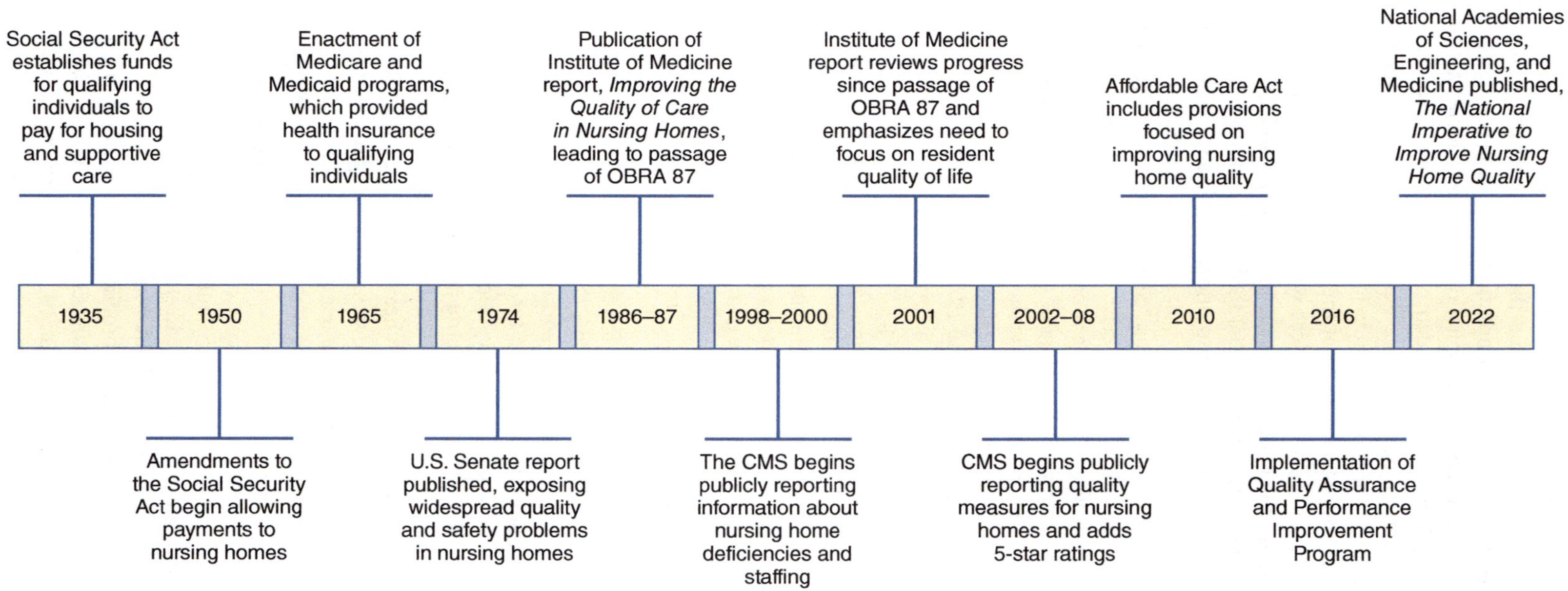

FIGURE 3.2. Important milestones in the development of nursing home quality and safety.

CMS, Centers for Medicare & Medicaid Services; OBRA, Omnibus Budget Reconciliation Act.

not foresee the implications of this policy decision, namely, that Medicaid would play a major role in institutionalizing long-term care. Although the majority of Medicaid-covered long-term care is now delivered in HCBS, Medicaid remains the largest payer of long-term care in nursing homes (Chidambaram & Burns, 2024). Medicare too became a major source of nursing home revenue. Under Medicare, short-term posthospital recovery (postacute care) became reimbursable in "extended care facilities," which included nursing homes. Over time, nursing homes have played an increasing role in postacute care delivery. Today, most nursing homes provide Medicare-covered postacute services in addition to long-term care.

The Social Security Act and establishment of the Medicare and Medicaid programs, as well as continued medicalization of the health services system, led to a dramatic rise in the number of nursing homes throughout the United States during the 1960s and 1970s. Nursing homes, as well as state-run mental hospitals and residential facilities for individuals with intellectual and developmental disabilities, were designed as institutions (Goffman, 1961). Early nursing homes, many of which still exist, were modeled after rural, state-run hospitals. Environmental features such as long, narrow hallways; tile floors; florescent lighting; and shared resident rooms—features designed to maximize efficiency—emphasized the "institutional feel" of these facilities. Care structures and processes also reinforced an "enclosed, formally administered way of life" (Goffman, 1961, p. 11), thus stripping residents of their autonomy. Residents typically had no choice about when to get up in the morning, take showers, or have meals.

The institutionalization of long-term care created serious consequences for residents, as well as for those who worked in these settings. The 1970s, for example, were marked by frequent exposés of egregious safety violations, as well as by abuse and neglect of residents of nursing homes and other institutional settings. Beginning in 1969, the U.S. Senate Special Committee on Aging held a series of hearings on nursing homes, resulting in roughly 1,300 pages of testimony and a 12-volume report entitled, "Nursing Home Care in the United States: Failure in Public Policy" (U.S. Senate, 1974). In 1975, Mary Mendelson exposed pervasive financial fraud associated with the "tender loving care" nursing homes purported to deliver (Mendelson, 1975). A primary concern was that public resources were going to private organizations—many driven by profit—to provide care to vulnerable members of society. There was overwhelming evidence that many facilities were not providing this care well. Concerns persist about the influence of private business interests on the quality and safety of nursing homes. Research has shown, for example, that for-profit nursing homes typically provide lower quality of care to residents than their nonprofit counterparts (Braun et al., 2021; Comondore et al., 2009). About two-thirds of U.S. nursing homes today are for-profit organizations, many part of large corporate chains. However, it should be noted that for-profit facilities generally care for more Medicaid residents, whereas not-for-profit facilities tend to care for more private-pay residents. This can influence quality of care.

In response to the evidence of gross mistreatment of nursing home residents and misuse of public funds, the government clamped down on nursing homes with extensive regulations. Today, the nursing home sector remains one of the most heavily regulated industries in the United States. Although there is widespread agreement that government oversight of nursing homes is needed, critics of the strict regulatory environment for nursing homes argue that it stifles innovation and creates too much emphasis on mere compliance with regulations, at the expense of more meaningful quality improvement (QI). Critics further argue that the regulatory orientation reinforces more focus on protection and safety at the expense of resident autonomy and quality of life. For example, concerns about residents falling (which could negatively impact a nursing home's health inspection results or quality measures) could lead staff to discourage residents from getting up and walking, thus limiting their mobility and independence.

In 1972, the Long-Term Care Ombudsman program was established as a demonstration program in four states (National Ombudsman Resource Center [NORC], 2023). In 1975, amendments to the 1965 Older Americans Act expanded the program to all states. Since that time, Long-Term Care Ombudsmen have played an important role in nursing homes, assisted living facilities, and other sites of long-term care (LTC) delivery. Specifically, the Ombudsmen provide education and training on residents' rights, investigate complaints, mediate conflicts, and work with nursing home resident and family councils to strengthen the voice of residents and family members in facility operations.

Nursing Home Reform

As part of a broader agenda aimed at loosening market restrictions across a range of sectors, then President Ronald Reagan attempted to deregulate nursing homes in the early 1980s. The National Citizen's Coalition for Nursing Home Reform and other consumer advocates led a public outcry against the proposed deregulation (Braithwaite et al., 2007; Hawes, 1987). Although many nursing home advocates recognized limitations with an overreliance on regulations, there was too much evidence of poor care in nursing homes—and too much at stake—to substantially loosen or eliminate regulations, which were developed to protect adults who were extremely vulnerable. To broker a compromise between groups who wanted more and less regulation of nursing homes, Representative Henry Waxman from California proposed that all changes to existing regulations be tabled until a comprehensive study of nursing home quality could be completed. Waxman's proposal led to the establishment, in 1983, of the IOM Committee on Nursing Home Regulations, comprised of national experts on nursing home quality.

The recommendations were included in the resulting IOM report, *Improving the Quality of Care in Nursing Homes* (IOM, 1986), and led to the passage of the Omnibus Budget Reconciliation Act of 1987 (often referred to as "OBRA 87"), including the Nursing Home Reform Act. The legislation marked an important step in defining quality standards for nursing homes. It also affirmed that nursing home residents have fundamental rights, including the right to freedom from abuse and neglect, the right to be treated with dignity, and the right to self-determination, among other rights (IOM, 1986). Table 3.1 lists nursing home resident rights. Additionally, the OBRA 87 legislation led to the creation of a set of assessment and care guidelines focused on improving resident care. For example, OBRA 87 established requirements that nursing homes provide nursing, dietary, and pharmaceutical services (structural measures) and that residents receive periodic and comprehensive assessments (process measures).

In 2001, another IOM report was published, *Improving the Quality of Long-Term Care* (Wunderlich & Kohler, 2001), which reviewed progress made since the OBRA 87 legislation. The

TABLE 3.1 Nursing Home Resident Rights

Federal law guarantees nursing home residents with important rights, including the right to:	
	Freedom from discrimination
	Freedom from abuse and neglect
	Privacy
	Be free of restraints
	Be treated with respect
	Exercise rights as a U.S. citizen
	Receive appropriate medical care
	Information about services and fees
	Participate in activities
	Spend time with visitors
	Participate in resident groups
	Manage one's own money
	Make complaints

report concluded that, although notable gains had been made in nursing home quality in the 15 years since the 1986 IOM report, there was still a need for substantial QI. Importantly, the report identified the need to prioritize resident quality of life, build organizational capacity in nursing homes to implement needed quality and safety changes, and strengthen the LTC workforce, which was at that time comprised primarily of unlicensed individuals who often lacked the training and compensation to provide high-quality care. Although nursing home care is still provided primarily by unlicensed personnel, a result of OBRA 87 is increased training and continuing education requirements for caregiving staff. For example, it mandated nursing assistant certification after completion of a standardized training program, ongoing competency evaluation of nursing assistants, and mandated states to maintain a certified nursing assistant registry (Kelly, 1989).

Nursing home reform (OBRA 87) has a significant role in the current emphasis on care quality, quality measurement, and QI in nursing homes. It aimed to standardize definitions of quality and require facilities to report those objective, standardized measures to reimbursement agencies for public accountability. Although the tenets of OBRA have evolved over time, the legislation remains foundational to our current view of nursing homes as professional caregiving settings with accountability to provide the public with a high standard of care. For example, mandated implementation of the Minimum Data Set (MDS), a resident-specific assessment tool that is required annually and at other pivotal times for each resident to monitor resident status, changes, and outcomes for care planning and reimbursement, forms the basis of many of the current quality indicators and is the direct result of the policy changes initiated in OBRA 87.

Quality Assurance and Quality Improvement: From Manufacturing to Long-Term Care

Quality assurance (QA) aims to prevent quality failures and assure that the determined quality standard is achieved and maintained. The QA approach to quality management grew out of the industrial manufacturing sector. During World War II, it became increasingly important that newly developed manufacturing standards were achieved to maintain the safety of military equipment. An initial and inefficient approach to QA was to inspect each item individually. To create more efficient inspection processes, manufacturers began using protocols, random sampling, and other statistical techniques to monitor product quality. Gradually, the techniques of QA made their way into other sectors, including education, healthcare, and LTC. The OBRA 87 legislation, for example, established the requirement that nursing homes maintain a QA committee, which met quarterly and focused on identifying and addressing quality and safety issues with the goal of assuring safe, adequate care was provided to residents. A 2003 report by the U.S. Department of Health and Human Services (HHS)Office of Inspector General found that most nursing homes met federal requirements related to QA committees (e.g., in frequency of meetings and composition of QA committees). However, the report also identified major challenges that limited the effectiveness of nursing home QA committees, including limited knowledge among committee members related to "conducting QA work," and ongoing staffing challenges in nursing homes, such as inadequate staffing levels and high staff turnover, which limited the amount of time and effort available to put toward QA activities.

Although QA remains an important aspect of nursing home quality and safety requirements, an important limitation is that QA processes tend to focus on achieving compliance and maintaining the current status quo rather than understanding how underlying structures or processes may be contributing to quality problems or changing processes to continually improve. Consequently, there is little opportunity for organizational learning or growth. According to former CMS administrator and founder of the Institute for Healthcare Improvement, Dr. Donald Berwick, QA reinforces a "minimum standards" framework (Berwick, 1989, 2008). Nursing home administrators, for example, devote considerable resources to ensuring compliance with state and federal regulations to avoid legal or financial consequences. Consequently, there is often little room for innovation unless there are immediate and direct regulatory or financial implications.

Frustration with QA's limited impact on improving quality outcomes led to the development of more comprehensive approaches to monitor and address quality issues. Initially referred to as "total quality management" (TQM) and later as "continuous quality improvement" (CQI—or simply QI), these approaches focused on modifying organizational processes with the aim of continually innovating product or service delivery. Techniques such as the "plan-do-study-act" cycle and "root cause analysis" were developed with the goal of involving broad layers of the organization in continually examining and improving their performance. Organizational learning and teamwork are fundamental to QI. Thus, the process of implementing QI may help develop organizational capacity for ongoing performance improvement (Werner & Konetzka, 2010).

As with QA, industrial manufacturers were the first to systematically implement QI. After observing success with QI in the manufacturing sector, healthcare organizations began adopting QI in the mid-1980s. During the late 1980s and 1990s, the methods of QI spread quickly throughout the healthcare industry, particularly in hospitals. An early question was whether QI was appropriate for health and LTC settings, given the complexity of healthcare delivery relative to industrial manufacturing. The National Demonstration Project in Quality Improvement in Health Care showed that healthcare organizations could effectively implement the principles and techniques of QI and that improvements in costs and clinical outcomes could be attained, even relatively quickly (Berwick et al., 1990). The demonstration also showed, however, that QI implementation was less consistent in healthcare than in the manufacturing sector, an expected finding given the individual variation between persons in all roles within a healthcare facility and the less predictable nature of the human response relative to machine responses to input. Even with external support and technical assistance, the demonstration found the implementation of QI was inconsistent across sites. Outcomes of QI, thus, were mixed. Other early research on nursing home QI showed that QI implementation varied widely across facilities and that QI processes had an inconsistent impact on care outcomes (Berlowitz et al., 2003). In addition to the already mentioned challenges related to organizational capacity and staffing, another major challenge for nursing homes at the time was a lack of reliable data and consistent quality metrics to target in QI efforts, a factor that is much improved for today's nursing home providers and administrators, who despite that challenging nature of quality measurement have a number of well-developed data sources to draw upon to identify problems and evaluate solutions.

Establishing a Foundation for More Systematic Quality Improvement in Nursing Homes

The movement to improve healthcare quality was expanding and there was growing emphasis on increasing the transparency of care quality provided—in hospitals, clinics, and nursing homes. On the heels of OBRA 87, researchers at the University of Wisconsin began developing and testing a set of quality measures for use in nursing homes (Zimmerman et al., 1995). The quality measures were based on information collected by nursing home personnel through the MDS. Data from the MDS also formed the basis for calculating the reimbursements provided to nursing homes by Medicare and Medicaid for the care they delivered to residents, as well as being the primary data source for multiple quality indicators.

Beginning in 1998, the CMS began publicly reporting information about nursing home regulatory deficiencies in an early version of Nursing Home Compare (now Care Compare), a web-based public report card for all nursing homes certified by Medicare and/or Medicaid (Konetzka et al., 2021). The goals of Nursing Home Compare were to provide an incentive for nursing homes to improve the quality of care they provided and provide members of the public with information to help them make choices about where to receive nursing home care when needed. In 2000, Nursing Home Compare was expanded to include information about nurse staffing levels. The first measures reported on Nursing Home Compare were limited by their focus primarily on structural and process aspects of quality (information about staffing levels and regulatory deficiencies), rather than care outcomes. Currently, Care Compare includes information about staffing levels (structure), performance on quality indicators (process, outcome), and health inspection reports (structure, process, outcome), taking a multifaceted approach to evaluating quality.

In 2002, the federal government initiated the Nursing Home Quality Initiative. The Initiative expanded the public reporting of quality information for nursing homes to include 10 of the quality measures developed by the Wisconsin research team. The quality measures included indicators of care outcomes for postacute residents (four measures) and LTC residents (six measures) and focused primarily on adverse outcomes, such as pressure ulcers and urinary tract infections. Table 3.2 includes the CMS's currently used quality measures.

The 2003 report by the Inspector General of the HHS (mentioned earlier) noted that most nursing homes reported using the new publicly reported quality measures as the primary data source for their QA/QI work. Because of their importance in the regulatory health inspection process and online public ratings, most nursing home QI efforts continue to focus on the CMS quality measures. However, several states, including Minnesota, Michigan, and Ohio, have developed other quality indicators for nursing homes, which may take higher precedence as QI targets in those states depending on how reimbursement incentives are structured. Minnesota, for example, has developed its own online nursing home report card, which includes numerous quality indicators related to clinical care and resident quality of life. Case Study 3.1 highlights the Minnesota Performance-Based Incentive Payment Program (Minnesota PIPP), a state initiative

TABLE 3.2 Current Quality Measures for Nursing Homes

QUALITY MEASURE (% OF RESIDENTS WHO WERE OR HAD. . .)	NURSING HOME POPULATION	
	SHORT-STAY	LONG-STAY
Increased need for ADL assistance		X
Worsened ability to walk independently		X
Catheter inserted and left in bladder		X
Physically restrained		X
Urinary tract infection		X
Fall with major injury		X
Bowel or bladder incontinence (new or worsened)		X
Lost too much weight		X
Depressive symptoms		X
Used an antianxiety or hypnotic medication		X
Self-reported moderate to severe pain	X	X
Pressure ulcer/injury	X	X
Received an antipsychotic medication	X	X
Hospitalized/Rehospitalized	X	X
ED visit	X	X
Assessed/Appropriately given the flu vaccine	X	X
Assessed/Appropriately given the pneumococcal vaccine	X	X
Discharge function score (better than expected)	X	

ADL, activities of daily living.

Source: Data from Centers for Medicare & Medicaid Services, (2024, July 1). *Quality measures.* https://www.cms.gov/medicare/quality/nursing-home-improvement/quality-measures

Case Study 3.1 Multicomponent State Initiative to Promote Nursing Home Safety

Background

Various organizational and policy strategies have focused on improving care quality and safety in nursing homes. Many of these initiatives, however, have had limited or short-lasting impacts. Beginning in 2007, the state of Minnesota launched the Minnesota PIPP. The program leverages multiple strategies to promote improved nursing home quality with the goal of creating broader and sustained positive impacts on nursing home quality. The program has been nationally recognized for its innovative approach.

Program Components

- Financial incentives are given to participating nursing homes for improving targeted quality metrics through a pay-for-performance mechanism.
- Public reporting of quality-related information is used in a state-developed public report card for nursing homes, which includes a range of indicators related to quality of care and resident quality of life.
- Close collaboration occurs between state program personnel and nursing home leaders throughout the QI process. For example, the state provides technical support and guidance in using data, identifying evidence-based strategies to target specific quality areas (e.g., resident falls or hospital readmissions), and using established QI techniques (such as root cause analysis).
- Mechanisms to facilitate collaboration and peer learning across nursing homes in the state are promoted. For example, the state has sponsored conferences where nursing home personnel can exchange information about their QI projects.

Outcomes

- An external evaluation found that nursing homes participating in Minnesota PIPP demonstrated greater improvement in a composite measure of care quality than nursing homes that did not participate in the program (Arling et al., 2013).
- Interviews with nursing home staff implementing QI projects through the Minnesota PIPP often described learning new skills, seeing positive results related to their QI efforts, and being more satisfied with their jobs (Abrahamson et al., 2015; Davila et al., 2016).
- The state has been recognized nationally for its high-quality long-term services and supports "system," including in the state's nursing homes (see, for example, https://ltsschoices.aarp.org/scorecard-report/2023).

Case Study Discussion Questions

1. How do the components of the Minnesota PIPP relate to some of the approaches to improving nursing home quality and safety outlined in this chapter?
2. Thinking about the findings of the 2022 National Academies of Sciences, Engineering, and Medicine (NASEM) report and nursing home reforms put forth by the Biden–Harris administration, what other strategies could state or federal government agencies use to promote quality and safety in nursing homes?

(*continued*)

Case Study 3.1 Multicomponent State Initiative to Promote Nursing Home Safety (*continued*)

For Further Reading

- Abrahamson, K., Miech, E., Davila, H. W., Mueller, C., Cooke, V., & Arling, G. (2015). Pay-for-performance policy and data-driven decision making within nursing homes: A qualitative study. *BMJ Quality & Safety*, *24*(5), 311–317. https://doi.org/10.1136/bmjqs-2014-003362
- Arling, G., Cooke, V., Lewis, T., Perkins, A., Grabowski, D. C., & Abrahamson, K. (2013). Minnesota's provider-initiated approach yields care quality gains at participating nursing homes. *Health Affairs*, *32*(9), 1631–1638. https://doi.org/10.1377/hlthaff.2013.0294
- Castle, N. G., & Ferguson, J. C. (2010). What is nursing home quality and how is it measured? *The Gerontologist*, *50*(4), 426–442. https://doi.org/10.1093/geront/gnq052
- Davila, H., Abrahamson, K., Mueller, C., Inui, T. S., Black, A. G., & Arling, G. (2016). Nursing assistant perceptions of their role in quality improvement processes in nursing homes. *Journal of Nursing Care Quality*, *31*(3), 282–289. https://doi.org/10.1097/NCQ.0000000000000170

using a multipronged approach to promote nursing home QI, including financial incentives for achieving quality goals, public reporting of quality information, and technical assistance.

The Nursing Home Quality Initiative also began requiring CMS-sponsored Quality Improvement Organizations (QIOs) to work with nursing homes to develop and implement strategies to improve care quality and safety. This requirement was intended to address ongoing evidence that most nursing homes lacked the internal capacity to effectively implement QI. For example, important activities of the QIOs include promoting QI in nursing homes and offering resources, training, and other technical assistance. One strategy has involved QI collaboratives, often focused on specific QI initiatives in nursing homes (e.g., reduction of unnecessary use of antipsychotic medications or reduction of hospital readmissions). In addition to being led by CMS QIOs, other QI collaboratives have been initiated by state agencies, LTC provider associations, the federal government, and independent groups of nursing homes. For example, Case Study 3.2 demonstrates an innovative and effective nonpharmacologic approach to improving the quality of care for dementia patients in nursing homes by reducing the reliance on psychotropic medications. An additional strategy has been to target QIO resources toward those nursing homes most in need of improvement in key areas such as restraint use or pressure ulcers, a strategy which has been criticized for taking too narrow a view of a quality by focusing on a single quality criterion, instead of a comprehensive multifaceted selection approach (Stevenson & Mor, 2009).

In 2008, the CMS expanded Nursing Home Compare to include a 5-star composite rating. Specifically, the CMS began rating each nursing home from 1 (lowest quality) to 5 (highest quality) based on information related to three performance domains (each of which also received a separate 5-star rating): (1) regulatory health inspections (conducted by states and the CMS), (2) nurse staffing levels, and (3) the quality measures. The regulatory health inspections receive the most weight in the 5-star ratings. Deficiencies received by facilities for violations received during their regulatory health inspections can range from minor environmental issues (e.g., dust on a fan) to serious deficiencies, which include deficiencies that are likely to cause—or that do cause—harm to residents (e.g., serious injury, impairment, or death). Often, facilities must pay fines ("civil monetary penalties") for deficiencies they receive which, depending on the severity of the violation, can be sizable. Nursing homes must also develop and submit a plan of correction related to deficiencies they receive. In extreme cases, a facility can be placed on "special status," which requires heightened regulatory oversight, or forced to close because of ongoing evidence of poor or inadequate care provided to residents.

Case Study 3.2 Nonpharmacologic Approach to Reducing Use of Psychotropic Medications

Background

Overuse of psychotropic medications (e.g., antianxiety and antipsychotic medications) among nursing home residents, particularly those with dementia, is a documented quality problem and policy priority for the CMS.

Initiative

A medium-sized nonprofit nursing home chain wanted to reduce the unnecessary use of antipsychotic medications among their residents with dementia. A QI nurse developed a QI approach to address this problem, primarily by relying on principles of person-centered care and nonpharmacologic strategies. After piloting the QI project and seeing success at one nursing home, the organization rolls out the initiative to several other nursing homes.

The Main Components of the Quality Improvement Project

- Identify residents with dementia in the nursing home who are taking antipsychotic medications, but whose quality of life may be negatively affected by unnecessary use of these medications.
- Engage an interdisciplinary team (e.g., nurse, nursing assistant, social worker, activities/ recreational therapy staff) to develop a personalized life story for each resident. The life story included the residents' interests, prior daily routines, vocational history (e.g., they were a farmer), and other information about their life and individual preferences (e.g., food they enjoy, family members who visit, etc.)
- Develop an individualized care and activity plan for each resident based on their biography and creative nonpharmacologic approaches. Examples of activities include aromatherapy, cooking, art, walking, and games, among others.

Outcomes

- All 15 nursing homes that implemented the QI project reported a reduction in use of psychotropic medications among residents with dementia.
- Staff reported other positive outcomes, including greater social engagement among participating residents, improved resident independence in daily activities, and decreased incidence of resident symptoms of anxiety and distress.

Case Study Discussion Questions

1. The primary outcome targeted in this QI project was use of psychotropic medications. Thinking about the CMS quality measures (Table 3.2), are there other measures you think could be positively affected through this initiative?
2. Can you think of technology-related interventions that could potentially be adapted to help residents with dementia remain active and engaged so antipsychotic medications may be less necessary?

For Further Reading

- Abrahamson, K., Davila, H., Kirk, L., Garavito, G. A., & Mueller, C. (2021). Can a nursing home psychotropic reduction project be successfully implemented in assisted living? *Journal of Applied Gerontology*, *40*(9), 1071–1079. https://doi.org/10.1177/0733464820948328

Although the specific quality measures publicly included in the 5-star rating calculations have evolved somewhat over time, the measures have remained focused on adverse clinical outcomes. One of the ongoing concerns with the quality measures is that most are based on information reported by nursing home personnel. Thus, many have argued, they are open to manipulation or "gaming" by nursing home providers. For example, many nursing homes have improved their quality measure scores more than they have the regulatory health inspection or staffing components of their public ratings (Han et al., 2018). To strengthen the quality measures, the CMS has added several measures that are based on Medicare claims data, such as rehospitalizations and ED visits, rather than staff-reported information. Further, the CMS has modified how nursing home staffing data are compiled so they reflect more objective information (i.e., payroll-based information instead of staff-reported information). Although evidence shows that nursing home ratings do not always accurately reflect care quality, research has also demonstrated that high and low ratings likely represent a meaningful difference in care quality (Konetzka et al., 2021). Thus, there is likely a real difference in the quality of care provided in nursing homes with 1- and 5-star ratings, although many 3- and 4-star nursing homes are likely to have similar care quality.

Passage of the Affordable Care Act (ACA) in 2010 instituted an additional nursing home QI initiative entitled the Quality Assurance and Process Improvement (QAPI) program. The QAPI directs nursing home providers to address QI systematically, comprehensively, and with the use of data. Within nursing homes, QAPI programs are directed by facility administrators and a multidisciplinary QAPI committee. Facilities are required to address the five elements of QAPI: QAPI design and scope; establishment of QAPI governance within the facility; feedback, data systems, and monitoring; conduction of performance improvement projects; and systematic evaluation and action based upon findings. The objective of QAPI is to improve the quality of care and resident quality of life within facilities, and the program requires nursing homes to be accountable for a number of process measures such as data collection and committee activities related to the five elements. More research and evaluation are needed to elucidate the impact of QAPI on outcomes.

CHALLENGES, OPPORTUNITIES, AND FUTURE DIRECTIONS

The Movement Toward Person-Centered Care

The movement toward person-centered care (often referred to as "patient-centered care" in the broader healthcare context) in LTC has taken place over several decades and involved efforts by consumer advocates, LTC providers, professional associations, and state and federal government agencies. Unlike the early orientation of nursing homes, which focused on maximizing efficiency and control, person-centered care involved a reorientation toward care structures and processes that are driven by the preferences, needs, and experiences of those receiving LTC in nursing homes, assisted living facilities, and other LTC settings. The initial calls for person-centered care go back to the nursing home reform movement of the 1970s and 1980s. For example, the OBRA 87 legislation required nursing homes to develop individualized care plans (i.e., person-centered care plans) for all their residents. Although OBRA 87 led to important advances in the quality of care provided to nursing home residents, it fell short of achieving the level of change many advocates hoped for. For example, advocates argued that the standardized care assessments instituted after OBRA 87 emphasized clinical aspects of resident care over their overall quality of life (Koren, 2010).

In the late 1990s, ongoing efforts by consumer advocates led to the birth of the nursing home "culture change" movement, which promoted individualized care, empowered staff, created more "homelike" nursing home environments, and ensured that the voices of residents were heard in decisions affecting them. The culture change movement, which continues today, represents a broad shift toward person-centered care. Table 3.3 outlines key structural and process components of nursing home culture change. The culture change movement has led to important changes in many nursing homes. For example, many facilities have adopted process changes such as flexible mealtimes, greater food choice, and improved activities programming. Many nursing homes have also instituted structural changes. For example, many nursing homes have implemented some

TABLE 3.3 Structural and Process Components of Nursing Home Culture Change

DOMAIN	EXAMPLE STRUCTURE COMPONENT	EXAMPLE PROCESS COMPONENT
Activities	• Adding space for resident activities (e.g., outdoor gardens, bird aviaries in common areas within facility) • Engaging volunteers to assist with activities for residents	• Adding more activities (e.g., on weekends) and more varied activities to address interests of different residents
Daily routines	• Hiring a part-time staff person to assist with morning routines	• Allowing residents to decide when to get up in the morning, when to bathe, etc.
Environment	• Designing the building in a "homelike" style (e.g., private bedrooms, warm paint colors, fireplaces, plants, etc.)	• Engaging residents and families in personalizing space, such as by creating "memory boxes" outside of residents' rooms
Food/meals	• Creating dining spaces for small groups of residents (vs. a large dining hall)	• Providing residents with food options for snacks and meals
Relationships	• Adding small sitting areas for residents and their visitors to spend time	• Welcoming families and members of the community to visit frequently; scheduling events to "bring people in"
Staffing	• Providing staff training and support (e.g., related to delivering person-centered care, implementing quality improvement activities, etc.)	• Scheduling the same staff members to work on a particular unit so they know individual residents and their preferences better

level of consistent staffing (i.e., assigning the same staff members to work with specific residents to strengthen relationships between staff and residents, as well as staff's knowledge of each resident's unique care preferences and needs).

Further, many nursing homes have made some environmental modifications that are consistent with nursing home culture change. Relatively easy environmental changes include using warm-toned paint, carpeting, and furniture colors; creating "memory boxes" outside residents' rooms to highlight who each resident is as a unique person; and integrating plants and animals into the facility (e.g., bird aviaries). A number of specific culture change initiatives, such as Green House nursing homes, the Eden Alternative, and Small House nursing homes, have aimed to institute multiple aspects of culture change by recreating the vision of what a nursing home is and creating homelike care facilities that remove the institutional aspects of care. For example, meals are prepared and provided family style at a kitchen table, staff eat and engage with residents throughout the day, and the physical facilities are designed to resemble a family home without long hallways, nursing stations, and medication carts. There is evidence that the Green House and similar models can improve the quality of care and life for nursing home residents (Williams & Joshi, 2023).

Early research found that most nursing home experts considered the principles of nursing home culture change "the ideal" (Miller et al., 2008). Further, many nursing home administrators reported adopting elements of culture change in their facilities (Doty et al., 2008). Although research on the impact of nursing home culture change on resident outcomes remains limited, some research suggests implementation may reduce certain types of regulatory deficiencies (Lepore et al., 2020) and positively impact resident quality of life and family satisfaction (Duan et al., 2020).

After several years of development, in 2010 the CMS implemented a revised resident screening and assessment tool (the MDS 3.0) that shifted resident assessments from administrative records and staff observations to hearing directly from residents about their needs and preferences (Saliba & Buchanan, 2008). The MDS 3.0 also improved assessments related to mood, cognition, pain, and residents' preferences related to daily routines and activities. These changes to the MDS have led to greater attention to understanding and fulfilling resident preferences (Abbott et al., 2018; Van Haitsma et al., 2014) and better identification of residents' care needs.

The shift to person-centered care has increased the focus on quality of life, which is a key outcome centered on the individual's experience in receiving services. Essential aspects of quality of life in nursing homes include dignity and respect, emotional well-being, physical comfort, relationships, enjoyment of food and meals, social integration, independence, mood, and autonomy or self-determination (Kane et al., 2003). Efforts to understand residents' views on nursing home quality and develop ways to assess their care experiences and quality of life first emerged during the person-centered care and nursing home reform movements in the 1980s. In a foundational study, the National Citizen's Coalition for Nursing Home Reform sponsored a series of discussions to elicit nursing home residents' perspectives on how nursing home quality should be defined and measured (National Citizens' Coalition for Nursing Home Reform, 1985). Discussion sessions were held in 15 cities and involved over 450 residents of 150 nursing homes. As a result of this work and related initiatives, by 2007 a total of 50 tools had been developed to assess the care satisfaction or quality of life of nursing home and assisted living residents (Castle, 2007).

In recent years, there has been an increasing focus on assessing person-reported outcomes, including the experiences of patients, residents, and families with the care they receive. Minnesota and Ohio were the first states to systematically assess and report the experience of nursing home residents (quality of life in Minnesota; satisfaction in Ohio; Kane et al., 2003; Straker et al., 2007). Today, however, person-report outcome measures have become more common. Several states, for example, have adopted CoreQ measures as part of routine quality monitoring of their state Medicaid programs. The CoreQ is a set of five measures developed to assess residents' and families' satisfaction with care received in SNFs and assisted living facilities (Castle et al., 2021). CoreQ measures are also increasingly used in nursing home QI efforts. Although the CMS Care Compare rating system has been widely criticized for lacking a standardized, publicly reported measure of consumer experience to supplement the other metrics included in the 5-star ratings, that will likely soon change. The CMS has proposed a rule that SNFs be required to collect data from short-stay nursing home residents via the CoreQ Short Stay Discharge survey for residents.

The Affordable Care Act: Integration and Differentiation in Long-Term Care

The 2010 ACA included numerous provisions focused on improving nursing home quality, including requirements related to greater information transparency (e.g., about nursing home ownership and staffing), staff training (e.g., related to dementia care and the prevention of resident abuse), background check requirements for nursing home staff, and the establishment of compliance and ethics programs in nursing homes.

After a period of development and testing, in 2016 the ACA began requiring nursing homes to develop QAPI programs. The QAPI program was developed to integrate the QA and QI approaches to quality. Through QAPI, nursing homes are required to implement ongoing QI activities focused on clinical care, resident choice, and resident quality of life. As part of QAPI, the CMS encourages nursing home staff to engage residents and families in QI activities within the facility. For example, staff could solicit input from residents and families on areas they view as priorities for improvement, such as environmental features of the facility, activities for residents, food, or interactions with staff. Feedback could also be sought on the impact of improvement initiatives, particularly efforts focused on resident choice and quality of life.

The ACA also introduced broader, systemwide reforms that impacted nursing homes, particularly through relationships with hospitals. For example, the ACA instituted financial penalties for hospitals with high rates of hospital readmission. Further, the ACA encouraged healthcare organizations to form accountable care organizations and to adopt bundled payment models. The goal of these models is to improve patient outcomes and lower costs by promoting improved coordination and shared responsibility across healthcare settings. For example, a person hospitalized with pneumonia may be at high risk for rehospitalization after hospital discharge. Yet, the desire to lower hospital costs encourages shorter hospital stays and earlier discharge. Consequently, as hospitals have patients hospitalized for shorter periods, nursing homes (SNFs—those that provide Medicare-reimbursed postacute care) have played a growing role in posthospital recovery. Consequently, incentives were created for nursing homes to differentiate themselves from other nursing homes as high-quality providers to attract more postacute hospital referrals. Growing competition among nursing homes has also led many facilities to provide specialized services: dementia care, hospice and palliative care, and specific types of posthospital recovery, such as cardiac care.

COVID-19 and Renewed Calls for Nursing Home Reform

In 2020, the Committee on the Quality of Care in Nursing Homes began work on a comprehensive examination of nursing home quality. Commissioned by the NASEM (formerly the IOM, which produced the 1986 and 2001 nursing home quality reports), the committee began its work during the COVID-19 pandemic, which brought intense public attention to nursing homes. With high death rates among residents and disproportionate impacts on staff, these facilities became a central focus in daily news headlines. (Cronin & Evans, 2022; Grabowski & Mor, 2020). Suddenly, long-standing challenges facing nursing homes—inadequate staffing, insufficient training and infection control expertise, crowded conditions—became public and urgent.

The Committee's work led to an extensive report on the current state of nursing home quality and safety. The report, *The National Imperative to Improve Nursing Home Quality* (NASEM, 2022), concluded that major changes are needed to the financing, delivery, and regulation of nursing homes in the United States, and that "immediate action to initiate fundamental changes is necessary" (p. 495). The report included seven overarching goals to achieve high-quality nursing home care, each with specific recommendations (see Table 3.4 for a list of the goals with examples).

TABLE 3.4 Key Goals From the 2022 NASEM Report

GOAL	RECOMMENDATION (EXAMPLES)
1. Provide comprehensive, equitable care that maximizes residents' health, safety, and quality of life.	1B. Government agencies and other organizations should support research and demonstration projects to identify, develop, and test promising models of care.
2. Strengthen the workforce by supporting more training and appropriate compensation.	2A. Recruit and retain staff through more competitive wages and benefits.
3. Increase transparency and accountability related to ownership and finances.	3B. Create a mechanism to ensure information on nursing home ownership and financing is publicly available.
4. Develop a better system for financing nursing home care.	4D. Increase Medicaid reimbursement rates to support better staffing and higher quality of care.
5. Improve QA systems to effectively monitor and address quality concerns.	5B. Develop and test strategies to improve the effectiveness of QA processes.
6. Expand quality measurement capabilities and QI processes.	6A. Add resident and family experience ratings to the online Care Compare reporting system.
7. Ensure all nursing homes adopt health information technology.	7A and C. Provide resources to support widespread adoption of health information technology.

QA, quality assurance; QI, quality improvement.

Source: Adapted from National Academies of Sciences, Engineering, and Medicine. (2022). *The national imperative to improve nursing home quality: Honoring our commitment to residents, families, and staff.* National Academies Press. https://doi.org/10.17226/26526

TABLE 3.5 Biden-Harris Administration Reforms to Improve Nursing Home Quality

AREA OF REFORM	SPECIFIC INITIATIVES
1. Ensuring taxpayer dollars support nursing homes that provide safe, adequate, and dignified care	• Establish a minimum nursing home staffing requirement. • Reduce resident room crowding. • Strengthen the Skilled Nursing Facility Value-Based Purchasing Program (SNF-VPB). • Reinforce safeguards against unnecessary medications and treatments.
2. Enhancing accountability and oversight	• Adequately fund inspection activities. • Beef up scrutiny on more of the poorest performing facilities. • Expand financial penalties and other enforcement sanctions. • Increase accountability for chain owners of substandard facilities. • Provide technical assistance to nursing homes to help them improve.
3. Increasing transparency	• Create a database of nursing home owners and operators. • Improve transparency of facility ownership and finances. • Enhance nursing home Care Compare. • Examine the role of private equity.
4. Creating pathways to good-paying jobs with the free and fair choice to join a union	• Ensure nurse aide training is affordable. • Support state efforts to improve staffing and workforce sustainability. • Launch national Nursing Career Pathways Campaign.
5. Ensuring pandemic and emergency preparedness in nursing homes.	• Continued COVID-19 testing in long-term care facilities. • Continued COVID-19 vaccinations and boosters in long-term care facilities. • Strengthen requirements for on-site infection preventionists. • Enhance requirements for pandemic and emergency preparedness. • Integrate pandemic lessons into nursing home requirements.

Source: The White House. (2022, February 28). *Fact sheet: Protecting seniors by improving safety and quality of care in the nation's nursing homes.* https://www.whitehouse.gov/briefing-room/statements-releases/2022/02/28/fact-sheet-protecting-seniors-and-people-with-disabilities-by-improving-safety-and-quality-of-care-in-the-nations-nursing-homes

The devastating impact of COVID-19 on nursing homes also led the Biden administration to initiate numerous reforms targeting nursing home quality and safety (The White House, 2022). Many of these reforms overlap with recommendations included in the 2022 NASEM report and address five broad areas (Table 3.5 outlines specific initiatives associated with each of these areas):

1. Ensure federal funding supports nursing homes that provide safe, adequate and dignified care.
2. Enhance accountability and oversight.
3. Increase transparency.
4. Create pathways to good-paying jobs with the free and fair choice to join a union.
5. Ensure pandemic and emergency preparedness in nursing homes.

SUMMARY

Nursing homes have been heavily shaped by federal policies and programs (e.g., Social Security Act, Medicare and Medicaid, ACA). Some important gains have been made in nursing home quality and safety over time. Nursing home residents have more direct input into their care needs and preferences (e.g., through care assessments and "culture change" initiatives) and there is growing focus on residents' quality of life. Use of certain harmful practices has been reduced (e.g., overuse of antipsychotic medications among residents with dementia, physical restrains) and many nursing homes and hospitals have become more integrated, which has contributed to growing specialization among nursing homes, as well as improved outcomes, such as lower rates of rehospitalization. Considerable challenges to nursing home quality and safety remain, however, which the COVID-19 pandemic highlighted. Many nursing homes are understaffed, staff often do not receive the training and support they need, and there are inequities in the quality of care available to nursing home residents based on where they live, or their race and ethnicity. Although new policy reforms have been initiated, more substantial change will be needed to ensure nursing home residents consistently receive care that is both high quality and safe.

END-OF-CHAPTER RESOURCES

DISCUSSION QUESTIONS

1. How do pay-for-performance policies impact decision making processes in nursing homes?
2. What is the history of nursing home quality improvement and how has it evolved over time?
3. What factors contribute to resident satisfaction in nursing homes?
4. How do government regulations and inspections impact nursing home care quality in the United States?
5. What are some of the key challenges facing nursing homes and long-term care facilities in the United States today?
6. What ethical concerns arise in the provision of care in nursing homes and long-term care facilities, and how can these concerns be addressed?

SPRINGER PUBLISHING CONNECT™

A robust set of instructor resources designed to supplement this text is located at http://connect.springerpub.com/content/book/978-0-8261-4935-0. Qualifying instructors may request access by emailing textbook@springerpub.com.

REFERENCES

Abbott, K. M., Heid, A. R., Kleban, M., Rovine, M. J., & Van Haitsma, K. (2018). The change in nursing home residents' preferences over time. *Journal of the American Medical Directors Association*, *19*(12), 1092–1098. https://doi.org/10.1016/j.jamda.2018.08.004

Abrahamson, K., Miech, E., Davila, H. W., Mueller, C., Cooke, V., & Arling, G. (2015). Pay-for-performance policy and data-driven decision making within nursing homes: A qualitative study. *BMJ Quality & Safety*, *24*(5), 311–317. https://doi.org/10.1136/bmjqs-2014-003362

Arling, G., Cooke, V., Lewis, T., Perkins, A., Grabowski, D. C., & Abrahamson, K. (2013). Minnesota's provider-initiated approach yields care quality gains at participating nursing homes. *Health Affairs*, *32*(9), 1631–1638. https://doi.org/10.1377/hlthaff.2013.0294

Berlowitz, D. R., Young, G. J., Hickey, E. C., Saliba, D., Mittman, B. S., Czarnowski, E., Simon, B., Anderson, J. J., Ash, A. S., Rubenstein, L. V., & Moskowitz, M. A. (2003). Quality improvement implementation in the nursing home. *Health Services Research*, *38*(1 Pt 1), 65–83. https://doi.org/10.1111/1475-6773.00105

Berwick, D. M. (1989). Continuous improvement as an ideal in health care. *New England Journal of Medicine*, *320*(1), 53–56. https://doi.org/10.1056/NEJM198901053200110

Berwick, D. M. (2008). The science of improvement. *Journal of the American Medical Association*, *299*(10), 1182–1184. https://doi.org/10.1001/jama.299.10.1182

Berwick, D. M., Godfrey, A. B., Roessner, J., Plsek, P. E., & Garvin, D. A. (1990). *Curing health care: New strategies for quality improvement: A report on the national demonstration project on quality improvement in health care.* Jossey-Bass Publishers.

Braithwaite, J., Makkai, T., & Braithwaite, V. A. (2007). *Regulating aged care: Ritualism and the new pyramid.* Edward Elgar Publishing.

Braun, R. T., Jung, H. Y., Casalino, L. P., Myslinski, Z., & Unruh, M. A. (2021, November). Association of private equity investment in US nursing homes with the quality and cost of care for long-stay residents. *JAMA Health Forum, 2*(11), e213817. https://doi.org/10.1001/jamahealthforum.2021.3817

Castle, N. G. (2007). A review of satisfaction instruments used in long-term care settings. *Journal of Aging & Social Policy, 19*(2), 9–41. https://doi.org/10.1300/J031v19n02_02

Castle, N. G., & Ferguson, J. C. (2010). What is nursing home quality and how is it measured? *The Gerontologist, 50*(4), 426–442. https://doi.org/10.1093/geront/gnq052

Castle, N. G., Gifford, D., & Schwartz, L. B. (2021). The CoreQ: Development and testing of a nursing facility resident satisfaction survey. *Journal of Applied Gerontology, 40*(6), 629–637. https://doi.org/10.1177/0733464820940871

Chidambaram, P., & Burns, A. (2024, January 5). *A look at nursing facility characteristics between 2015 and 2023.* KFF. https://www.kff.org/medicaid/issue-brief/a-look-at-nursing-facility-characteristics

Comondore, V. R., Devereaux, P. J., Zhou, Q., Stone, S. B., Busse, J. W., Ravindran, N. C., Burns, K. E., Haines, T., Stringer, B., Cook, D. J., Walter, S. D., Sullivan, T., Berwanger, O., Bhandari, M., Banglawala, S., Lavis, J. N., Petrisor, B., Schünemann, H., Walsh, K., … Guyatt, G. H. (2009). Quality of care in for-profit and not-for-profit nursing homes: Systematic review and meta-analysis. *British Medical Journal, 339*, b2732. https://doi.org/10.1136/bmj.b2732

Cronin, C. J., & Evans, W. N. (2022). Nursing home quality, COVID-19 deaths, and excess mortality. *Journal of Health Economics, 82*, 102592. https://doi.org/10.1016/j.jhealeco.2022.102592

Davila, H., Abrahamson, K., Mueller, C., Inui, T. S., Black, A. G., & Arling, G. (2016). Nursing assistant perceptions of their role in quality improvement processes in nursing homes. *Journal of Nursing Care Quality, 31*(3), 282–289. https://doi.org/10.1097/NCQ.0000000000000170

Donabedian, A. (1966). Evaluating the quality of medical care. *The Milbank Memorial Fund Quarterly, 44*(3), 166–206. https://doi.org/10.2307/3348969

Doty, M. M., Koren, M. J., & Sturla, E. L. (2008, May 1). *Culture change in nursing homes: How far have we come? Findings from the Commonwealth Fund 2007 National Survey of Nursing Homes.* Commonwealth Fund. https://www.commonwealthfund.org/publications/fund-reports/2008/may/culture-change-nursing-homes-how-far-have-we-come-findings

Duan, Y., Mueller, C. A., Yu, F., & Talley, K. M. (2020). The effects of nursing home culture change on resident quality of life in US nursing homes: An integrative review. *Research in Gerontological Nursing, 13*(4), 210–224. https://doi.org/10.3928/19404921-20200115-02

Goffman, E. (1961). *Asylums: Essays on the social situations of mental patients and other inmates.* Anchor Books.

Grabowski, D. C., & Mor, V. (2020). Nursing home care in crisis in the wake of COVID-19. *Journal of the American Medical Association, 324*(1), 23–24. https://doi.org/10.1001/jama.2020.8524

Han, X., Yaraghi, N., & Gopal, R. (2018). Winning at all costs: Analysis of inflation in nursing homes' rating system. *Production and Operations Management, 27*(2), 215–233. https://doi.org/10.1111/poms.12804

Hawes, C. (1987). Nursing home reform and the politics of long-term care. *PS: Political Science & Politics, 20*(2), 232–241. https://doi.org/10.2307/419160

Institute of Medicine, Committee on Nursing Home Regulation. (1986). *Improving the quality of care in nursing homes.* National Academies Press.

Institute of Medicine, Committee on Quality of Health Care in America. (2001). *Crossing the quality chasm: A new health system for the 21st century.* National Academies Press. https://doi.org/10.17226/10027

Kane, R. A., Kling, K. C., Bershadsky, B., Kane, R. L., Giles, K., Degenholtz, H. B., Liu, J., & Cutler, L. J. (2003). Quality of life measures for nursing home residents. *The Journals of Gerontology Series A: Biological Sciences and Medical Sciences*, 58(3), M240–M248. https://doi.org/10.1093/gerona/58.3.M240

Kelly, M. (1989). The Omnibus Budget Reconciliation Act of 1987: A policy analysis. *Nursing Clinics of North America, 24*(3), 791–794. https://doi.org/10.1016/S0029-6465(22)01539-0

Konetzka, T. R., Yan, K., & Werner, R. M. (2021). Two decades of nursing home compare: What have we learned? *Medical Care Research and Review, 78*(4), 295–310. https://doi.org/10.1177/1077558720931652

Koren, M. J. (2010). Person-centered care for nursing home residents: The culture-change movement. *Health Affairs, 29*(2), 312–317. https://doi.org/10.1377/hlthaff.2009.0966

Lepore, M. J., Lima, J. C., & Miller, S. C. (2020). Nursing home culture change practices and survey deficiencies: A national longitudinal panel study. *The Gerontologist, 60*(8), 1411–1423. https://doi.org/10.1093/geront/gnaa063

Mendelson, M. A. (1975). *Tender loving greed.* Random House.

Miller, E. A., Booth, M., & Mor, V. (2008). Assessing experts' views of the future of long-term care. *Research on Aging, 30*(4), 450–473. https://doi.org/10.1177/0164027508316607

National Academies of Sciences, Engineering, and Medicine. (2022). *The national imperative to improve nursing home quality: Honoring our commitment to residents, families, and staff.* The National Academies Press. https://doi.org/10.17226/26526

National Citizens' Coalition for Nursing Home Reform. (1985). *A consumer perspective on quality of care: The residents' point of view.* https://theconsumervoice.org/uploads/files/issues/resident_pers.pdf

National Ombudsman Resource Center. (2023). *The national long-term care Ombudsman Resource Center. Program history.* https://ltcombudsman.org/about/about-ombudsman/program-history

Office of Inspector General. (2003). *Quality assurance committees in nursing homes* (Report #OEI-01-01-0090). U.S. Department of Health and Human Services. https://oig.hhs.gov/oei/reports/oei-01-01-00090.pdf

Saliba, D., & Buchanan, J. (2008, April). *Development and validation of a revised nursing home assessment tool: MDS 3.0.* Centers for Medicare and Medicaid Services. https://www.cms.gov/Medicare/Quality-Initiatives-Patient-Assessment-Instruments/NursingHomeQualityInits/downloads/MDS30FinalReport.pdf

Stevenson, D. G., & Mor, V. (2009). Targeting nursing homes under the quality improvement organization program's 9th statement of work. *Journal of the American Geriatrics Society, 57*(9), 1678–1684. https://doi.org/10.1111/j.1532-5415.2009.02401.x

Straker, J. K., Ejaz, F. K., McCarthy, C., & Jones, J. A. (2007). Developing and testing a satisfaction survey for nursing home residents: The Ohio experience. *Journal of Aging & Social Policy, 19*(2), 83–105. https://doi.org/10.1300/J031v19n02_05

U.S. Senate. (1974). *Nursing home care in the United States: Failure in public policy.* U.S. Government Printing Office.

Van Haitsma, K., Abbott, K. M., Heid, A. R., Carpenter, B., Curyto, K., Kleban, M., Eshraghi, K., Duntzee, C. I., & Spector, A. (2014). The consistency of self-reported preferences for everyday living: Implications for person-centered care delivery. *Journal of Gerontological Nursing, 40*(10), 34–46. https://doi.org/10.3928/00989134-20140820-01

Watson, S. D. (2009). From almshouses to nursing homes and community care: Lessons from Medicaid's history. *Georgia State University Law Review, 26*(3), Article 13. http://digitalarchive.gsu.edu/gsulr/vol26/iss3/13

Werner, R. M., & Konetzka, R. T. (2010). Advancing nursing home quality through quality improvement itself. *Health Affairs, 29*(1), 81–86. https://doi.org/10.1377/hlthaff.2009.0555

The White House. (2022, February 28). *FACT SHEET: Protecting seniors by improving safety and quality of care in the nation's nursing homes.* https://www.whitehouse.gov/briefing-room/statements-releases/2022/02/28/fact-sheet-protecting-seniors-and-people-with-disabilities-by-improving-safety-and-quality-of-care-in-the-nations-nursing-homes

Williams, C., & Joshi, A. (2023). The Greenhouse model of nursing home care: A scoping review. *Journal of Applied Gerontology, 43*(7), 803–813. https://doi.org/10.1177/07334648231216005

Wunderlich, G. S., & Kohler, P. O. (Eds.). (2001). *Improving the quality of long-term care.* National Academies Press. https://doi.org/10.17226/9611

Zimmerman, D. R., Karon, S. L., Arling, G., Clark, B. R., Collins, T., Ross, R., & Sainfort, F. (1995). Development and testing of nursing home quality indicators. *Health Care Financing Review, 16*(4), 107–127. https://www.ncbi.nlm.nih.gov/pmc/articles/PMC4193525

CHAPTER 4

REGULATORY FRAMEWORK AND COMPLIANCE IN LONG-TERM CARE

Pamela Nadash

Learning Objectives

After completing this chapter, each learner will be able to:

- Understand the history and background of long-term services and supports (LTSS), and how that has led to the regulatory structure we see today.
- Comprehend how the payment sources for LTSS—primarily, the Medicaid program—have influenced the availability, structure, and quality of LTSS.
- Understand the role of states in not only administering the Medicaid program, which shapes the service infrastructure for LTSS, but also in licensing and certifying LTSS providers.
- Gain insight into how the regulatory structure for nursing homes raises key issues in ensuring quality and safety in LTSS, including the adequacy of staffing, regulatory oversight mechanisms, and the role of data collection and reporting.
- Gain an understanding of how expanded access to home- and community-based services poses new regulatory challenges given the wide range of service types and settings.

INTRODUCTION

Understanding the history of long-term services and supports (LTSS) is critical to understanding its regulation—most importantly, understanding how the role of government has grown over time in paying for and overseeing the range of services and settings that comprise LTSS. While the term *government* implies a unified entity, in fact many different governmental entities are involved in LTSS regulation, with the most important split being between federal and state responsibilities. This fragmentation of responsibility is largely due to the different payment sources for LTSS—Medicaid, Medicare, and private pay—as well as the many different types of professionals involved—each of which adheres to different state-specific licensing requirements. An historical perspective is central to understanding LTSS regulation because the sector was critically shaped by the dominance of nursing homes as the archetypal LTSS service—so much so that many people think only of nursing homes when they hear "long-term care" (LTC). Thus, the story of LTSS regulation is a story of an evolving set of strategies to protect nursing home residents and ensure that the government is getting value for money, as well as belated efforts to adapt those strategies in response to the increasing availability of LTSS outside of nursing home settings—which is in turn a response to the aging community's emphasis on aging in place, and the disability rights movement's view that the ability to live out one's life in the community is a human right.

HISTORY OF LONG-TERM SERVICES AND SUPPORTS

Historians trace the beginnings of government involvement in LTSS to the establishment of poorhouses (also known as almshouses) in early America, similar to those common in England during Elizabethan times. This "indoor relief" was meant for any person unable to support themselves, whether because of circumstance (widows and children) or illness or disability. Significant stigma was attached to relying on these institutions, which were operated according to the whims of the local communities that sustained them (Watson, 2009).

Only in the 20th century did this change, with the Depression era reducing stigma for those in need and increasing political support for more systematic ways of helping people. Backing for a stronger government role was epitomized by the passage of the Social Security Act in 1935, which not only identified specific groups deemed worthy of support and created distinctions among groups (especially between workers who made Social Security contributions and people who did not), but also set out a framework for how states and the federal government could work together in operating the various programs. This overall framework continues to govern Titles XVIII and XIX of the Act to this day—the Medicare and Medicaid programs, which were added in 1965 (Watson, 2009).

As life expectancy increased over the 20th century and older people became less impoverished (largely due to the new Social Security program), demand for care homes for older adults boomed. This set the stage for the growth of the nursing home industry, which grew from 1,037 facilities in 1930 to 17,455 in 1957 (Kaffenberger, 2001). This new industry successfully advocated for itself, gaining important concessions from government—such as loan guarantees from the Federal Housing Administration in 1959 and the 1960 Kerr–Mills Act (Medical Assistance for the Aged, PL 86–778, §601, 74 Stat. 924, 987), which dramatically expanded the nursing home industry in certain states as well as the role of government in funding it (Watson, 2009). But the most significant boost to the nursing home industry—a step that entrenched nursing homes as the default mode of LTSS—was when nursing home services were required under the Medicaid program.

Thus, the Medicaid program came to finance the majority of paid LTSS (e.g., 59% of nursing facility residents are now covered by Medicaid [Medicaid and CHIP Payment and Access Commission (MACPAC, 2023)]). States make the choice to participate in Medicaid and have considerable discretion in determining what the program covers and who may participate. However, to receive federal matching funds, states must meet certain federal requirements. These federal requirements constitute the baseline for state Medicaid programs; states may (and do) choose to exceed them. The matching funds represent a big incentive for state participation in Medicaid, one that is stronger for poor states than for wealthier ones. While states with high per capita incomes get only 50 cents from the federal government for every Medicaid dollar spent, less well-off states get more—as much as 77 cents on the dollar, in the case of Mississippi (KFF, 2023). Enhancing the matching rate is one way that the federal government can encourage states to expand their Medicaid offerings.

NURSING HOMES AND THE MEDICAID PROGRAM

The new Medicaid program placed considerable responsibility on states, both generally and with respect to nursing homes. Because nursing home care is a required service under the program, states are legally mandated to provide nursing home services to anyone meeting eligibility requirements. And, like any service covered under the Medicaid and Medicare programs (or, indeed, any health insurance plan), the service itself must meet various requirements in order to be reimbursed. Generally speaking, the federal government sets out the minimum requirements that providers must meet to receive Medicaid payments. States may add additional requirements and are responsible for monitoring and enforcing those requirements.

Coverage of nursing home care through the Medicaid program had another consequence: the medicalization of the nursing home experience. That is, it accelerated the shift in residential care from "old-age homes" to institutions that focus on residents' medical needs, largely due to the high cost of residential care. Not only were long-term nursing home stays excluded from the Medicare program because of their high cost, but policymakers also sought ways to limit access to the benefit once it became part of the Medicaid program. An important way to do this was by limiting access to those with high needs, rather than those needing custodial care only (D. B. Smith & Feng, 2010). Consequently, nursing home residents became ever more vulnerable: they were both poor (they had to be, to qualify for Medicaid) and experienced significant health challenges. The vulnerability of this population has thus played a large role in the evolving regulatory regime for nursing homes.

Exploitation and neglect of vulnerable residents has been constant throughout the history of nursing homes. Indeed, outrage about conditions in nursing homes led Congress to introduce further regulations only a few years after the launch of the Medicaid program, setting the precedent for incremental regulatory adjustments. Subsequently, evidence of problems with the quality of care in nursing homes continued to emerge over the 1970s and 1980s (Moss & Halamandaris, 1977; Vladeck, 1980), culminating in a 1986 Institute of Medicine (IOM) report that reviewed the state of nursing homes, concluding that it was too often seriously inadequate, and called for more robust regulation (IOM, 1986). This, in turn, led to the Nursing Home Reform Act, included in the Omnibus Budget Reconciliation Act (OBRA) of 1987, which established the basic framework for nursing home regulation that persists to this day (Table 4.1). More recently, the National Academies of Sciences, Engineering, and Medicine (NASEM) issued a 2022 report that in many ways parallels the IOM report, identifying serious concerns and proposing remedies (NASEM, 2022). Whether it similarly results in significant policy action is as yet uncertain.

TABLE 4.1 Landmarks in LTSS Regulation

YEAR	ACTION	IMPACT
1935	Social Security Act	Guaranteed income from Social Security spurred the development of private boarding homes targeted at older people, which evolved into nursing homes; the law also created a legal framework for cooperative federal/state programs
1950	Social Security Act Amendments	Created a public assistance program that allowed states to reimburse nursing homes for certain categories of medically needy individuals
1960	Kerr–Mills Act	Established Medical Assistance for the Aged, a means-tested grant program targeted at older adults that provided federal funds to states opting to provide a range of healthcare services, including nursing homes
1965	Title XVIII (Medicare) and XIX (Medicaid) of the Social Security Act	Created entitlements to certain LTC facilities—most importantly, made nursing homes a required service under the Medicaid program
1974	HCFA sets federal "Conditions of Participation"	Established 18 broadly written criteria that contain 90 more detailed standards of nursing home performance
1975	State plan person care services	Enabled states to offer personal care services as a Medicaid benefit
1981	Home- and community-based waivers (1915[c]) established	Enabled states to request waivers of Medicaid requirements from the federal government in order to offer a range of HCBS to individuals meeting a nursing home level of care
1986	IOM report on nursing home quality	Provided a comprehensive critique of the systems for regulating nursing homes, with extensive recommendations for reform
1987	OBRA 1987 (including the Nursing Home Reform Act)	Established a comprehensive regulatory structure for nursing homes

(*continued*)

TABLE 4.1 Landmarks in LTSS Regulation (*continued*)

YEAR	ACTION	IMPACT
1999	*Olmstead v. L.C* Supreme Court decision	Established that people needing LTSS have a right to live in the "least restrictive setting," providing a legal basis for the shift toward HCBS
2006	Home- and community-based waiver options (1915[i] and [j])	Enabled states to offer HCBS and participant-directed personal assistance services as state plan services
2022	National Academies of Sciences, Engineering, and Medicine report on nursing home quality	Issued an updated report on key issues in nursing home regulation and quality, along with comprehensive recommendations

HCBS, home- and community-based services; HCFA, Health Care Financing Administration (previous name for the current Centers for Medicare & Medicaid Services); IOM, Institute of Medicine; LTC, long-term care; LTSS, long-term services and support; OBRA, Omnibus Budget Reconciliation Act.

THE GROWING ROLE OF HOME- AND COMMUNITY-BASED SERVICES

Although the initial design of the Medicaid program favored nursing homes as the site of care for people needing LTSS, the program also contained provisions enabling states to offer some LTSS in the home. While some of these benefits were required components of the Medicaid program (e.g., the home health benefit, which covers the cost of skilled care in the home), other home- and community-based benefits were optional for states, such as the personal care benefit (which provides help with basic activities of daily living such as bathing, toileting, and the like). Over time, Congress introduced mechanisms (known as "waivers") that provide flexibility for states in how they can offer home- and community-based services (HCBS). These waivers allow states to target specific services to specific populations (such as people with traumatic brain injuries) and to place a cap on the number of people enrolled in the waiver—giving states an appealing level of control over waiver expenditures.

Despite the availability of these options, most states were slow to offer HCBS, in large part out of fear of spurring increased demand and its associated costs, although this picture varied widely by state. What changed all of this? In addition to the bad press associated with them, a civil rights argument against nursing homes emerged, promoted by the growing disability movement (Scotch, 2009; Watson, 2009). This focused on framing nursing homes as fundamentally restricting the liberty of people with disabilities, a perspective that was endorsed by the 1999 Supreme Court decision in *Olmstead v. L.C.* This groundbreaking decision found the unjustified segregation of people with disabilities in nursing homes to be a form of unlawful discrimination under the Americans with Disabilities Act (ADA).

LANDMARK LEGAL CASE: *OLMSTEAD V. L.C, 1999*

The case concerned two women, Lois Curtis and Elaine Wilson, who had mental illness and developmental disabilities and were admitted to the psychiatric unit in the state-run Georgia Regional Hospital for treatment. Although hospital staff stated that each was ready to leave for a community-based program, the women remained confined in the institution for several years after their treatment was concluded. They filed suit under the ADA for release from the hospital.

The Court held that this confinement to an institution was a form of unjustified segregation of persons with disabilities, thus violating Title II of the ADA. Indeed, the Court found that the law required that people with disabilities be served in "integrated settings" when these are medically appropriate, the individuals concerned desire such placement, and the resources for such a transfer are available. However, the state's financial constraints matter only where the state can demonstrate that allocation of resources to one patient will cause harm to others.

One way that states could meet the Olmstead requirements was to develop comprehensive working plans (known as Olmstead Plans) for placing qualified persons with disabilities in less restrictive settings. The requirement to develop such plans put pressure on states to holistically assess their HCBS infrastructure, aided by federal grant opportunities that supported "rebalancing" of LTSS systems to shift service provision away from institutions and toward community living.

Thus, the landmark *Olmstead* decision was not only critical in recasting "confinement to an institution" as a civil rights violation; it also provided the legal backing to push states to create more HCBS options. Ensuring compliance with the *Olmstead* requirement to provide care in the least restrictive setting has therefore become a central component of federal LTSS policy. It led to the "rebalancing" movement—the effort to establish a balance between HCBS and institutional LTSS (Figure 4.1). (It should be noted that the latter includes not only nursing homes, but also institutions serving individuals with intellectual disabilities and mental health facilities, which comprise 20% of institutional spending in the Medicaid program [Murray et al., 2021].) The rebalancing movement has been successful, overall. While 12% of Medicaid LTSS spending went toward HCBS in 1989, 30 years later that proportion has risen to 59%. However, like many aspects of the Medicaid program, this picture varies by state. In 2019, Mississippi was at the low end of the HCBS spending spectrum, with 33% of its Medicaid LTSS spending going toward HCBS. At the other end was Oregon, which spent 83% of its Medicaid LTSS money on HCBS (Murray et al., 2021).

This expansion of Medicaid funding for HCBS has meant that Medicaid now plays a significant role in a wide range of services. However, the range of services covered is yet another area of state variation. For example, the Medicaid program in the state of Oregon is noted for its use of adult foster homes—private homes that serve a small number of older adults (Lehning & Austin, 2010)—whereas California stands out for its use of self-directed services, where Medicaid enrollees who receive the personal care benefit hire independent providers (often family members) to provide support, rather than using aides employed by a home care agency or other entity (Whitenhill & Shugarman, 2011). In some states, Medicaid will pay for assisted living. And many states rely heavily on managed care plans to organize and deliver HCBS. This variety makes regulation challenging.

REGULATORY OVERLAP IN LONG-TERM SERVICES AND SUPPORT

The landscape of LTSS regulation can be confusing, given the host of entities that have a role in ensuring LTSS quality. Most important of these are the federal government, state Medicaid programs, provider licensing and certification entities, and state insurance regulators. This section discusses the many players involved.

The Role of Medicaid

Even though Medicaid is not the only source of funding for LTSS, Medicaid requirements have an outsized influence on the LTSS industry. Certainly, some people pay out of pocket for LTSS, while a small proportion (11% of people 65 or older) have a private insurance policy covering LTSS expenses (Johnson, 2016). (Remember that Medicare offers only very limited coverage.) However, because most providers rely on Medicaid—supplemented by Medicare as well as private-pay clients—for the survival of their businesses (despite Medicaid's low reimbursement rates), they must meet Medicaid and Medicare requirements. Take, for example, nursing homes. Only a quarter of residents pay for their own stay. About 13% are covered by the Medicare program for a short-term stay, while the remaining 62% are Medicaid recipients (Chidambaram, 2024).

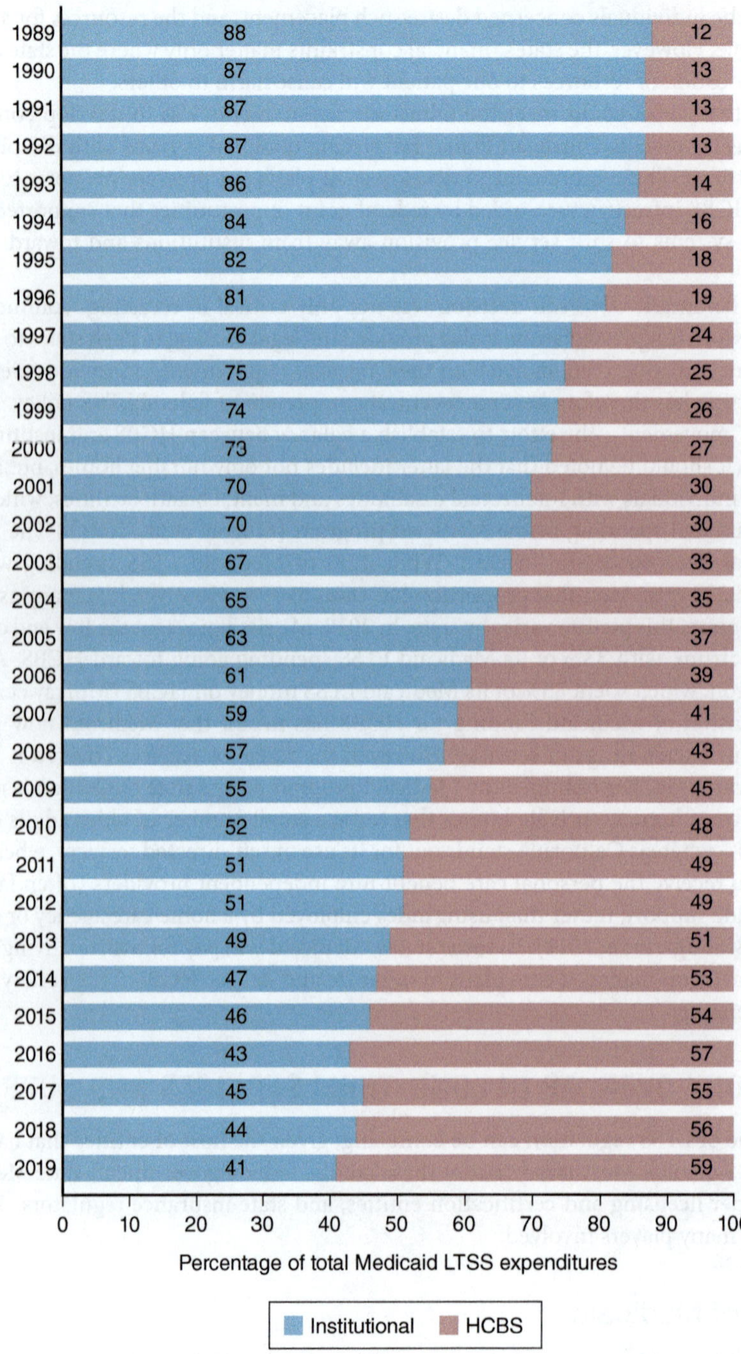

FIGURE 4.1. Medicaid HCBS and institutional LTSS expenditures as a percentage of total Medicaid LTSS expenditures.

HCBS, home- and community-based services; LTSS, long-term services and support.

Source: Adapted from Murray, C., Tourtellotte, A., Lipson, D., & Wysocki, A. (2021, December 9). *Medicaid long-term services and supports annual expenditures report: Federal fiscal year 2019.* Centers for Medicare & Medicaid Services. https://www.medicaid.gov/medicaid/long-term-services-supports/downloads/ltssexpenditures2019.pdf

Thus, meeting Medicaid (and Medicare) requirements is crucial for many LTSS providers, even where Medicaid is less important as a revenue stream. Accordingly, 98% of nursing homes are Medicare certified and 95% are Medicaid certified (National Center for Health Statistics, n.d.).

Licensing and Certification

An important state-level function is the licensing and certification of LTSS professionals, although this is typically delegated to independent professional organizations. For example, state licensing boards control what skilled providers such as RNs or PAs can and cannot do. This can have a significant impact on service delivery. For example, a perennial issue in LTSS is whether only nurses may perform certain tasks, such as administering medications—some state boards of nursing permit them to delegate that responsibility to unskilled staff (most often to certified nursing assistants, or CNAs, but also to personal care assistants working in the community), while others do not. At the same time, CNAs are governed by federal government rules setting out the tasks they may perform. For CNAs to legally administer medications, the state must expand their scope of practice.

Many states also try to control the number and distribution of nursing facilities in their state by requiring a "certificate of need" for those wishing to establish a new nursing home in the state. The goal is mostly to limit capacity due to the high costs of nursing home care and the potential for induced demand, due to the likelihood that any new facility will be heavily dependent on Medicaid. However, this regulatory tool also serves to ensure that the geographic distribution of nursing homes meets needs.

Level of Care

A critical issue in LTSS is ensuring that people are served in settings that have the capacity to keep them safe, by ensuring that providers offer the appropriate staffing, physical space, and procedures for individuals with a defined level of need. This has resulted in a plethora of service delivery categories, with requirements specific to each category. One of the more critical distinctions is between skilled nursing facilities (SNFs) and nursing facilities, which are both often referred to as nursing homes—unsurprisingly, as they are often housed in the same building. However, to be an SNF, a facility must offer a higher level of care, including an onsite physician and the ability to provide physical therapy and manage medical devices such as ventilators. This makes sense because the goal of a Medicare-reimbursed SNF stay is to help people recover following a hospitalization; thus, Medicare covers only 100 days, resulting in an average SNF stay of around a month—in contrast to the much longer stays typical of nursing homes.

Another important distinction is between nursing homes and assisted living facilities. People are sometimes surprised when an assisted living facility asks a resident to leave because of their declining health. However, from a regulatory perspective, the facility lacks the capacity to serve that person appropriately. Assisted living facilities are not required to have a nurse on staff, nor to ensure access to a physician. Accordingly, assisted living facilities are proscribed from serving people with significant care needs. Complicating this picture, however, is the creation of different categories of assisted living facilities, as discussed in the section on residential care facilities that follows.

The need for appropriate placement in nursing homes prompted the introduction of a screening tool, the Preadmission Screening and Resident Review (PASRR). This tool serves several functions: most importantly, it screens out people whose reason for admission is mental health needs. This tool responded to the concern that people who were deinstitutionalized would end up in nursing homes, which are not well placed to serve this population.

Managed Care

Medicaid-funded LTSS—in both nursing homes and the community—is increasingly being delivered through managed care organizations (MCOs). This landscape is complex: The types of insurance plans and the scope of their coverage varies widely. The services they deliver, however, are governed by contracts negotiated with states, which can strongly influence the LTSS that enrollees have access to and the nature of those services. For example, states may require that MCOs offer self-directed services (as Wisconsin does), or that they contract with community-based organizations for certain services (as Massachusetts does). Such insurance plans are also governed by the state entities that regulate insurance products; however, these regulatory agencies tend to focus on regulating commercial health insurance and Medicare Advantage plans that do not cover LTSS. Consequently, they may lack expertise in LTSS.

A further concern is the lack of accountability around managed LTSS. Only recently (2016) has the federal government required reporting specific to LTSS for MCOs, including whether beneficiaries receive the services and supports set forth in their care plans (Caldwell & Machledt, 2022). Required reporting elements focus mainly on process measures, with the only outcome measures assessing transitions to and from nursing homes (Centers for Medicare & Medicaid Services [CMS], 2024). Moreover, states vary widely in their levels of oversight.

NURSING HOME REGULATION

For better or for worse, the regulation of nursing homes remains the touchstone for LTSS regulation. Over the years, a range of approaches were taken to ensure the safety and well-being of residents, approaches that evolved over time. Initially, regulation focused on structural components of quality assurance. Eventually, the focus shifted more and more toward a focus on resident outcomes, publicizing information about nursing home quality, and creating incentives for high quality. The attempt to shine a light on nursing home quality and to reward good behaviors has meant that collecting meaningful, reliable, and accurate data is of paramount importance.

Staffing

A key structural component of nursing home quality is ensuring that facilities are well staffed—although what "well-staffed" means in practice has been constantly debated. To operate, facilities must have appropriate levels and types of staffing, and staff must meet all training requirements. Certain staffing levels are mandated by the federal government: Facilities must provide licensed nursing services (an RN or LPN) 24 hours a day, 7 days a week and have an RN on duty 8 hours/day, 7 days/week. Facilities must also appoint a director of nursing, have a full-time registered dietician on staff, and provide services that are "sufficient" to meet residents' needs.

However, such blanket requirements have long been seen as insufficient. Most importantly, they do not accommodate common variations among facilities, such as the number of beds and the range of conditions experienced by residents. Advocates therefore focus on staffing as a ratio of the hours staff work to the number of residents or beds in a facility—defined as "hours per resident day," or HPRD (although this metric fails to take residents' conditions into account). Until recently, no federal standard using HPRD existed, despite consistent advocacy and the recommendations of numerous government task forces and committees (as detailed in NASEM, 2022). Summarizing the consensus, a 2001 government report identified specific minimum staffing thresholds, recommending a daily minimum standard of 4.1 hours of total direct care nursing time per resident: 2.8 hours from CNAs, 0.75 hours from RNs, and 0.55 hours from LPNs/licensed vocational nurses.

As of April 2024, the Biden administration issued a final rule establishing a minimum staffing standard of 3.48 HPRD (although adjustments for resident acuity were not included). Another requirement, that nursing homes have at least one RN on site 24 hours a day, 7 days a week, has also been finalized; both of these requirements are being challenged in court by nursing home trade associations, who argue that the nationwide staffing crisis makes these requirements unrealistic.

State staffing regulations can, and do, exceed federal requirements. However, only the District of Columbia exceeds the CMS report's recommended level of 4.1 HPRD. Most other states fall short, and some states (18) fail to specify any standards for unskilled staff (Burns et al., 2023).

Regardless of the formal requirements, it is no secret that nursing homes are routinely understaffed but experience few sanctions, largely due to the widely acknowledged dearth of people willing to take on these difficult and often poorly paid jobs—and, some argue, due to profit taking by for-profit facility owners. Not only are nursing homes understaffed, they also tend to have high turnover among staff at all levels—including the highest levels of management—with predictable consequences for the quality of care.

Although the level of staffing is a perennial issue, so too are the types of training required for staff, with debates over the level of education required for nursing home administrators as well as the appropriateness of training for unskilled CNAs; while the federal requirement for CNAs is 75 hours of training, some states require more: Alaska, for example, requires 140 hours (Paraprofessional Healthcare Institute [PHI], n.d.). The desperate need for workers has, in some cases, meant that policymakers have sought to keep barriers to entry into the profession—that is, training requirements—low, despite calls for a minimum 120-hour requirement (IOM, 2008).

Assessments

A critical piece of the Nursing Home Reform Act was the requirement that residents be assessed upon admission and periodically thereafter. To do so, the federal government developed and mandated the use of the Resident Assessment Instrument (or RAI), which has been updated several times; the data derived from it comprise the Minimum Data Set (MDS).

Information from these assessments is used in several important ways. First, it is used for clinical assessment and to develop personalized plans of care, in consultation with an interdisciplinary team (including a physician, RN, and CNA). In addition, the data derived from assessments enables facilities to track their performance. These data are also reported to regulators for the purpose of oversight and, additionally, provide the public with information on nursing home performance. And lastly, the data are used to adjust Medicaid and Medicare reimbursement to reflect the complexity of residents' health conditions.

Clearly, a lot rides on these assessments, which have been critiqued from a number of angles. From the perspective of regulation, however, the biggest concerns are the built-in incentives for misreporting—specifically, the clear incentive to underreport unflattering information and to overreport the complexity of residents' health conditions in order to maximize reimbursement. However, efforts to increase the accuracy of data collection are limited by practical concerns—particularly the persistent issue of insufficient and poorly trained staff (Rahman & Applebaum, 2009).

State Surveys

A core element of nursing home oversight is the onsite survey, administered by state survey agencies. The agencies' responsibilities are to conduct periodic surveys, investigate complaints, take enforcement actions, and publicize survey results. Surveys must be unannounced and occur yearly, on average, or at least every 15 months. They may also be prompted by resident or family complaints.

Surveyors undertake a host of activities to assess whether a nursing home meets all regulatory requirements. Where a facility falls short, the surveyors issue "deficiencies" (called F-tags) that identify issues across a wide range of parameters. These fall into areas such as resident rights, quality of care, physical environment, and infection control and are graded to denote their scope (whether a deficiency is isolated, a pattern, or widespread) and severity (which ranges from "no actual harm with potential for minimal harm" to "immediate jeopardy to resident health or safety"). Upon completion of the survey, the survey agency issues a statement of deficiencies and develops a plan of correction with the facility, which it must make available to residents and their representatives. Moreover, these deficiencies become part of the public record and contribute to a nursing home's quality rating.

These activities require significant investments by states, as the work of survey teams is not easy. Most importantly, survey agencies must maintain a roster of trained, competent surveyors. However, this is often not the case: A 2022 study found that 31 survey agencies had vacancy rates of 20% or higher, with three having rates of 70% or higher. (Respondents indicated that these vacancies were long-standing and not pandemic related.) Even among well-staffed agencies, turnover was reported as high, impacting the quality of surveys. Consequently, 28% of American nursing homes have not been inspected for 16 months or more (as of May 2023), and one in nine has not been inspected in 2 years (Senate Special Committee on Aging, 2023).

Surveyors are critical in not only identifying issues, but also in ensuring that nursing homes address them—specifically, by determining whether a nursing home has implemented the correction plan developed following the identification of deficiencies. However, if a nursing home's problems are serious enough, it can receive a "special focus" designation, which triggers an additional set of requirements, including more frequent surveys. Facilities must show constant improvement on subsequent surveys or face enforcement actions including fines, denials of payment, and/or temporary management—or the ultimate sanction, termination from the Medicaid program.

This federal framework should lead to consistency in oversight across states. As noted, however, surveying practices vary widely—in large part due to a lack of commitment on the part of states, but also due to a lack of investment by the federal government. Indeed, a recent report from the Senate Special Committee on Aging noted that federal investment in state nursing home survey and certification functions has not increased significantly in a decade, rising only 2.5% since 2015 (Senate Special Committee on Aging, 2023).

This lack of investment in oversight has real consequences in terms of nursing home quality. Variations in quality across states are evident. Some research has been able to explicitly tie these variations in quality to a state's investment in regulatory oversight (Mukamel et al., 2012).

The limited commitment to enforcement means that nursing homes rarely suffer significant sanctions for poor performance. Indeed, the ultimate sanction for a nursing home's poor performance is closure, an option that may receive pushback from families who have no other feasible options for their family member—for example, in rural areas where the next nearest nursing home is several hours away. Closures have also been found to affect disadvantaged communities more heavily (Feng et al., 2011). Accordingly, this sanction is rarely used.

Another important recourse for residents is the state Long-Term Care Ombudsman Program. Its job is to advocate on behalf of nursing home residents by responding to complaints and reporting complaints data. These programs tend to be poorly staffed and rely heavily on volunteers, a resource that took a big hit due to the COVID-19 pandemic (Nelson & Netting, 2021). Nonetheless, Ombudsmen represent an important independent perspective on nursing home quality and concerns.

THE CHALLENGE OF REGULATING HOME- AND COMMUNITY-BASED SERVICES

For a regulatory system that is based on the nursing home model of service provision, the shift to HCBS poses significant challenges. Medicaid now covers HCBS that are provided in myriad ways to a wide range of populations. Moreover, those services were largely developed in less regulated environments, and may be paid for not just by government, but also out of pocket (including under-the-table arrangements) or, for the favored few, by LTC insurance. Given the widespread consensus about the weaknesses of nursing home regulation, coupled with the diversity of payment sources and provider types found among HCBS, it is not clear what a strong regulatory framework for HCBS would look like.

The Current Home- and Community-Based Services Regulatory Framework

Unlike LTSS delivered in controlled settings such as nursing homes, HCBS lack obvious oversight mechanisms. States have consequently struggled to develop ways to regulate this sector, a struggle that is made more difficult by the lack of a national framework for HCBS (such as that laid out for nursing homes in the Nursing Home Reform Act). In addition, the absence of a unified approach to data collection means that regulators lack the information needed to conduct meaningful oversight. Indeed, a 2012 review of state oversight concluded that seven of the 25 states selected had inadequate systems for ensuing quality of care (Office of Inspector General [OIG], 2012).

Meanwhile, states are under pressure to comply with the Olmstead mandate requiring that people who need LTSS be served in the least restrictive setting possible. To fund the array of services necessary to support people safely at home and in other community-based settings, states often use the Medicaid HCBS waiver mechanism: 277 waivers were in effect across 48 states as of 2018 (Musumeci et al., 2020). Such waivers enable states to offer services not included in the standard Medicaid benefit package, such as case management, personal care, adult day health, and/or respite services. In addition, states may waive requirements that apply to Medicaid benefits, such as the need to offer services "statewide" and the prohibition against capping enrollment in specific programs. Waivers also allow states to target services to certain populations, such as people with traumatic brain injury. Thus, while the use of Medicaid waivers has expanded access to HCBS, it has also led to wide variations in access based on geography, disability category, and other factors; waiting lists, which are not allowed for standard Medicaid benefits, are common in HCBS waiver programs, with a reported 820,000 on such lists in 2018 (Musumeci et al., 2020). In contrast, states offering personal care by including it under their State Plan (as 34 states do) must provide the benefit to all who are eligible. All states must offer Medicaid home health services, which are part of the standard benefit package.

The waiver application and renewal process therefore represents a primary mechanism for regulating HCBS. When applying for waivers, states must detail how they will meet federal requirements, which focus on three areas: service plans, health and welfare, and qualified providers; these mainly focus on processes measures. When states fail to meet these assurances, the CMS may implement a corrective action plan; onsite reviews are required at least once during each 3-to-5-year waiver period.

Another approach to improving oversight involves the adoption of uniform performance measures, as well as the data infrastructure necessary to support them. Compared to the significant reporting requirements for nursing homes, HCBS data requirements are currently limited and vary across states—indeed, one study found over 130 data collection instruments in use (Caldwell & Machledt, 2022)—hence the push for standardization and public reporting. In 2020, the CMS released a draft set of recommended quality measures for voluntary use by states, MCOs, and other entities engaged in administering and delivering HCBS—but these have a way to go before being implemented.

And lastly, as of March 2023, the CMS has implemented the HCBS Settings Rule. This Rule details basic rights pertaining to people receiving Medicaid HCBS (in line with the Nursing Home Bill of Rights required under the Nursing Home Reform Act), and aims to ensure their access to community living. It does so by outlining their right to control personal resources; be treated with privacy, dignity, respect, and freedom from coercion and restraint; decide what and when to eat; have visitors; be able to lock doors; and have the protections of a lease or other legally enforceable agreement. The rule also requires a person-centered process for planning HCBS. It remains to be seen whether these new expectations have an impact—and whether and how well they will be enforced.

Residential Care Facilities

A big challenge in HCBS is regulating the range of residential settings that is categorized—for want of a better term—as *residential care facilities*, which provide limited supports (personal care and routine nursing services) to people who do not meet a nursing home level of care. "Residential care" includes everything from high-end assisted living facilities operated by the hospitality industry to so-called "board and care" homes and adult foster homes operated by private individuals, although the term *assisted living* generally refers to larger facilities. It can also include settings with memory care units that cater to people with cognitive impairment. Consequently, regulation of these settings is extremely varied: One study identified 182 licensing classifications nationally, which could be combined in 350 different ways (L. Smith et al., 2021). In contrast to the nursing home industry, this sector does not rely heavily on Medicaid for reimbursement.

Although such settings must meet state-level licensure and certification requirements, they are not subject to the same level of regulation as nursing homes. Indeed, advocates for assisted living point to the failure of the regulatory approach to nursing homes as evidence supporting a different approach—although that different approach has yet to be articulated (Wilson, 2007). Meanwhile, the nursing home industry argues that the disparity in regulatory oversight is unfair, given the assisted living industry's incursion into the nursing home market and the resulting medical complexity of assisted living residents (see, for example, Han et al., 2017). However, the fact that assisted living facilities are not required to collect and report data on residents makes this argument hard to address—a nice catch-22: While such facilities are required to assess residents, no standardized tool is mandated and it is thus difficult to draw evidence-based conclusions about populations and outcomes. State licensing agencies do survey and report on licensed facilities, but the ability to access the reports varies across states. Another way of knowing what's going on in facilities is through Long-Term Care Ombudsmen, who are increasingly including such facilities into their scope of work, although the underinvestment in Ombudsmen offices limits their reach.

Self-Directed Services

This service category includes a range of state programs that allow Medicaid LTSS recipients to hire a person of their choosing (rather than use an agency employee) to provide personal care and other supportive services—and, in some cases, to purchase other goods and services that address their functional and other needs. The goal is to empower service recipients to make their own decisions about the types of supports they need, how they should be provided, and who should provide them. However, the option to self-direct also means that participants take on significant responsibilities: for example, they must ensure that workers are paid correctly. States have an interest in ensuring that participants in self-directed programs comply with relevant employment laws; to do so, states make financial management services available (and, in some cases, require participants to use them), which support participants in their employer-related duties and may be responsible for managing the budget on behalf of the participant.

States set different rules about who may be hired under self-directed programs. For example, some states may not allow certain family members (often, spouses) to be paid to provide support, or may require criminal background checks or certain types of training. Another area of concern is whether budget allocations are being used appropriately. To address the potential for fraud in HCBS, the 21st Century Cures Act (2016) has required electronic visit verification (EVV) for workers providing in-home services. Although the law pertains to all personal care and home health services under Medicaid, it can be particularly tricky to implement in self-directed programs, where the provider may be coresident and provide intermittent services.

Staffing

Many of the staffing issues pertaining to nursing homes also pertain to HCBS workers; for example, the ongoing workforce crisis has led states to keep barriers to entry into the profession low in order to attract and retain staff. Combined with low pay, the lack of training and preparation result in high turnover and low quality among direct care workers (DCWs). To address this, in 2024 the Biden administration set a rule (which is under review at the time of writing) stipulating that 80% of Medicaid payments for home health, homemaker, and personal care services be directed toward employee compensation, aiming to ensure better pay for these critical workers.

Making the picture more complex is the myriad of job categories and related requirements that govern DCWs—who are variously called personal care attendants, personal care aides, home care workers, homemakers, and more. This has led to calls for developing a national set of core competencies that would professionalize the role, enable workers to more easily move from job to job, and potentially customize training for different care roles, such as supporting individuals with intellectual disabilities. Currently, seven states set no training requirements at all for personal care aides (Campbell et al., 2020). In contrast, home health aides (whose duties tend to be more clinical in nature) frequently serve both Medicaid and Medicare home health patients and therefore need to comply with Medicare requirements (a minimum of 75 hours of training along with 12 hours of in-service training per year). In summary, regulation and oversight of the direct care workforce is a significant challenge for states, whose primary mechanism is licensing and certification.

The Gray Market in Long-Term Services and Support

Any discussion of LTSS regulation should not ignore the existence of a large unregulated market in LTSS. As we have noted in this chapter, regulation of LTSS depends heavily on the payer of services and on licensing and certification efforts. Where there is no payer except for the service recipient or their family, and where tasks are low-skill and providers are unlicensed (such as with many LTSS), oversight is particularly tricky. This is especially the case when workers are hired on an informal basis to work in the home and then paid off the books. The hidden nature of these relationships means that we lack hard data on the size of this gray market in LTSS and have even less information about the outcomes associated with it. One of the few studies to attempt to quantify the size of this gray market estimated that roughly a third of caregivers of people with dementia sought gray market care (Shih et al., 2022).

Another gray market is that of unlicensed care homes, defined as "homes offering room, board, and personal care that either fall outside the bounds of the state licensure requirements (i.e., legal unlicensed care homes) or violate state licensure requirements (i.e., illegal unlicensed care homes)" (Lepore et al., 2019, p. 50). Very little is known about these settings, but they appear to cater to a particularly vulnerable population (with high incidence of substance use disorder and/or mental illness) who resort to these settings due to their very low incomes (Lepore et al., 2019). Given the vulnerability of many LTSS recipients and high rates of reported fraud and abuse, this gray market in care represents a huge gap in our understanding of LTSS.

LOOKING FORWARD

Perhaps it is the aging of the population that has—finally—spurred action. Or maybe the COVID-19 pandemic has so starkly highlighted the weaknesses of the LTSS system that it has become harder to ignore. For whatever reason, the past few years have seen limited progress on some of the key issues identified in this chapter, at both the federal and state levels. This chapter has, however, outlined how challenging the issues are moving forward.

National Academies of Sciences, Engineering, and Medicine Report on Nursing Home Quality

One area of movement is seen in nursing home regulation. In 2022, the NASEM issued a comprehensive report highlighting the many significant issues around nursing home regulation (NASEM, 2022); it proposed a set of ambitious recommendations, which include enhanced staffing requirements, physical environment updates, ownership transparency and accountability, and survey regulation and oversight. The hope is that the report will result in meaningful policy action. Although no legislative action has ensued, the Biden administration has issued a series of executive orders (The White House, 2023a, 2023b): One of the most important concerns the commitment to set a federal minimum staffing standard for nursing homes—albeit one criticized as being too low by some.

Other important actions involve increasing oversight and accountability in nursing homes. One significant step was a commitment to greater transparency regarding the owners, operators, and management of nursing homes, which is critical for establishing legal accountability; for example, nursing homes would be required to disclose who provides administrative services or clinical consulting services to the nursing homes. Currently, complex contracting arrangements mask the role of various players (such as private equity) in nursing homes and make it difficult to hold entities accountable.

The Data Challenge

Another area where movement is occurring is in the collection of data to support oversight of LTSS, which depends heavily on good, reliable data. While the infrastructure for data on nursing homes is well-developed, the field has yet to develop an actionable strategy for collecting information to inform oversight of HCBS. Thus, movement toward standardizing and mandating collection of data will be important in ensuring the safety of HCBS consumers and the appropriate use of public funds.

However, both nursing homes and HCBS face the challenge that the people best placed to collect data are those who have the strongest incentives to misrepresent it, given the multiple uses for these data. It is therefore critical that government establishes independent means of collecting and verifying information; this requires greater investment in existing monitoring mechanisms such as state surveys of nursing homes—an issue raised in the NASEM report—as well as expansions of Ombudsmen programs to ensure they have adequate resources to cover a broader range of services. So, too, should managed care plans be required to report out information regarding members receiving LTSS through such plans.

SUMMARY

This chapter began by highlighting the historical context in which nursing homes became the default site for LTSS, a status that was reinforced with the establishment of Medicaid. Readers were taught to understand how the source of financing—whether from private individuals, Medicare, or Medicaid—plays a crucial role in shaping LTSS regulation. The chapter detailed the involvement of various entities in ensuring LTSS quality, including the federal government, state

Medicaid programs, state insurance regulators, and provider licensing bodies. It emphasized that state commitment, demonstrated through investment in infrastructure, oversight, and enforcement, is a significant determinant of LTSS quality. The increasing provision of LTSS via HCBS was discussed, highlighting the challenges in ensuring access and quality due to the wide range of services and providers involved. Lastly, the chapter underscored the importance of access to meaningful and reliable data, noting it as a critical challenge in LTSS oversight. This comprehensive exploration provided a detailed understanding of the multifaceted nature of LTSS regulation and the ongoing efforts to improve care quality and access.

END-OF-CHAPTER RESOURCES

DISCUSSION QUESTIONS

1. How do you think the history of nursing homes, with their origins as "poorhouses," has affected how we think about and regulate nursing homes today?
2. Is it a good or bad thing that states play such a critical role in overseeing LTSS? What are the advantages and disadvantages of state-level oversight?
3. What are the most important things that the federal government could do to improve the quality of LTSS?
4. Do you agree that it's a basic civil right for people to be able to live in the community if they so choose? Is it ever appropriate to place someone in a nursing home against their wishes?
5. What level of government oversight is appropriate for LTSS providers who don't receive government funds? For example, should private pay assisted living facilities be required to publicly report on the quality of care they deliver?

TOOLS FOR FURTHER LEARNING

- Campbell, S., Del Rio Drake, A., Espinoza, R., & Scales, K. (2020). *Caring for the future: The power and potential of America's direct care workforce*. Paraprofessional Healthcare Institute. https://www.phinational.org/caringforthefuture. This presents a compelling overview of the issues facing the most vulnerable component of the LTSS workforce.
- The National Academies of Sciences, Engineering, and Medicine. (2022). *The national imperative to improve nursing home quality: Honoring our commitment to residents, families, and staff* (p. 26526). National Academies Press. https://doi.org/10.17226/26526. This, contains a detailed overview of the regulatory challenges facing nursing homes today, along with important recommendations.
- Vladeck, B. C. (1980). *Unloving care: The nursing home tragedy*. Basic Books. This book documents the horrific state of many nursing homes in the United States prior to the passage of the Nursing Home Reform Act of 1987, playing an important role in raising awareness.
- Watson, S. D. (2009). From almshouses to nursing homes and community care: Lessons from Medicaid's history. *Georgia State University Law Review*, *26*(3), 937–969. https://readingroom.law.gsu.edu/cgi/viewcontent.cgi?article=2416&context=gsulr. This law review article contains a comprehensive and very readable history of the evolution of America's LTSS system.

REFERENCES

Burns, A., Chidambaram, P., Neuman, T., & Rudowitz, R. (2023, September 18). *What share of nursing facilities might meet proposed new requirements for nursing staff hours?* KFF. https://www.kff.org/medicaid/issue-brief/what-share-of-nursing-facilities-might-meet-proposed-new-requirements-for-nursing-staff-hours

Caldwell, J., & Machledt, D. (2022). Advancing policy and practice in Medicaid home and community-based services quality. *Frontiers in Rehabilitation Sciences, 3*, 876871. https://doi.org/10.3389/fresc.2022.876871

Campbell, S., Del Rio Drake, A., Espinoza, R., & Scales, K. (2020). *Caring for the future: The power and potential of America's direct care workforce.* Paraprofessional Healthcare Institute. https://www.phinational.org/caringforthefuture

Centers for Medicare & Medicaid Services. (2024). *Long-term services and supports (LTSS) quality measures: Technical specifications and resource manual.* https://www.medicaid.gov/medicaid/managed-care/downloads/mltss-tech-specs-res-manual.pdf?t=1712861368

Chidambaram, P. (2024, January 5). *A look at nursing facility characteristics between 2015 and 2023.* KFF. https://www.kff.org/medicaid/issue-brief/a-look-at-nursing-facility-characteristics

Feng, Z., Lepore, M., Clark, M. A., Tyler, D., Smith, D. B., Mor, V., & Fennell, M. L. (2011). Geographic concentration and correlates of nursing home closures: 1999-2008. *Archives of Internal Medicine, 171*(9), 806–813. https://doi.org/10.1001/archinternmed.2010.492

Han, K., Trinkoff, A. M., Storr, C. L., Lerner, N., & Yang, B. K. (2017). Variation across U.S. assisted living facilities: Admissions, resident care needs, and staffing. *Journal of Nursing Scholarship, 49*(1), 24–32. https://doi.org/10.1111/jnu.12262

Institute of Medicine. (1986). *Improving the quality of care in nursing homes.* National Academies Press. https://doi.org/10.17226/646

Institute of Medicine. (2008). *Retooling for an aging America: Building the health care workforce.* National Academies Press. http://www.ncbi.nlm.nih.gov/books/NBK215401

Johnson, R. W. (2016). *Who is covered by private long-term care insurance?* Urban Institute. https://www.urban.org/sites/default/files/publication/83146/2000881-Who-Is-Covered-by-Private-Long-Term-Care-Insurance.pdf

Kaffenberger, K. R. (2001). Nursing home ownership. *Journal of Aging & Social Policy, 12*(1), 35–48. https://doi.org/10.1300/J031v12n01_04

KFF. (2023). *Federal Medical Assistance Percentage (FMAP) for Medicaid and multiplier* [Dataset]. https://www.kff.org/medicaid/state-indicator/federal-matching-rate-and-multiplier

Lehning, A. J., & Austin, M. J. (2010). Long-term care in the United States: Policy themes and promising practices. *Journal of Gerontological Social Work, 53*(1), 46–63. https://doi.org/10.1080/01634370903361979

Lepore, M., Greene, A. M., Porter, K., Lux, L., Vreeland, E., Hawes, C., Lepore, M., Greene, A. M., Porter, K., Lux, L., & Vreeland, E. (2019). Unlicensed care homes in the United States: A clandestine sector of long-term care. *Journal of Aging & Social Policy, 31*, 49–65. https://doi.org/10.1080/08959420.2018.1485397

Medicaid and CHIP Payment and Access Commission. (2023, January). *Estimates of Medicaid nursing facility payments relative to costs.* https://www.macpac.gov/wp-content/uploads/2023/01/Estimates-of-Medicaid-Nursing-Facility-Payments-Relative-to-Costs-1-6-23.pdf

Moss, F. E., & Halamandaris, V. J. (1977). *Too old, too sick, too bad: Nursing homes in America.* Aspen Systems.

Mukamel, D. B., Weimer, D. L., Harrington, C., Spector, W. D., Ladd, H., & Li, Y. (2012). The effect of state regulatory stringency on nursing home quality. *Health Services Research, 47*(5), 1791–1813. https://doi.org/10.1111/j.1475-6773.2012.01459.x

Murray, C., Tourtellotte, A., Lipson, D., & Wysocki, A. (2021, January 7). *Medicaid long-term services and supports annual expenditures report: Federal fiscal years 2017 and 2018.* Centers for Medicare & Medicaid Services. https://www.medicaid.gov/medicaid/long-term-services-supports/downloads/ltssexpenditures-2017-2018.pdf

Musumeci, M., Watts, M. O., & Published, P. C. (2020, February 4). *Key state policy choices about Medicaid home and community-based services* (Issue Brief-9296-02). KFF. https://www.kff.org/report-section/key-state-policy-choices-about-medicaid-home-and-community-based-services-issue-brief

National Academies of Sciences, Engineering, and Medicine. (2022). *The national imperative to improve nursing home quality: Honoring our commitment to residents, families, and staff* (p. 26526). National Academies Press. https://doi.org/10.17226/26526

National Center for Health Statistics. (n.d.). *Data from the 2020 National Post-Acute and Long-Term Care Study*. Retrieved Feburary 17, 2024, from https://www.cdc.gov/nchs/npals/webtables/overview.htm

Nelson, H. W., & Netting, F. E. (2021). A COVID reset: The future of the Long-Term Care Ombudsman Program and its volunteer advocates. *Journal of Gerontological Social Work, 65*(4), 465–471. https://doi.org/10.1080/01634372.2021.1980479

Office of Inspector General. (2012). *Oversight of quality of care in Medicaid home and community-based services waiver programs* (OEI-02-08-00170). U.S. Department of Health & Human Services.

Paraprofessional Healthcare Institute. (n.d.). *Nursing assistant training requirements by state* [dataset]. Retrieved February 17, 2024, from https://www.phinational.org/advocacy/nurse-aide-training-requirements-state-2016

Rahman, A. N., & Applebaum, R. A. (2009). The nursing home Minimum Data Set assessment instrument: Manifest functions and unintended consequences—Past, present, and future. *The Gerontologist, 49*(6), 727–735. https://doi.org/10.1093/geront/gnp066

Scotch, R. K. (2009). "Nothing about us without us": Disability rights in America. *OAH Magazine of History, 23*(3), 17–22. https://doi.org/10.1093/maghis/23.3.17

Senate Special Committee on Aging. (2023). *Uninspected and neglected: Nursing home inspection agencies are severely understaffed, putting residents at risk*. U.S. Senate. https://www.aging.senate.gov/imo/media/doc/UNINSPECTED%20&%20NEGLECTED%20-%20FINAL%20REPORT.pdf

Shih, R. A., Friedman, E. M., Chen, E. K., & Whiting, G. C. (2022). Prevalence and correlates of gray market use for aging and dementia long-term care in the U.S. *Journal of Applied Gerontology, 41*(4), 1030–1034. https://doi.org/10.1177/07334648211023681

Smith, D. B., & Feng, Z. (2010). The accumulated challenges of long-term care. *Health Affairs, 29*(1), 29–34. https://doi.org/10.1377/hlthaff.2009.0507

Smith, L., Carder, P., Bucy, T., Winfree, J., Brazier, J. F., Kaskie, B., & Thomas, K. S. (2021). Connecting policy to licensed assisted living communities, introducing health services regulatory analysis. *Health Services Research, 56*(3), 540. https://doi.org/10.1111/1475-6773.13616

21st Century Cures Act, Pub. L. No. 114-255, 130 Stat. 1033 (2016).

Vladeck, B. C. (1980). *Unloving care: The nursing home tragedy*. Basic Books.

Watson, S. D. (2009). From almshouses to nursing homes and community care: Lessons from Medicaid's history. *Georgia State University Law Review, 26*(3), 937–969. https://readingroom.law.gsu.edu/cgi/viewcontent.cgi?article=2416&context=gsulr

The White House. (2023a, April 18). *FACT SHEET: Biden-Harris administration announces most sweeping set of executive actions to improve care in history*. https://www.whitehouse.gov/briefing-room/statements-releases/2023/04/18/fact-sheet-biden-harris-administration-announces-most-sweeping-set-of-executive-actions-to-improve-care-in-history

The White House. (2023b, September 1). *FACT SHEET: Biden-Harris administration takes steps to crack down on nursing homes that endanger resident safety*. https://www.whitehouse.gov/briefing-room/statements-releases/2023/09/01/fact-sheet-biden-harris-administration-takes-steps-to-crack-down-on-nursing-homes-that-endanger-resident-safety

Whitenhill, K., & Shugarman, L. R. (2011). *Medicaid-funded home- and community-based services* (Technical Brief Series 9; Long-Term Care Fundamentals). The SCAN Foundation. https://www.thescanfoundation.org/sites/default/files/ltc_fundamental_9_0.pdf

Wilson, K. B. (2007). Historical evolution of assisted living in the United States, 1979 to the present. *Gerontologist, 47*, 8–22. https://doi.org/10.1093/geront/47.supplement_1.8

PART II

QUALITY AND SAFETY PRACTICE IN LONG-TERM CARE

CHAPTER 5

QUALITY ASSURANCE AND PERFORMANCE IMPROVEMENT

Sandi J. Lane

Learning Objectives

After completing this chapter, each learner will be able to:

- Understand the principles of the Quality Assurance and Performance Improvement (QAPI) program in healthcare organizations.
- Analyze the scope of a QAPI plan and how it integrates the care and service areas of an organization.
- Evaluate the role of leadership and governance in fostering a culture of openness and transparency in QAPI.
- Recognize the importance of feedback, data systems, and monitoring in informing performance improvements in healthcare organizations.
- Analyze the steps of the PDSA (Plan-Do-Study-Act) cycle and how they can be applied in the context of QAPI.

INTRODUCTION

Quality care and services are essential to improve individual health and outcomes, as well as provide the highest practicable physical, mental, and psychosocial well-being for residents. Quality assurance (QA) and performance improvement (PI) processes are mutually reinforcing aspects of quality management. When used in tandem, they create the Quality Assurance and Performance Improvement (QAPI) program required by the Centers for Medicare & Medicaid Services (CMS) as the foundation for nursing home quality improvement programs. QAPI is a proactive, ongoing, organized, data-driven method of not only improving quality but also doing business to achieve optimum outcomes (CMS, 2023). QAPI tools and approaches are used in all aspects of nursing home operations to identify gaps in systems and opportunities for improvement, develop action plans, and to continuously monitor effectiveness. This chapter covers the five strategic elements that create the framework of the QAPI program, the contents of the QAPI plan, the facility assessment, and PI models and tools.

HISTORY AND BACKGROUND

Prior to 2016, the CMS required nursing homes to have a Quality Assessment and Assurance (QAA) program. The QAA provision of 42 CFR, Part 483.75(g) specified the members of the committee, how often they met, and ways to develop plans of action to correct any identified quality deficiencies. The weakness of the rule was the lack of details and specifications for the methods to implement the QAA regulations (CMS, 2023).

In March 2010, the Affordable Care Act was passed by Congress and provisions in Section 6102(c) significantly expanded the level and scope of required QA and improvement activities through identification and correction of quality deficiencies through continuous improvement processes. The provision states that the CMS is to establish and implement a QAPI program for nursing homes that includes development of standards, technical assistance, and best practices for nursing homes to meet the QAPI standards (CMS, 2023).

A demonstration project was launched in 2011, through a CMS contract with the University of Minnesota and Stratis Health. The project included 17 nursing homes from four states to identify and assess the best practices for helping nursing homes improve their QA and improvement processes. These findings, along with comments and feedback from consumers, providers, and other stakeholders, provided the foundation for the creation of the QAPI tools and resources (CMS, 2012). An acceptable QAPI program provides a systematic, comprehensive, data-driven approach to quality care and services (Lake Superior Quality Innovation Network, 2016). The demonstration project guided the CMS in writing the "Reform of Requirements for Long-Term Care Facilities" released in October of 2016. Leaders who embrace and promote the QAPI approach were believed to be able to prevent adverse events, promote safety and quality, and reach a higher level of quality than with the previous QAA program (Lake Superior Quality Innovation Network, 2016).

UNDERSTANDING QUALITY ASSURANCE AND PERFORMANCE IMPROVEMENT: AN OVERVIEW

QAPI brings together two separate approaches to quality management, QA and PI. These different approaches, when used in tandem, create a systematic and comprehensive approach to care and services.

- QA is considered a retrospective review to identify trends, or patterns of problems. The collection of resident incidents (e.g., falls, infections, wounds), for example, can be a QA risk management function. It is often used as a regulatory quality standards approach assuring that care meets a threshold to comply with regulations (CMS, n.d.-b; Joshi et al., 2023).
- PI is a proactive effort to improve the overall quality of an organization including such items as clinical, satisfaction, safety, and financial measures by focusing on processes and systems on a continuous basis. It is more than a set of projects or activities, but a leadership philosophy guided by mental models that leaders adopt and use. Used in nursing homes, PI aims to improve processes in healthcare delivery, resident care, and quality of life (CMS, n.d.-b; Joshi et al., 2023).

When combined, QA and PI form QAPI, where aspects of QA, such as meeting standards, review of data, and inspections, are combined with aspects of PI, such as continuous review and improvement, prevention, and a systems approach. QAPI involves all levels of care and services within the nursing home. It is not the responsibility of one person or a committee; rather, it involves all staff, residents, and their families. Through active participation, QAPI uses a continuous data-driven approach to identify opportunities for improvement and the corrective actions needed to meet goals and improve performance (CMS, n.d.-b).

THE FIVE ELEMENTS FOR FRAMING QUALITY ASSURANCE AND PERFORMANCE IMPROVEMENT IN NURSING HOMES

The framework for QAPI is the five building blocks or strategic elements of the nursing home's QAPI program. These interrelated elements are then used for developing, implementing, and sustaining the QAPI program. As shown in Figure 5.1, the interrelated elements are (a) design and scope; (b) governance and leadership; (c) feedback, data systems, and monitoring; (d) PI projects; and (e) systematic analysis and systemic action (CMS, 2023). The QAPI program should be specific to the nursing home with its design and scope addressing the full range of

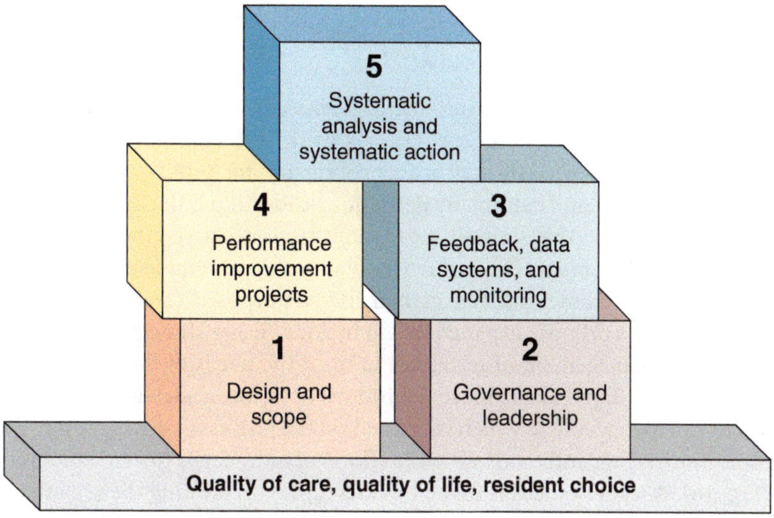

FIGURE 5.1. Building blocks of QAPI.

QAPI, Quality Assurance and Performance Improvement.

Source: Centers for Medicare & Medicaid Services. (n.d.). *QAPI at a glance: A step by step guide to implementing quality assurance and performance improvement (QAPI) in your nursing home.* Retrieved December 7, 2023, from https://www.cms.gov/medicare/provider-enrollment-and-certification/qapi/downloads/qapiataglance.pdf

services provided by the nursing home. In order to do this, the nursing home must complete an annual facility assessment. The QAPI program should always include clinical care, quality of life, and resident choice, with a fully implemented program to include all systems of care and all departments (QAPI, 2022).

The design and scope focus on safety and high-quality care while assuring resident autonomy and choice. The QAPI program is integrated into the responsibilities of nursing home leadership to establish the culture, designate resources, and identify persons involved in leading the QAPI program. This includes developing the leadership and nursing home–wide training on QAPI, ensuring that staff are provided time to participate in QAPI projects and the necessary equipment is available for use when needed. This also creates a culture of openness, teamwork, and psychologic safety (QAPI, 2024).

The nursing home will have systems in place to obtain data from multiple sources for monitoring care and services. Feedback systems should include input from staff, residents, families, and other stakeholders to monitor organization-wide processes, systems, and outcomes. This includes not only evaluating outcomes against benchmarks or organizational targets but also investigating adverse events and action plans to prevent their reoccurrence (QAPI, 2022).

The QAPI program will address the process for conducting a performance improvement project (PIP). A PIP is used to examine and improve a specific service or process identified as a priority needing attention. The nursing home must include in their QAPI program a systematic approach to how potential projects or topics (PIPs) will be identified. It will designate the data systems being monitored as well as the input from residents, staff, families, and other stakeholders (QAPI, 2022).

The QAPI program designates a systematic approach to evaluate organizational processes and systems and to determine when an in-depth analysis is needed to understand the processes and outcome. The thorough and structured approach evaluates the potential processes, policies, and procedures that contribute to the outcomes or problems (QAPI, 2022).

The five interrelated elements are the framework for developing the nursing home's QAPI written plan. It is based on the facility assessment, which indicates the full range of services provided, resident needs, and the nursing home's quality issues and opportunities for improvement (CMS, n.d.-b).

LEADERSHIP AND GOVERNANCE FOR QUALITY ASSURANCE AND PERFORMANCE IMPROVEMENT

For QAPI to be successfully embedded into the organization's culture, leadership must guide the culture change through visionary influence. Leaders work with their governing body (if they are not-for-profit) or corporate office (if they are a proprietary, for-profit) to develop the organization's mission, vision, values, and culture. By definition, leadership is the influential act among and between people to act in ways that support the organization's mission, vision, and goals, including change. Daft defines *leadership* as "an influence relationship among leaders and followers who intend real changes and outcomes that reflect their shared purposes" (Daft, 2023, p. 4). The definition Ledlow and Stephens propose expands this to include "using strategic systems, the collective action of people, and management of resources to meet the needs of the external environment" (Ledlow & Stephens, 2018, p. 14). As these definitions describe, leadership is a relationship with other people; it is not management, which is defined as "the process of getting things done through and with people by directing and motivating the efforts of individuals toward common objectives" (Dunn, 2021, p. 16). A leader's focus is much broader and is on creating the organization's culture and strategic systems for high performance and goal achievement (Ledlow & Stephens, 2018).

An organization's culture is its guide to behaviors and actions. Culture is the shared values and norms held by the organizational members on how the organization should act and conduct business. The values and norms of the organization shape the behaviors of individuals and guide their relationships and communication with others, including what is considered acceptable versus not acceptable behaviors and actions. The leader plays a critical role in creating a healthy organizational culture through their actions, behaviors, and expectations. A healthy organizational culture is one where people feel valued, commit themselves to the organization's goals, feel safe to speak up and contribute, and are creative and respectful of each other (Daft, 2023). Leaders can use a healthy organizational culture to bring staff, residents, families, and other stakeholders together to embrace QAPI processes and value QAPI as key to their performance outcomes and success.

Table 5.1 provides examples of how a leader can create a culture of openness and high performance, and embed QAPI into the organization's daily operations and actions.

Leaders and the governing body designate the person(s) responsible for developing the QAPI plan, assure that adequate resources (e.g., staff time, financial resources, and technical training) are made available for QAPI tasks and projects, and provide facility-wide training on QAPI.

TABLE 5.1 Tools to Create a Culture of Openness and High Performance
Maintain an open-door policy and desire to learn from all staff, residents, families, and key stakeholders.
Create a culture supported by processes that promote communication across shifts, disciplines, and departments.
Develop an environment of psychologic safety so all staff, residents, families, and key stakeholders can bring concerns forward without fear of punishment.
Monitor the current culture, and look for gaps in expected culture and actual norms and behaviors.
Model the expectation of PI in all operations to support resident safety, autonomy, and choice.
Create an environment for teams to communicate, build relationships, and work toward the same goals.
Create teams with a purpose and set team guidelines and supports.

PI, performance improvement.

Source: Data from Daft, R. L. (2023). *The leadership experience* (8th ed.). Cengage; Lake Superior Quality Innovation Network. (2016). *QAPI written plan how-to guide.* Centers for Medicare & Medicaid Services. https://www.cms.gov/medicare/provider-enrollment-and-certification/qapi/downloads/qapi-plan-how-to-guide.pdf

Leaders and the governing body create policies that support QAPI processes including a culture of safety, quality, resident's rights and choice, and respect, while ensuring a balance between safety and resident-centered rights and choice (QAPI, 2022).

Leaders establish a committee often called the QAPI steering committee that has the overall responsibility for developing and maintaining the QAPI plan and its activities. The QAPI steering committee members include the administrator, director of nursing, and participants from across the organization who can inform the committee about their department and/or discipline. The organization's QAA committee can become the QAPI steering committee, with some meeting times and membership adjustments. The QAPI steering committee annually reviews the facility assessment and adjusts the QAPI plan to meet the needs of the organization and the residents it serves, reviews organizational data and outcomes, charters teams to work on specific topics/problems identified, and establishes priorities for PIPs (CMS, n.d.-b; QAPI, 2022).

THE WRITTEN QUALITY ASSURANCE AND PERFORMANCE IMPROVEMENT PLAN

The QAPI plan serves as the organization's guide to a comprehensive and data-driven PIP. QAPI regulations mandate that a written plan be developed and reviewed annually, or otherwise as needed, to reflect the organization's evolving needs and commitment to a culture of continuous improvement (QAPI, 2022). Before writing the purpose statement for the QAPI plan, the organization's mission, vision, and guiding principles should be reviewed to ensure alignment with the organization's overall purpose, goals, and culture.

In the following paragraphs, we refer to the "QAPI Written Plan How-To Guide" created by the Lake Superior Quality Innovation Network (2016). This guide provides a comprehensive list of resources for developing a QAPI plan, including guides, worksheets, checklists, and tools that cover topics such as purpose and guiding principles, measure/indicator collection and monitoring plans, prioritization, goal setting, data sources, and PIPs.

The foundation of the QAPI plan is the *purpose statement*, which outlines what the organization aims to achieve (Daft, 2023). This purpose should align with the organization's mission, vision, and guiding principles, often incorporating language from these elements. The purpose statement should describe the organization's continuous efforts to monitor and improve key performance indicators and demonstrate the interconnectedness of the QAPI plan with the organization's values and culture. Additionally, it should specify who reviews and updates the QAPI plan, how updates are communicated, and the dissemination plan for these updates.

The CMS has provided five key strategic elements that serve as the foundation for an effective Quality Assurance and Performance Improvement (QAPI) program. These *five elements* are: (1) design and scope; (2) governance and leadership; (3) feedback, data systems, and monitoring; (4) PIPs; and (5) systematic analysis and systemic action. Together, these elements create a strategic framework for developing, implementing, and sustaining a QAPI program. In addition to these elements, it is essential to develop *guiding principles* that reflect the organization's beliefs and philosophy concerning QAPI. The CMS suggests nine guiding principles that should be considered when crafting a QAPI plan. These principles guide what the organization does, why it does it, and how it achieves its objectives.

For example, a guiding principle for the *design and scope* element might be: The organization's comprehensive QAPI plan addresses all aspects of operations and guides day-to-day operations and decision-making.

For the *governance and leadership* element, a guiding principle might be: The organization's leadership team and governing body foster a culture of openness, transparency, and psychologic safety that supports employee reporting of concerns, near misses, errors, or problems.

For the *feedback, data systems, and monitoring* element, a guiding principle could be: The organization bases decisions on input from various data sources and input from staff, residents, and families to monitor processes and outcomes.

For the *PIPs* element, a guiding principle might be: The organization provides the support and resources necessary to conduct PIPs and implement changes to improve care and services across all service areas.

Finally, for the *systematic analysis and systemic action* element, a guiding principle might be: The organization supports and resources the development and maintenance of staff proficiency in PI techniques.

The *scope* of the QAPI plan provides an overview of how the care and services areas of the organization are integrated into the QAPI plan, the operational policies and procedures used to guide performance, and how the organization will address key issues using the best available evidence in its decisions. It outlines the operations, policies, and services that can impact clinical care and services, resident choice and quality of life, and transitions of care. The organization uses the completed facility assessment to determine the service and/or care areas offered by the organization and the unique needs of the different resident populations. The intent is not to list each diagnosis but to garner sufficient information to determine common diagnoses and conditions that will be used to determine resources to meet the needs of the different resident populations. Examples of services include dementia care, hospice, long-term care, memory care, postacute care, rehabilitation services, and transitional care.

The facility assessment also includes facility and community risk factors, which are incorporated into the QAPI plan to ensure these risk factors are addressed (QAPI, 2022). As indicated, the QAPI program, plan, and processes are the responsibility of the leadership team and governing body. The leadership team, in coordination with the governing body, is responsible for determining who oversees various aspects of the QAPI plan, activities, processes, outcomes, and the communication plan. This ensures that key stakeholders (e.g., director of nurses, administrator, governing body) and the community at-large, including staff, residents, and families, are informed of QAPI activities, processes, and outcomes.

The QAPI plan will outline the leadership support and financial resources allocated to the QAPI processes, including a budget and provisions for direct care staff (i.e., nursing assistants, nurses) to have their assignments covered while they participate in QAPI activities. Additionally, the QAPI plan should specify the frequency of budget reviews to assure that resources remain available to support QAPI activities and implementation of improvement plans as they evolve over time (QAPI, 2022).

The QAPI plan will specify the data systems and monitoring process from across the organization's departments and services that will be used by the organization to develop and monitor performance. Healthcare organizations including nursing homes have a wealth of information and data available to them to effectively improve performance; increase resident safety; monitor staff competency; and review resident, family, and staff satisfaction, along with other key performance indicators the organization needs to establish an effective data system and monitoring plan and the requisite processes. Figure 5.2 provides an example of how the data systems and monitoring processes can be organized and documented. Examples of data sources include CMS quality metrics and CASPER (Certification **A**nd **S**urvey **P**rovider **E**nhanced **R**eports) reports, internal QAA measures (e.g., infection control, falls, medical errors), abuse, neglect and mistreatment reports, resident and staff satisfaction surveys, and state survey results.

PIPs are in-depth focused efforts to identify the causes of specific problems or systemic issues within a facility. The QAPI plan outlines the organization's policies and procedures for conducting PIPs to improve care and services. This includes the reasons for conducting PIPs and how potential topics will be identified and prioritized.

The QAPI steering committee will develop a systematic methodology that considers data from across the organization's services and departments, as well as input from residents, families, staff, and other stakeholders, to determine how a PIP is selected (QAPI, 2022). Potential areas of concern include high-risk (e.g., wound care, weight loss), high-volume (e.g., newly admitted residents), and problem-prone areas (e.g., incident reports, resident/family complaints) that impact the quality of care, quality of life, resident choice, and resident outcomes.

Data sources	Data collection frequency	Benchmarks to analyze this data source	Who will analyze the data?	Data analysis frequency	Data will be communicated with	Communicate data analysis via	Frequency of communication
Suggestions	• *Weekly* • *Monthly* • *Quarterly* • *Annually*	• *Applicable clinical guidelines* • *Identified best practices* • *National data* • *Corporate data* • *State data* • *Facility-identified performance indicators/goals* • *Thresholds/targets*	• *HR* • *Leadership team* • *QAPI committee*	• *Weekly* • *Monthly* • *Quarterly* • *Annually*	• *Board members* • *Caregivers* • *Community* • *Executive leadership* • *Families* • *Residents* • *Volunteers*	• *Board meetings* • *Bulletin boards* • *Dashboards* • *Newsletters* • *Posters* • *QAPI interdisciplinary meetings* • *Staff meetings*	• *Weekly* • *Monthly* • *Quarterly* • *Annually*
Choose a data source							
Choose a data source							

Suggested data sources:

- Advanced care planning audits
- CMS quality measures (long stay; short stay)
- Case mix
- CASPER report
- Community activities
- Consistent assignment
- Discharged resident surveys
- Drug regimen review summary
- Falls
- Family satisfaction
- Fire safety deficiencies
- Infection prevention and control program
- Info from providers, physicians, contractors, vendors
- Licensed nurse staff hours/resident day
- Medication administration audits
- Medication errors
- Medication room audits
- Near misses (incidents w/out serious harm)
- Nursing assistant staff hours/resident day
- Occupancy rates
- Performance indicators
- Rehospitalization rates
- Resident council minutes
- Resident satisfaction surveys
- Revenue payer sources mix
- Staff retention
- Staff satisfaction
- State survey results
- Staff turnover
- Volunteer hours
- Other

FIGURE 5.2. Data sources for performance monitoring.

CASPER, Certification and Survey Provider Enhanced Reports; CMS, Centers for Medicare & Medicaid Services; HR, human resources; QAPI, Quality Assurance and Performance Improvement.

Source: Lake Superior Quality Innovation Network. (2016). *QAPI written plan how-to guide.* Centers for Medicare & Medicaid Services. https://www.cms.gov/medicare/provider-enrollment-and-certification/qapi/downloads/qapi-plan-how-to-guide.pdf

The QAPI plan specifies how PIP team members will be selected, who will lead the team, and the documentation and communication process. When implementing a PIP, the organization must consider factors such as alignment with the mission, vision, and guiding principles; the need for training; costs; resource availability; and feasibility. Once the PIP topic is determined and the team assembled, a project charter should be developed. This charter sets the goals, scope, timing, milestones, and team roles and responsibilities, helping the team stay focused on the PIP objectives and individual contributions to the PIP and the QAPI steering committee.

Each PIP is a learning experience that encourages team member contributions and improved organizational performance, supporting quality resident care and staff satisfaction. The QAPI plan designates the processes for conducting research, gathering data, using data analysis tools/methods, documenting findings, selecting PI tools (e.g., root cause analysis [RCA]), and reporting and communicating results.

The QAPI steering committee monitors the progress of PIPs through a systematic reporting process supported by formalized documentation, ensuring a structured approach to documentation and communication (Lake Superior Quality Innovation Network, 2016).

The QAPI plan includes a description of the systematic approach to data collection, organization, analysis, interpretation, and reporting results. The goal of this process is to identify the root causes of problems, concerns, or negative trends; understand the systems involved; and determine how to address the identified issues. A systematic approach provides a consistent, well-documented framework for the process and helps identify potential unintended consequences of proposed changes. This approach considers all involved systems and how a change in one system could impact another (Spath, 2022). For example, when addressing the issue of residents receiving cold food, the organization must consider not only nutrition services but also nursing, therapy, and activities as systems or departments affected by changes in nutrition services processes.

The implementation processes should be clearly stated in the QAPI plan, including how policies and procedures will be updated to prevent future events and the roles and responsibilities of individuals or departments involved in the change processes. A communication plan is essential for informing various stakeholders of the changes and specifying the training individuals will need to perform new or modified tasks, ensuring compliance and adherence from staff, residents, and families (Spath & DeVane, 2023).

The organization should be prepared for roadblocks and pushback from different stakeholder groups and have processes in place to address them (Joshi et al., 2023). A communication plan should explain why the change is necessary, how the decision for the change was made, the steps to implement the new process, and the evaluation approach.

THE FACILITY ASSESSMENT

The phase II requirements of the revised federal nursing home regulations, along with the updated interpretative guidelines, came into effect on November 28, 2017. These regulations require that nursing homes "conduct and document a facility-wide assessment to determine what resources are necessary to care for its residents competently during both day-to-day operations (including nights and weekends) and emergencies" (Facility Assessment, 2024). This assessment is mandated to be reviewed and updated at least annually or when substantial changes occur within the nursing home. The facility assessment comprises three parts: the resident population, the nursing home's resources, and a facility-based and community-based risk assessment.

The assessment of the resident population includes the number of residents, their physical and cognitive disabilities, types of diseases, overall acuity, and other relevant information used in determining their care needs. Additionally, such items as staff competencies necessary for resident care; as well as the physical environment including equipment, services, and building layout, must be considered when providing care and services to the residents. Some examples include a memory care unit that provides care for residents with dementia and dementia-related disorders; equipment for obese residents; and ethnic, cultural, or religious considerations affecting care and services (Facility Assessment, 2024).

In the facility resources assessment, all buildings, physical structures, equipment (both medical and nonmedical), vehicles, provided services such as rehabilitation therapies (physical, occupational, and speech), and pharmacy are evaluated. This includes a comprehensive listing and description of all personnel, including contracted staff and volunteers, noting their education, training, and necessary competencies. Furthermore, third-party contracts, agreements, and memorandum for equipment and services are to be listed for both day-to-day operations and emergencies. The nursing home's digital technology resources such as electronic medical records, and their sharing capability, are included (Facility Assessment, 2024).

The third component involves facility-based and community-based risk assessment, utilizing an all-hazards approach. This approach required, since 2014, developing a continuity of operations business plan, collaborating with local emergency preparedness agencies, and analyzing the vulnerabilities specific to the facility for each identified hazard (Director of Survey and Certification Group, 2014). Facilities are encouraged to use resources such as the National Preparedness System by the Federal Emergency Management Agency (FEMA; 2020) and tools provided by the Agency for Healthcare Research and Quality (AHRQ; n.d.). The Centers for Disease Control and Prevention's *All-Hazards Preparedness Guide* (Office of Public Health Preparedness and Response, 2012) and the facility-based and community-based risk assessment and plan developed for emergency preparedness compliance can serve as the third component of the facility assessment (Lake Superior Quality Innovation Network, 2016).

APPLYING QUALITY MANAGEMENT IN COMPLEX SYSTEMS

To implement any aspect of the QAPI plan effectively for evaluating and improving processes, one must acknowledge the complexity inherent in an organization and the individuals within them. *Systems thinking* offers a method to comprehend the complexity, emphasizing the interrelatedness of processes and tasks. It provides a framework for understanding the interrelatedness of the parts rather than the things acting in silos, looking for patterns of change and the interconnectedness of the tasks and activities to create the organization in its environment. Healthcare organizations, in particular, are marked by complexity due to the numerous variables interacting in diverse ways (Spath, 2022).

For example, consider the diversity among the workforce providing care in the nursing home. From traditionalists to Millennials, each generation cares for residents with a multitude of conditions and needs, ranging from cognitive impairments to mobility challenges (Bahnemann et al., 2018). This diversity results in countless potential interactions between staff and residents, each with its own set of outcomes, contributing to dynamic complexity where actions may yield vastly different results in different parts of the system (Spath, 2022).

Dynamic complexity poses challenges to implementing changes as it requires assessing system behaviors and interrelated parts and modifying behaviors at the systemic level (Binbasioglu & Zychowicz, 2023). For example, during the COVID-19 pandemic, healthcare organizations faced severe staff shortages, exacerbated by factors such as illness, death, fear, and mandatory stay-at-home rules (Lane et al., 2023). Hiring contract staff to address shortages inadvertently led to increased labor costs and further staff migration to contract positions (Yang & Mason, 2022).

Understanding systems and their dynamics is imperative for successful change implementation. An often-used metaphor, the iceberg or triangle, illustrates how visible aspects of the organization's behavior represent events and patterns, while underlying aspects—behaviors, relationships, culture, and values—drive these events (Hassmiller Lich & Kuhlberg, 2020). For instance, analyzing staffing challenges reveals key system variables such as attendance policies (e.g., scheduling, sick, late, overtime), infection prevention measures, and organizational culture, which collectively influence staff behavior and contribute to systemic structures (Spath, 2022).

Administrators and leadership must grasp the interrelatedness of system variables to redesign systems effectively and achieve desired outcomes, such as reduced reliance on contract staff and improved work environment quality (Spath, 2022). Delving below the surface to make systemic changes entails questioning why current results occur and investigating organizational structures, cultures, information flow, and historical data (Hassmiller Lich & Kuhlberg, 2020).

STRATEGIES TO MAKE SYSTEMIC CHANGES

Strategies that leaders can employ to identify the systems and processes within their organizations and make systemic changes include understanding the history of their organization, being aware of mental models, and using double-loop learning. The current work in an organization is influenced by its previous workings and operations—its history (Spath, 2022). For instance, a nursing home with a history of leaders who create a caring environment and spend time engaging with staff and residents will foster a common understanding of the organization's workings and culture. This builds trust and encourages staff to share information with leadership, contributing to improvement initiatives (Lane et al., 2023). In contrast, a nursing home with frequent changes in leadership and staff will have a history of inconsistency and unknowns, making it difficult for new leadership to build relationships and make improvements due to the prevailing belief that "this leader is only temporary too" (Carnahan & Unroe, 2022). Strategies for new leaders to understand the history and perspective of the staff include discussing significant events, observing patterns, listening to staff interactions, asking staff to share their experiences, and learning about them as individuals (Daft, 2023).

Mental models are deeply ingrained assumptions that guide one's thinking about a situation, problem, or the world. These models can interfere with the ability to see the root causes of problems (Daft, 2023). For example, a mental model about the work ethic of BabyBoomers versus Millennials (people born between 1981 through 1996) could cloud judgment. Viewing BabyBoomers as hard working and loyal and Millennials as lacking commitment and entitled can limit a leader's ability to engage all workers and improve performance. Acknowledging these mental models allows individuals to adopt more constructive models. For instance, in the staffing crisis example from the iceberg metaphor, a leader who understands their mental model of the workforce and implements human resources policies that support Millennials' desire for flexible scheduling and learning opportunities, as well as policies that reward the hardworking Baby Boomers, encourages broader workforce participation (Graystone, 2019).

Conflicting mental models among individuals in an organization can be a source of conflict. For example, a model of "transparency builds trust" encourages staff to share information, including errors and near misses, whereas a model of "information is power" discourages communication. Leaders can overcome these challenges by discussing their viewpoints, assumptions, and mental models to establish a common understanding among the team (Graystone, 2019).

Double-loop learning "is a process that involves behavioral changes resulting from cognitive changes, including modifying deeply held values, beliefs, and assumptions" (Auqui-Caceres & Furlan, 2023, p. 17). This type of learning can transform an organization into a learning organization by questioning its values, assumptions, and governing variables, leading to changes in actions, behaviors, practices, norms, and routines. However, double-loop learning should not be used for all problem inquiries due to its time burden, as well as the commitment required for open reflection and dialogue (Auqui-Caceres & Furlan, 2023). Efforts to evaluate "why do we do things this way?" will benefit from double-loop learning processes. Investigating the mental models and assumptions held by organizational members and learning new frameworks are necessary to sustain proposed changes. For example, improving recruitment and retention of a nursing home requires leadership to ask "Why do we recruit this way?" and "Is there a better way to retain staff?" This involves assessing the cognitive component of recruitment and retention, as well as the behaviors involved in interviewing, onboarding, and monitoring staff engagement (Carnahan & Unroe, 2022).

TEAMS AND TEAMWORK

Teams and teamwork are a core element of a QAPI program (QAPI, 2022). Teams should be established based on their assigned tasks and be comprised of members with the requisite knowledge. While management literature identifies different types of teams, QAPI teams have a specific purpose. The QAPI steering committee is a standing committee responsible for the QAPI program and its efforts (QAPI, 2022).

Required members of the committee include the director of nurses, the medical director or their designee, three nursing home leaders (such as the administrator, owner, board member, or department leader), the infection control and prevention officer, and other staff as determined necessary for the QAPI program. The QAPI steering committee determines the PIP to be implemented and the members of each PIP team. Each team should have a clear purpose for its establishment, with defined roles and responsibilities for each member (QAPI, 2022).

The team leader is responsible for creating an atmosphere of psychologic safety, ensuring that each member has a voice and feels safe contributing to the team's work (Daft, 2023). Team members need to be trained on data collection tools and techniques, analysis processes, and other PI tools such as RCA and Plan-Do-Study-Act (PDSA) cycles. While each team member is not expected to be proficient in data collection and analysis, they should receive enough training to contribute to evaluating findings and potential solutions. For instance, nursing assistants and environmental services staff may not be proficient with statistical process control methods, but they possess valuable knowledge about how work is completed on their units and how to implement new processes. When evaluating options and completing rapid-cycle analysis, these staff members provide feedback based on their experiences and institutional knowledge. Best practice is to share the findings with the team in a way that all team members can understand the data and the root cause(s) of an issue (CMS, n.d.-b).

Teams with all new members will need time to get to know each other. Leaders should consider facilitating icebreaker activities to help the team move from the formation stages (forming and storming) to performing. Leaders can also assist by helping with the team charter and explaining the organization's mission, vision, and values. Some teams may include residents or family members to provide a care recipient's perspective (CMS, n.d.-b).

DATA SOURCES AND DATA COLLECTION

QAPI is a data-driven process, and each individual organization will determine what data is important for evaluating their quality of care and services, resident quality of life, and organizational systems and processes.

Examples of in-house resident data sources include adverse events, near misses, falls, care plan audits, weight-loss, and medication audits. Data collected and analyzed during monthly meetings such as infection prevention and control data, meeting minutes, care plan meeting notes, identified concerns, drug regimen review, and resident and family council minutes allow leaders to identify trends and take necessary actions. Input from staff, residents, families, and others should be documented and included in performance assessments.

Examples of staffing data include staff satisfaction, recruitment, retention, turnover data, staff hours per resident day, and nursing staff consistent assignment. The organization should also incorporate CMS quality measures (long-stay and short-stay), CASPER report, payroll-based journal report data, performance indicators, and state survey and fire safety survey reports.

Administrative data sources include daily census and occupancy rates, actual versus planned budget, monthly profit and loss statements, revenue sources and payor mix, annual capital budget, and days in collection. The facility assessment contains a wealth of data that can be used in conjunction with other sources to evaluate organizational systems, interrelated processes of care and services, quality of life, resident autonomy, and operations.

Adverse events, near misses, and reports of abuse, neglect, or maltreatment should be thoroughly investigated using RCA methodology to identify the actual cause(s) of the incident (QAPI, 2022). Data sources for these events may include residents, staff, family members, or others such as volunteers or contractors. Other sources of data include the medication administration record, resident care plan, pharmacist and registered dietitian reports, activity attendance records, environmental services plan or records, infection prevention and control reports, and staffing assignments. In addition to filing the required reports to the designated agencies, the organization will use PI tools and techniques to investigate and implement policies and processes to prevent incidents from reoccurring (QAPI, 2022).

The data collected must be stored in a manner that allows the organization to evaluate trends and benchmark against established metrics. The organization should establish a data storage plan indicating the frequency and method of data collection and where and how it will be stored. Resident clinical data is part of the medical record and the care plan, but storing some information only in the medical record (e.g., weight loss, falls, and infections) does not allow for assessing trends over time. Data collection systems should facilitate easy transfer of information between locations with minimal opportunity for human error and duplicative work. Many electronic health record systems have report generation options that allow some sources of data to be used for benchmarking and trending. Other data, such as complaints, incident reports, and adverse event reports, will need to be collected and stored in a manner that allows for aggregation and analysis to meet the organization's needs (Spath & DeVane, 2023).

The organization will set targets or benchmarks for various performance elements. These targets should align with the mission, vision, and guiding principles of the organization and support continuous PI. Benchmarks can be set by reviewing national and state data, corporate or governing board metrics, clinical guidelines, evidence-based best practices, and organizational goals. The organization determines the frequency of reviewing outcomes against the set benchmarks and the process for communicating the findings and actions to be taken when benchmarks are not met (CMS, n.d.-b; Spath & DeVane, 2023).

PERFORMANCE IMPROVEMENT MODELS

Once an area for improvement has been identified, steps must be taken to identify the causes and implement measures to correct or eliminate them. A systematic PIP ensures that all team members are informed and provides the structure and steps toward a common goal. The process should follow the cycle of measurement, assessment, and improvement (Spath & DeVane, 2023). Specifically, measurement involves utilizing organizational data to assess actual versus expected performance. Improvement is planned when gaps are identified.

One commonly used approach is the PDSA cycle, originally developed by Shewhart (1939) and later modified by W. Edwards Deming (Best & Neuhauser, 2005). The steps in the cycle are outlined in Table 5.2.

TABLE 5.2 Steps in a PDSA Cycle

STAGES	ACTIONS TAKEN
Plan	State the objectives. Identify what needs to be improved. Identify the processes that need to be changed. State the plan to make the changes including who, what, when, and where. State the data that will be collected to evaluate the changes made.
Do	Implement the changes that were planned. Document all findings. Collect data to evaluate changes made and outcomes.
Study	Analyze the data collected. Evaluate whether expected outcomes occurred or not. Summarize and log the outcomes and identify lessons learned.
Act	If outcomes were not as expected, repeat the cycle. If outcomes were successful, implement in another unit—wider scale. Predict larger scale results.

Source: Adapted from Spath, P. L., & DeVane, K. A. (2023). *Introduction to healthcare quality management* (4th ed.). Health Administration Press.

TABLE 5.3 PDSA Cycle for Resident Falls

STAGES	ACTIONS TAKEN
PLAN	
Objective	To reduce the number of resident falls
Plan	Resident assessments will be done on all new admissions and residents who have had a change in status within 8 hours of admission or assessment indicating a change in status. Assessments will be completed by an RN.
Expected results	Residents will experience fewer falls. Assessments will identify residents at risk of falling and staff will implement measures to protect residents from falls.
Measures	Staff should monitor resident falls, falls committee meeting minutes, and resident assessments for new admissions and residents who have experienced a change in status.
DO	
	For 2 months, monitor resident falls, the falls committee meeting minutes, and resident assessments for new admissions and residents who experienced a change in status.
STUDY	
	Two residents experienced falls. The falls committee minutes showed that the falls reports were reviewed, and processes were put in place for both residents to prevent falls. Nine residents were admitted during the 2 months, assessments were completed on all nine within 8 hours, two were at risk of falling, and processes were put into place for each. Some success was made; repeat the cycle for 4 more months.
ACT	
Evaluate	Two residents fell during the 2 months. Repeat the cycle for 4 more months. Assessment nurse should search for best practices in fall prevention. Ask a pharmacist to review new admissions and residents who have experienced a change in status for medications that can contribute to falls. Review falls reports and interview nursing assistants who care for the residents.
Implement	Repeat the cycle, adding the input from the pharmacist and nursing assistants. Review findings on best practices for preventing falls.

Source: Adapted from Spath, P. L., & DeVane, K. A. (2023). *Introduction to healthcare quality management* (4th ed.). Health Administration Press.

With each repetition of the cycle, the team gains a deeper understanding of the process and its interrelated components. Table 5.3 provides an example of a PDSA cycle applied to reduce resident falls.

Rapid cycle improvement (RCI) utilizes multiple PDSA cycles in succession to achieve improvement goals (Spath & DeVane, 2023). This process has been successfully implemented by various organizations, including the Institute for Healthcare Improvement and the Quality Improvement Organizations (QIO) conducting Medicare quality initiatives.

For instance, consider an organization with a goal to improve recruitment and retention by 20% within the next year. The leadership team forms a PIP to explore ways to increase new hires and reduce staff turnover. They identify four opportunities to test using successive PDSA cycles: provide a mentor for at least 60 days for all new hires, offering $20 per day for each day the mentor spends training the mentee. A $100 bonus is awarded if the new hire stays for 90 days, and an additional $200 bonus is given for referring a friend who remains employed for 6 months. Figure 5.3 depicts these four ideas being trialed.

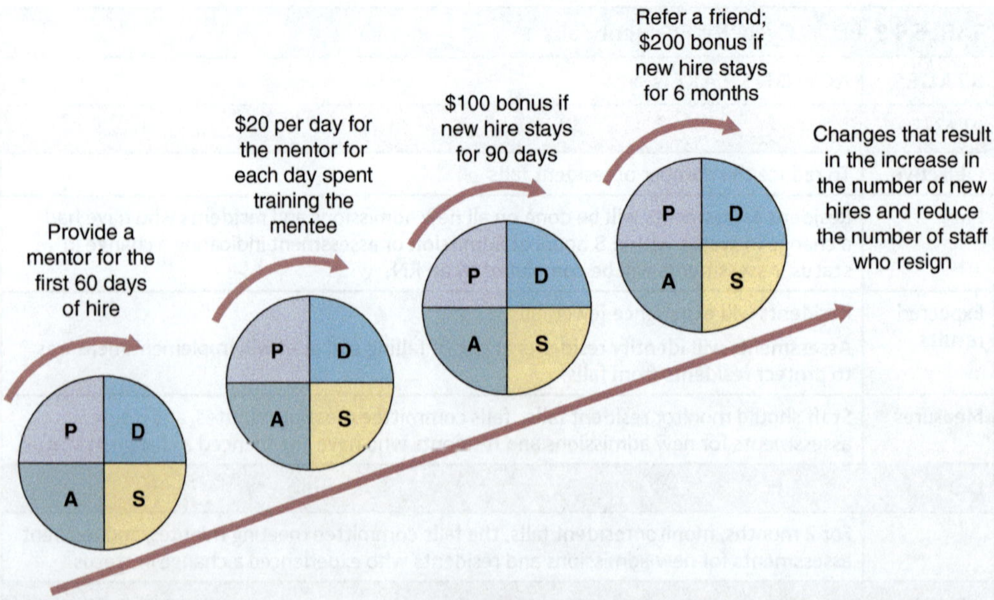

FIGURE 5.3. PDSA rapid cycle to increase staff and reduce turnover.
PDSA, Plan, Do, Study, Act.
Source: Data from Lake Superior Quality Innovation Network. (2016). *QAPI written plan how-to guide.* Centers for Medicare & Medicaid Services. https://www.cms.gov/medicare/provider-enrollment-and-certification/qapi/downloads/qapi-plan-how-to-guide.pdf

Lean is a PI model designed to eliminate inefficiencies that impact organizational performance. Originating in the Japanese automobile industry, Lean is credited to Womack and Jones in 2003 for its implementation by Toyota (Spath & DeVane, 2023). These concepts are now widely used by healthcare organizations to evaluate their operations, eliminate unnecessary steps and errors, and improve efficiency. Lean consists of five core principles:

1. *Value:* Understand how customers define value.
2. *Value stream or resident journey:* Map out the current steps in the process to identify waste.
3. *Processes flow without interruption:* Align processes to eliminate waste, adjust for demand to avoid batching or queuing, and create a smooth flow of care.
4. *Let the customer pull services:* Synchronize people, information, and supplies to be ready when the resident is.
5. *Strive for perfection:* Continuously improve processes over time to deliver the highest quality.

Lean thinking requires a culture shift where leaders spend time learning about the organization by observing work processes and listening to empowered employees, residents, and other stakeholders. It fosters an inclusive culture where leaders and employees collaborate to identify and eliminate waste, adding value to the system (Ellis, 2020).

Six Sigma is an improvement system aimed at reducing variation and eliminating defects in organizational processes. It is a data-driven approach based on Shewhart's statistical process control philosophy, aiming for no more than 3.4 defects per million opportunities, with a goal of zero defects (Pruitt et al., 2021). Using statistical processes and tools, leaders can assess and understand the process fluctuations, predict outcomes, and, when outcomes are unsatisfactory, use tools to identify influencing factors (Spath, 2022). For example, the falls committee can analyze a year's worth of data and, using statistical process control charts, evaluate variation in fall rates overtime and begin the improvement process.

Organizations using Six Sigma often follow the five steps of DMAIC methodology: Define, Measure, Analyze, Improve, and Control. These steps are similar to the PDSA cycle, but with a focused use of data and statistical tools to evaluate variation (Joshi et al., 2023). Understanding variation is critical to improve defects. Common cause variation occurs within a statistically controlled system due to chance events, such as a snowstorm or flu outbreak. Attempting to change processes due to these events can worsen outcomes (Joshi et al., 2023). Special cause variation, on the other hand, indicates that a process is not in statistical control and requires investigation and corrective action (Spath, 2022). For instance, if a falls analysis shows special cause variation, the falls committee or PIP should delve into the data to determine the underlying causes and actions needed.

Combining the Lean with Six Sigma allows organizations to improve efficiency by eliminating waste and standardizing work while leveraging Six Sigma's statistical analysis tools. This integrated *Lean Six Sigma model* helps address weaknesses in both approaches, ensuring changes are made efficiently and correctly. Lean alone does not necessarily provide error-free performance, and Six Sigma alone does not necessarily lower costs associated with the process inefficiencies (Spath, 2022). This combined model proved valuable during the COVID-19 pandemic when healthcare organizations were forced to rapidly revise work processes to protect staff and residents (Gillespie, 2021).

RCA is a structured process used by PIP teams to identify the root causes of untoward events or outcomes. It identifies breakdowns in processes and systems and determines how to prevent future events. The goal of RCA is to discover what happened, why it happened, and how to prevent it from recurring (CMS, n.d.-b; Spath &DeVane, 2023). A thorough RCA includes identifying human and related factors, underlying processes and systems, cause-and-effect relationships, risks, and potential process improvements (Veterans Health Administration National Center for Patient Safety, 2020). The RCA begins with establishing a timeline of events, identifying contributing factors, and digging deeper to find root causes. Once identified, corrective action and process changes can be implemented and tested (Joshi et al., 2023). PIPs should select actions that change the system to prevent reoccurrence (CMS, n.d.-b). Measures to determine success should be established alongside the actions (Spath & DeVane, 2023).

Failure mode and effectiveness analysis (FMEA) is a proactive structured approach to assessing risk before an adverse event occurs. FMEA identifies and analyzes potential failures in healthcare processes to reduce or eliminate risks to patient safety (Spath, 2018). The model asks three key questions: "What could go wrong?", "What will be the result if something goes wrong?", and "What needs to be done to prevent a bad result?" (Spath & DeVane, 2023, p. 209). FMEA is commonly used in high-risk processes such as medication administration, resident transfers, and fall prevention. The PIP team begins by creating a flowchart of the process, identifying potential failure modes at each step. The team then prioritizes critical failures based on frequency, severity of harm, and detectability (Tewfik, 2021). Figure 5.4 illustrates this process using an example of fall prevention.

PERFORMANCE IMPROVEMENT TOOLS

PI tools are essential for organizations to understand work processes and identify the root causes of outcomes. According to the American Society for Quality (ASQ), a process is defined as "a set of interrelated work activities that transform inputs into outputs" (ASQ, n.d.). Understanding the process is a prerequisite for improvement. One commonly used tool for documenting process steps is a flowchart such as Figure 5.4. In a flowchart, the steps or activities of the process are

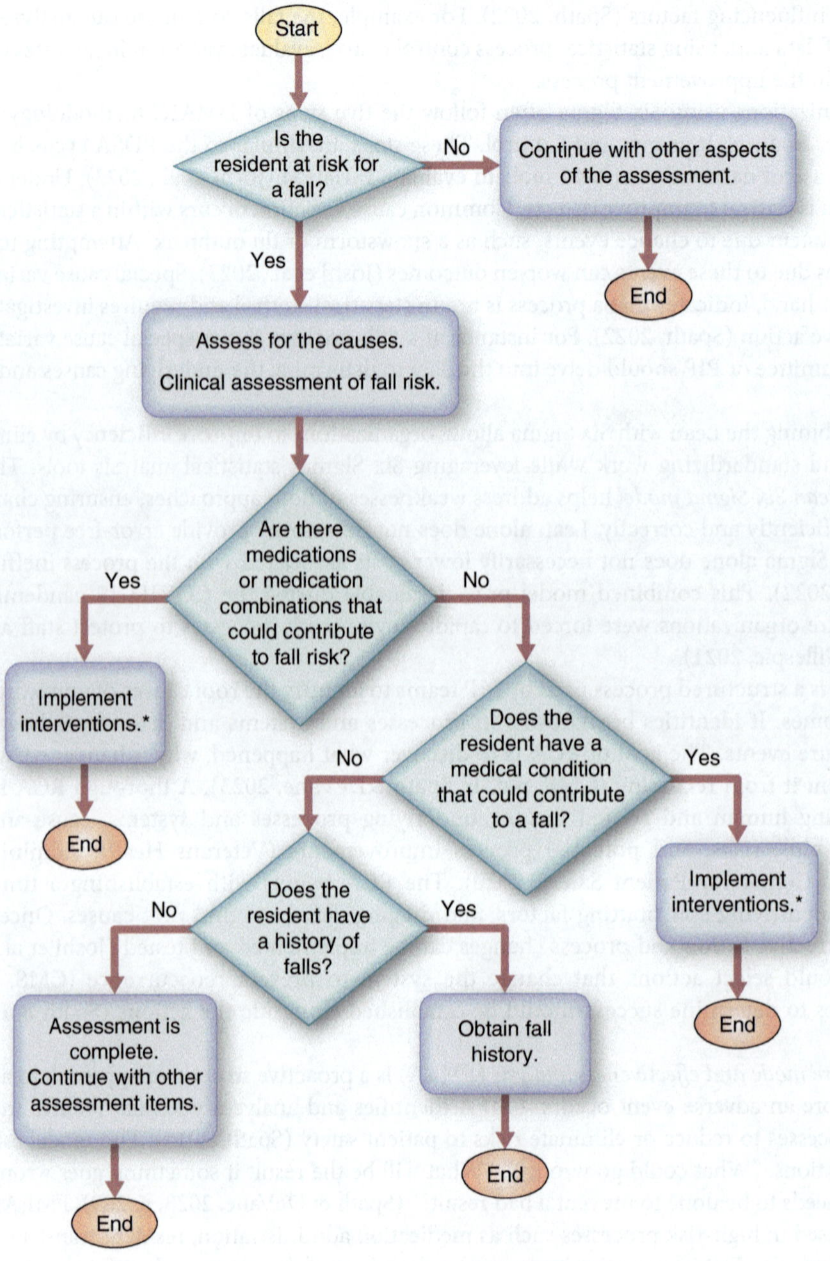

FIGURE 5.4. Inbound resident fall risk assessment process.

Source: Data from Centers for Medicare & Medicaid Services. (n.d.). *Flowchart guide*. Retrieved January 15, 2024, from https://www.cms.gov/Medicare/Provider-Enrollment-and-Certification/QAPI/downloads/FlowchartGuide.pdf

depicted using different shaped symbols, typically starting with an oval symbol to denote the start or end of the process. These symbols are then connected with arrows to show links and direction. Each step is represented within a square or rectangle, while decision points are typically depicted within diamonds. These decision points guide the actions and flow of the chart. For example, if the question "Is the new resident at risk for falls?" yields a "Yes" response, the flowchart would direct the review of the fall risk reduction and management policy. Conversely,

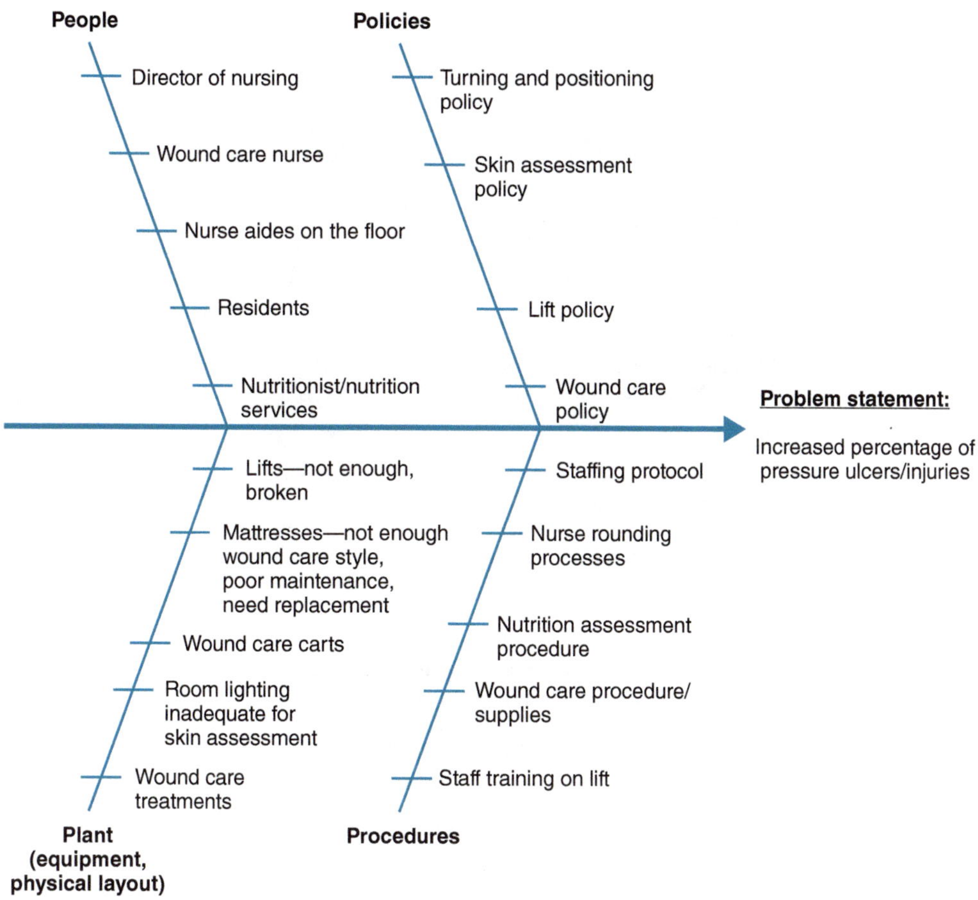

FIGURE 5.5. Fishbone diagram for root cause analysis.

Source: Data from Centers for Medicare & Medicaid Services. (n.d.). *How to use the fishbone tool for root cause analysis.* Retrieved January 21, 2024, from https://www.cms.gov/Medicare/Provider-Enrollment-and-Certification/QAPI/downloads/FishboneRevised.pdf

if the response is "No," the flowchart would proceed to the next step of the new resident admission assessment (CMS, n.d.-a).

Cause-and-effect diagrams, also known as Ishikawa or fishbone diagrams, are invaluable tools for identifying the multitude of causes behind a problem or objective. Named after Kaoru Ishikawa, the Japanese quality management specialist who created it, the diagram resembles a fishbone, hence its alternative moniker. In the process, teams typically engage in brainstorming sessions to categorize and organize the causes into various groups. Common categories include the four Ms (methods, manpower, materials, and machinery) or the four Ps (policies, procedures, people, and plant). Crucially, crafting a clear problem statement is vital for the successful identification of contributing causes (Spath & DeVane, 2023). The fishbone diagram provides a structured framework for the team to gain a comprehensive understanding of the systems and processes contributing to the problem (Figure 5.5).

Another method of uncovering causes is the "five whys" technique, which involves repeatedly asking "Why?" to drill down through the symptoms and pinpoint the root causes of the problem. This approach compels the team to move beyond surface-level observations and explore the underlying conditions contributing to the outcome. Figure 5.6 illustrates how a nursing home used this method to determine the root cause of a resident's fall, resulting in a serious injury during a transfer from a wheelchair to a bed (CMS, n.d.-b).

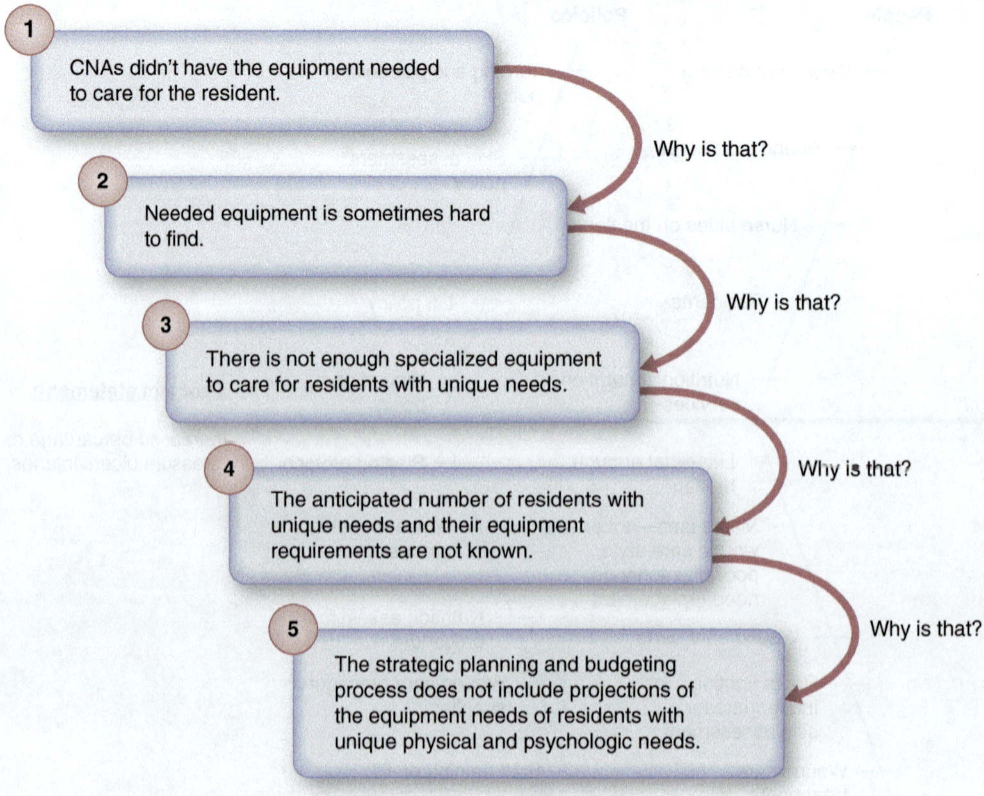

FIGURE 5.6. "Five whys" technique to identify the root causes.

CNAs, certified nursing assistants.

Source: Centers for Medicare & Medicaid Services. (n.d.). *Guidance for performing root cause analysis (RCA) with performance improvement projects (PIPs)*. Retrieved January 28, 2024, from https://www.cms.gov/medicare/provider-enrollment-and-certification/qapi/downloads/guidanceforrca.pdf

SUMMARY

QAPI is a structured format for self-assessment of organizational performance that incorporates processes of systems thinking and dynamic complexity. It requires a proactive and continuous approach that is organized and data-driven to evaluate all aspects of nursing home operations to identify gaps in systems and opportunities for improvement. Nursing homes are complex organizations with many interconnected systems and processes that need to be accounted for when evaluating an outcome or a trend in operations. The QAPI plan is a comprehensive document that guides the QAPI program, sets priorities, and defines how PIP teams will be created. Nursing home leadership—administrators, governing bodies, and owners—lead the QAPI program and ensure resources are available to evaluate, analyze, and improve performance. Leaders are also responsible to ensure organization-wide QAPI training is provided on a continuous basis and that PIP membership includes staff, residents, and family members most familiar with the processes. QAPI activities need to be well-documented and guided by evidence-based PI models and tools.

END-OF-CHAPTER RESOURCES

DISCUSSION QUESTIONS

1. What is the value of combining QA with PI to create QAPI, and why can it improve a nursing home's overall performance?
2. How would you set benchmarks for PIPs for pressure ulcers, weight loss, falls, and staff turnover?
3. How are the five elements of the QAPI framework interconnected, and why does each element play a critical role in a quality QAPI program?
4. During morning rounds, if a certified nursing assistant (CNA) observes a resident with bruises on her right arm that were not there yesterday when she went home at 3:00 p.m. and reports the bruises to the nurse, who then notifies the director of nursing, what steps will the nursing team take to conduct an RCA?
5. As a new administrator, how would you create a culture of openness and high performance?
6. How would you create a PDSA cycle to increase resident participation in bingo?
7. If you are leading a PIP on an increase in nosocomial infections in your nursing home, which PI tool would you select, and how would you determine the potential causes of the increase in infections?
8. After completing the annual facility assessment last week, you are reviewing the report to determine your priority PIPs for the quarter. What process would you use to prioritize PIPs?
9. What is leadership's role in the development of the QAPI plan and program?
10. What is the role of the QAPI steering committee?

SPRINGER PUBLISHING CONNECT™

A robust set of instructor resources designed to supplement this text is located at http://connect.springerpub.com/content/book/978-0-8261-4935-0. Qualifying instructors may request access by emailing textbook@springerpub.com.

REFERENCES

Agency for Healthcare Research and Quality. (n.d.). *Topic: Emergency preparedness*. Retrieved November 18, 2023, from https://www.ahrq.gov/topics/emergency-preparedness.html

American Society for Quality. (n.d.). *Quality glossary—P*. Retrieved December 26, 2023, from https://asq.org/quality-resources/quality-glossary/p

Auqui-Caceres, M.-V., & Furlan, A. (2023). Revitalizing double-loop learning in organizational contexts: A systematic review and research agenda. *European Management Review, 20*(4), 741–761. https://doi.org/10.1111/emre.12615

Bahnemann, S., Bryant-Mandler, J., Knutson, A., & Yost, J. (2018). Strategies for managing workforce generations that work. *Management in Healthcare, 3*(1), 82–91. https://doi.org/10.69554/MNAT7051

Best, M., & Neuhauser, D. (2005). W Edwards Deming: Father of quality management, patient and composer. *Quality and Safety in Healthcare, 14*(8), 137–145. https://doi.org/10.1136/qshc.2005.015289

Binbasioglu, M., & Zychowicz, E. J. (2023). Healthcare complexity: Redesigning care with systems modeling. *Issues in Information Systems, 24*(3), 181–194. https://doi.org/10.48009/3_iis_2023_116

Carnahan, J. L., & Unroe, K. T. (2022). Prioritizing nursing home staff and leadership consistency to improve quality. *Journal of the American Geriatric Society*, *70*(9), 2472–2473. https://doi.org/10.1111/jgs.17938

Centers for Medicare & Medicaid Services. (n.d.-a). *Flowchart guide*. Retrieved January 15, 2024, from https://www.cms.gov/Medicare/Provider-Enrollment-and-Certification/QAPI/downloads/FlowchartGuide.pdf

Centers for Medicare & Medicaid Services. (n.d.-b). *Guidance for performing root cause analysis (RCA) with performance improvement projects (PIPs)*. Retrieved December 18, 2023, from https://www.cms.gov/medicare/provider-enrollment-and-certification/qapi/downloads/guidanceforrca.pdf

Centers for Medicare & Medicaid Services. (2012, June 29). *Quality Assurance and Performance Improvement (QAPI) in nursing homes: Activities related to QAPI implementation* [Memo # 12-38-NH]. https://www.cms.gov/medicare/provider-enrollment-and-certification/surveycertificationgeninfo/policy-and-memos-to-states-and-regions-items/survey-and-cert-letter-12-38

Centers for Medicare & Medicaid Services. (2023, September 6). *QAPI description and background*. https://www.cms.gov/Medicare/Provider-Enrollment-and-Certification/QAPI/qapidefinition

Daft, R. L. (2023). *The leadership experience* (8th ed.). Cengage.

Director of Survey and Certification Group. (2014, February 28). *Survey and certification emergency preparedness initiative: S&C emergency preparedness checklist revision* [Letter]. U.S. Department of Health & Human Services, Centers for Medicare & Medicaid Services. http://www.cms.gov/Medicare/Provider-Enrollment-and-Certification/SurveyCertificationGenInfo/Downloads/Survey-and-Cert-Letter-14-12.pdf

Dunn, R. T. (2021). *Dunn and Haimann's healthcare management* (11th ed.). Health Administration Press.

Ellis, L. D. (2020, November 13). *The importance of adopting a lean mindset and culture for health care organizations*. Harvard Medical School, Trends in Medicine. https://postgraduateeducation.hms.harvard.edu/trends-medicine/importance-adopting-lean-mindset-culture-health-care-organizations

Facility Assessment, 42 C.F.R. § 483.71 (2024, August 30). https://www.ecfr.gov/current/title-42/chapter-IV/subchapter-G/part-483

Federal Emergency Management Agency. (2020, July 31). *National preparedness system*. https://www.fema.gov/emergency-managers/national-preparedness/system

Gillespie, L. (2021). Hospital safety improvements will outlast COVID-19. *Modern Healthcare*, *51*(3), 8–9. https://www.modernhealthcare.com/patient-care/hospital-safety-improvements-will-outlast-covid-19

Graystone, R. (2019). How to build a positive, multigenerational workforce. *Journal of Nursing Administration*, *49*(1), 4–5. https://doi.org/10.1097/NNA.0000000000000698

Hassmiller Lich, K., & Kuhlberg, J. (2020). Engaging stakeholders in mapping and modeling complex systems structure to inform population health research and action. In Y. Apostolopoulos, K. Hassmiller Lich, & M. K. Lemke (Eds.), *Complex systems and population health: A primer* (pp. 119–134). Oxford University Press.

Joshi, M. S., Ransom, S. B., Ransom, E., & Nash, D. B. (2023). *The healthcare quality book: Vision, strategy, and tools* (5th ed.). Health Administration Press.

Lane, S. J., Liu, D., & Rados, R. (2023). Post-acute and long-term care leaders' perspectives on leading during COVID-19. *Journal of Applied Gerontology*, *42*(11), 2179–2188. https://doi.org/10.1177/07334648231188282

Lake Superior Quality Innovation Network. (2016). *QAPI written plan how-to guide*. Centers for Medicare & Medicaid Services. https://www.cms.gov/medicare/provider-enrollment-and-certification/qapi/downloads/qapi-plan-how-to-guide.pdf

Ledlow, G. R., & Stephens, J. H. (2018). *Leadership for health professionals: Theory, skills, and applications* (3rd ed.). Jones & Bartlett Learning.

Office of Public Health Preparedness and Response. (2012, September 18). *All-hazards preparedness guide*. Centers for Disease Control and Prevention. https://stacks.cdc.gov/view/cdc/12007

Pruitt, Z., Smith, C. S., & Pérez-Ruberté, E. (2021). *Healthcare quality management: A case study approach*. Springer Publishing Company.

Quality Assurance and Performance Improvement, 42 C.F.R. § 483.75 (2022). https://www.govinfo.gov/content/pkg/CFR-2022-title42-vol5/pdf/CFR-2022-title42-vol5-sec483-75.pdf

Shewhart, W. A. (1939). *Statistical method from the viewpoint of quality control.* Dover Publications.

Spath, P. L. (2018). *Introduction to healthcare quality management* (3rd ed.). Health Administration Press.

Spath, P. L. (2022). *Applying quality management in healthcare: A systems approach* (5th ed.). Health Administration Press.

Spath, P. L., & DeVane, K. A. (2023). *Introduction to healthcare quality management* (4th ed.). Health Administration Press.

Tewfik, G. (2021). Proactive perioperative risk analysis: Use of failure mode and effects analysis (FMEA). *Anesthesia Patient Safety Foundation Newsletter, 36*(1), 17–20. https://www.apsf.org/wp-content/uploads/newsletters/2021/3601/APSF3601.pdf

Veterans Health Administration National Center for Patient Safety. (2020, October 20). *Guide to performing a root cause analysis.* https://www.patientsafety.va.gov/docs/RCA_Guidebook_10212020.pdf

Womack, J., & Jones, D. (2003). *Lean thinking: Banish waste and create wealth in your corporation* (2nd ed.). Free Press.

Yang, Y. T., & Mason, D. J. (2022, January 28). *COVID-19's impact on nursing shortages, the rise of travel nurses, and price gouging.* Health Affairs Forefront. https://doi.org/10.1377/forefront.20220125.695159

CHAPTER 6

ASSESSING LONG-TERM CARE QUALITY AND SAFETY: THE ROLE OF PUBLIC REPORT CARDS

Marcelo Coca Perraillon and Huiwen Xu

Learning Objectives

After completing this chapter, each learner will be able to:

- Understand the origin of public reporting of quality in nursing homes.
- Name the data sources used to evaluate quality measures in nursing homes and the different types of report cards.
- Evaluate the challenges of measuring quality of care.
- Understand the challenges of empirically evaluating the impact of public reporting of quality measures.
- Understand the evolution of the five-star ratings and unintended consequences.

INTRODUCTION

The quality of care in nursing homes has long been a concern for policymakers and families considering long-term care or postacute services. A landmark Institute of Medicine (IOM) report in 1986 concluded that despite extensive government regulation the quality of care and life in many nursing homes [was] not acceptable (IOM, 1986). Among other recommendations, the IOM called for more effective government regulation to ensure better quality of care and for a system to obtain standardized data on residents. The data system aimed to provide information for both nursing home management and government regulatory agencies to reorient the regulatory system from "facility-centered" to "resident-centered" and "outcome-oriented" (IOM, 1986). In response to the IOM report, the Centers for Medicare & Medicare (CMS) created the Minimum Data Set (MDS; Mor, 2005). The MDS contains data from comprehensive assessments of residents' functional capabilities that permit nursing home staff to identify health problems and create a plan of care. Federal regulation mandates that nursing homes certified by the CMS should conduct these assessments upon admission, quarterly, annually, at discharge, or if there is a considerable change in the health status of a resident.

MDS provided the necessary data to launch the Nursing Home Compare (NHC), a website created by the CMS to publicly report nursing homes' quality metrics along with other information like health inspection surveys. The ultimate goal of public reporting is to improve the quality of care in nursing homes, although the mechanism is indirect. The rationale is that if consumers use public reporting and choose nursing homes of better quality, then nursing homes have more incentives to improve the quality of care to attract (or not lose) residents. This rationale, despite being intuitive, depends on assumptions about the clarity and usability of public reporting, patients' and families' ability to choose nursing homes of better quality, and the incentives that public reporting provides to nursing homes.

This chapter aims to describe the historical evolution of Nursing Home Care Compare (NHCC) and to evaluate the empirical evidence regarding the success of public reporting to improve the quality of care in nursing homes. We first review the evolution of NHCC, from quality metrics to a five-star system. We then review the most important empirical evidence regarding the changes that NHCC induced in both consumers and nursing homes. We also discuss the unintended consequences of public reporting, many of which are a result of strategies used by nursing homes to increase ratings without improving the quality of care or the barriers faced by patients in choosing nursing homes.

Throughout this chapter, we use the term *consumer* to refer to patients, families, or other caregivers—the agents that choose a nursing home, which can also be discharge planners and physicians who provide care to patients. We use the term *report cards* as the more general term to refer to public reporting, but as we explain in the next section, public reporting in nursing homes has taken several forms over time.

CREATION OF NURSING HOME COMPARE

In 1998, the CMS introduced the first version of *public reporting* in nursing homes with a website that reported nursing home regulatory deficiencies for all CMS-certified nursing homes, which account for over 95% of all facilities in the country (National Center for Health Statistics [NCHS], 2004). The website was expanded in 2000 to include information on nursing homes' staffing levels. In 2002, it was expanded again to include quality measures. The 2002 change marked the start of the website that was known as NHC. The 2002 release was also accompanied by an advertising campaign and is thus considered the launch of public reporting in nursing homes. Before 2002, however, a 7-month pilot program tested the implementation of quality measures in six states (Kissam et al., 2003).

The NHC site published information on the characteristics of nursing homes, such as ownership status, size, Medicare/Medicaid participation, and health-related deficiencies resulting from on-site inspections of nursing homes, which occur every 9 to 15 months (Xu et al., 2022). NHC also included 10 clinical quality measures; six of them measured quality for long-stay residents with chronic care needs and four measured quality for patients in postacute care with skilled needs. The quality measures were expressed as the percentage of residents in a nursing home with some event deemed indicative of good care. The 2002 measures included the percentage of residents with pressure ulcers (separately for high- and low-risk patients), loss of ability in basic daily activities, infections, pain, physical restraints, and excessive weight loss (Grabowski & Town, 2011; Werner et al., 2012). Other measures were added and removed over the years. NHC was discontinued on December 1, 2020, and has been succeeded by Care Compare, which can be accessed at Medicare's Care Compare (www.medicare.gov/care-compare).

At the end of 2023, the reported information included quality measures for short-stay and long-stay residents based on the MDS and claims data, some of which are part of new ratings as described in the text that follows. Some measures reported include Skilled Nursing Facility (SNF) Value-Based Purchasing Program metrics, related to 30-day readmission rates, and several measures on staffing like turnover rates. Table 6.1 lists the quality measures by short-and long-stay and whether they are part of the ratings.

COMPOSITE RATINGS

In December 2008, the CMS made a significant change to NHC. It released a composite summary rating for nursing homes using a star system. Nursing homes were assigned up to five stars, from one star indicating quality "much below average" to five stars indicating quality "much above average." Thus, the new NHC website allowed consumers to rank and compare nursing homes in their area in a simpler manner. With the 2002 version, consumers were only able to compare nursing homes using selected quality measures and other information reported in NHC, but they were

TABLE 6.1 Quality Measures by Short- and Long-Stay Residents and Inclusion in Five-Star Ratings

QUALITY MEASURE	SHORT STAY	LONG STAY	PART OF RATINGS
Percentage of short-stay residents who were re-hospitalized after a nursing home admission	Yes	No	Yes
Percentage of short-stay residents who have had an outpatient ED visit	Yes	No	Yes
Percentage of short-stay (long-stay) residents who got antipsychotic medication for the first time	Yes	Yes	Yes
Percentage of SNF residents with pressure ulcers/ pressure injuries that are new or worsened*	Yes	No	Yes
Percentage of long-stay residents experiencing one or more falls with major injury	No	Yes	Yes
Percentage of short-stay residents who improved in their ability to move around on their own	No	No	Yes
Rate of successful return to home or community from an SNF	Yes	No	Yes
Percentage of short-stay residents who needed and got a flu shot for the current flu season	Yes	Yes	No
Percentage of healthcare personnel who got a flu shot for the current season[a]	Yes	Yes	No
Percentage of short-stay residents who needed and got a vaccine to prevent pneumonia	Yes	No	No
Percentage of SNF residents whose medications were reviewed and who received follow-up care when medication issues were identified	Yes	No	No
Percentage of SNF residents (long-stay) who experience one or more falls with major injury (during their SNF stay)	Yes	Yes	No
Percentage of SNF residents whose functional abilities were assessed, and functional goals were included in their treatment plan	Yes	No	No
Percentage of residents who are at or above an expected ability to care for themselves at discharge	Yes	No	No
Percentage of residents who are at or above an expected ability to move around at discharge	Yes	No	No
Change in residents' ability to care for themselves	Yes	No	No
Change in residents' ability to move around	Yes	No	No
Percentage of SNF healthcare personnel who completed COVID-19 primary vaccination series	Yes	No	No
Rate of potentially preventable hospital readmissions 30 days after discharge from an SNF	Yes	No	No
Percentage of infections patients got during their SNF stay that resulted in hospitalization	Yes	No	No
Medicare Spending Per Beneficiary (MSPB) for residents in SNFs	Yes	No	No

(continued)

TABLE 6.1 Quality Measures by Short- and Long-Stay Residents and Inclusion in Five-Star Ratings (*continued*)

QUALITY MEASURE	SHORT STAY	LONG STAY	PART OF RATINGS
SNF 30-Day All-Cause Readmission Measure	Yes	No	No
Number of hospitalizations per 1,000 long-stay resident days	No	Yes	Yes
Number of outpatient ED visits per 1,000 long-stay resident days	No	Yes	Yes
Percentage of long-stay residents with a urinary tract infection	No	Yes	Yes
Percentage of long-stay residents who have or had a catheter inserted and left in their bladder	No	Yes	Yes
Percentage of long-stay residents whose ability to move independently worsened	No	No	Yes
Percentage of long-stay residents whose need for help with daily activities has increased	No	No	Yes
Percentage of long-stay residents who were physically restrained	No	Yes	No
Percentage of long-stay low-risk residents who lose control of their bowels or bladder	No	Yes	No
Percentage of long-stay residents who lose too much weight	No	Yes	No
Percentage of long-stay residents who have symptoms of depression	No	Yes	No
Percentage of long-stay residents who got an antianxiety or hypnotic medication	No	Yes	No

*Only used in SNF reporting program.

Note: Please be aware that the inclusion of quality measurements may change over time. For the most up-to-date information of this table, refer to the latest user guide from the CMS.

CMS, Centers for Medicare and Medicaid; SNF, skilled nursing facility.

Source: Centers for Medicare & Medicaid Services. (2024, July). *Design for Care Compare nursing home five-star quality rating system: Technical users' guide.* https://www.cms.gov/medicare/provider-enrollment-and-certification/certificationandcomplianc/downloads/usersguide.pdf

not able to compare a summary of the information available on the website. Because the objective of the five-star rating is to compare nursing homes on domains that apply to all residents, the new five-star ratings were not calculated separately for long- and short-stay residents. From the start of the development of the five-star rating system, the CMS wanted to use only the existing information on NHC, incorporating all the dimensions available into summary stars, although not all the information available on NHC was included in the composite ratings (C. Williams et al., 2010).

Besides the overall number of stars, the new website showed separate five-star ratings for health inspections, staffing, and quality measure domains. The number of stars is based on the distribution of raw scores for each of the rating domains, of which the health inspection domain is the most important in determining the overall number of stars. The health inspection rating was based on a modified version of the Special Focus Facility algorithm developed to identify nursing homes that had a greater number of quality problems (Castle & Engberg, 2010; CMS, 2024). The algorithm assigned points to health inspection deficiencies based on unannounced on-site inspections. The points depended on the scope of the violation (isolated, pattern, or widespread) and its severity. Violations that cause no harm with the potential for minimal harm received no points. Stars were then assigned according to the percentiles of the distribution of health inspection scores at the state level. Within a state, the top 10% of nursing homes with the lowest scores received five stars, while 20% of nursing homes with the highest scores received one star. The remaining 70% were equally divided among two, three, and four stars.

Stars for the staffing domain were based on case-mix adjusted measures of staffing levels. At the time of the on-site health inspection, nursing homes self-reported their total staffing hours over the 2 weeks prior. When NHC was launched, the CMS did not verify the accuracy of the self-reported data, although it performed checks to identify facilities with unreliable staffing or resident census data (C. Williams et al., 2010). Total staffing hours were converted to staff hours per resident per day, adjusted for case-mix of patients (i.e., disease severity), relying upon the Resource Utilization Groups (RUG) system developed for prospective payment. The final score a nursing home received depended on its self-reported staffing levels compared to the expected national average. Stars were assigned based on both the distribution of this score and thresholds that were determined a priori by a study of staffing levels and quality of care (Kramer, 2001). Importantly, thresholds were set at the national level and were held constant over several years. Thus, contrary to the health inspection domain, the percentage of nursing homes that could achieve high ratings was not held constant. In the inspection domain, only 10% of nursing homes could receive five stars.

In December 2018, the CMS started to use the Payroll-Based Journal staffing data to calculate staffing levels, replacing the self-reported data. In July 2022, the CMS revised the methodology for calculating the staffing ratings. It is now based on six measures that attempt to capture staffing levels (total and per resident) and the percentage and number of nursing staff and administrators that leave a facility over 12 months (turnover). These changes were designed to more objectively measure staffing status in nursing homes (CMS, 2024).

For the quality measures domain, a score was originally calculated using a subset of 10 quality measures. Instead of using the most recent value available for each quality measure, a weighted average of the last three-quarters of data was calculated, where the weights were a function of the number of residents who were eligible for each of the measures. Points were calculated based on quintiles of the weighted quality measure and summed across the 10 measures. Stars were then assigned based on the distribution of summed points, much like the health inspection stars. However, the thresholds were set at the national rather than state level and were not changed for many years, much like the staffing domain. Thus, the percentage of top-rate facilities could increase over time. Currently, quality measures are based on both MDS and claims data and include more measures as described in Table 6.1. As with the first release of the five-star system, not all quality measures reported on NHC are part of the five-star ratings.

The overall number of stars a nursing home received followed a hierarchical set of rules, which is still in place with some modifications. The starting point is the health inspection number of stars. If the number of stars in the staffing domain is five stars, then one star is added, while one is subtracted if the staffing domain is one star. Another star is added or subtracted if the quality domain is five or one, respectively. Nursing homes with poor ratings in the quality domains (one star) cannot be upgraded by more than one star based on the staffing domain (CMS, 2024).

Several features of the way the information was summarized to create the five-star ratings are worth noting. First, the health inspection rating became the most important domain in determining the overall number of stars. The CMS wanted the health inspection domain to play a dominant role in determining the overall number of stars because inspections were deemed more objective than self-reported information (CMS, 2008, 2024; C. Williams et al., 2010). Second, the number of nursing homes that could receive high ratings was constrained by the health inspection domain, since only 10% of nursing homes could receive five stars. However, no constraints existed for the staffing and quality measures. Third, two domains, staffing and quality metrics, were originally based on self-reported data, which had the potential to be more easily manipulated. Fourth, the risk adjustment in the health inspection and quality domains was not extensive, although several measures are risk-adjusted. Thus, not all the components of the ratings are adjusted to consider differences in resident characteristics that may be associated with outcomes that result in lower ratings, perhaps independently of quality of care. Facilities that house more severe cases or residents that are difficult to care for may get penalized. Finally, the description of the algorithm highlights the difficulty faced by the CMS when summarizing vast amounts of information to rank nursing homes: Many decisions must be made that are somewhat arbitrary, which can result in different ratings. Framed in terms of Donabedian's framework, the five-star system summarized measures of structure, process, and outcomes, with a heavy emphasis on processes as determined by health inspections (Castle & Ferguson, 2010).

EVALUATING THE IMPACT OF NURSING HOME PUBLIC REPORTING

Studies evaluating the impact of nursing home public reporting usually take two points of view: the impact on consumers and the impact on nursing homes. Since the goal of public reporting is to motivate consumers to choose high-quality nursing homes, a clear metric of success is to evaluate whether consumers changed their behavior and chose better-quality facilities after its release. From the point of view of nursing homes, studies have evaluated whether they improved the quality of care or merely enhanced their ratings without actual improvement in care.

Regardless of the perspective, evaluating the causal impact of NHC is challenging. Public reporting was implemented at the population level, with all nursing homes receiving a rating and no control group for comparison, except for the pilot program before its 2002 launch. Therefore, evaluating the causal impact of the ratings on both consumers' and nursing homes' behavior requires quasi-experimental research designs. Other research designs, such as qualitative studies and surveys, provide supportive information about mechanisms for observed changes but do not permit ascertaining cause and effect.

The following sections summarize the most relevant studies evaluating the effect of NHC on consumer and nursing home behavior. For a comprehensive literature review, we recommend Konetzka et al. (2021). Early studies of the first version of NHC took advantage of the pilot study, using nonpilot states as a comparison. Evaluating the validity of these ratings is also of great policy importance since ratings that do not reflect the true quality of care can mislead consumers. We discuss evidence from studies attempting to ascertain the quality of the information provided and the strategies used by nursing homes to improve ratings. Additionally, we discuss research on the unintended consequences of NHC, particularly whether it increased disparities in access to high-quality nursing homes.

In more recent years, studies have begun focusing on the effects of NHCC (introduced in 2020), with further emphasis on the validity of the updated quality metrics (Chen et al., 2023) and their impact on both consumer behavior and nursing home operations (Sanghavi & Chen, 2023; Winter et al., 2022).

CONSUMER RESPONSE

The sparse evidence on consumer response to the initial release of public reporting was not conclusive, with surveys of families showing that NHC played a small role in consumers' decision process. Grabowski and Town (2011) studied the initial release leveraging the pilot implemented in six states using a difference-in-difference research design to compare the pilot states to the nonpilot states before and after the initial release of public reporting. They found no significant effect of NHC on market share for most of the quality measures. Werner et al. (2012) used an instrumental variable approach, also in part leveraging the staggered release in six states, to study the choice of nursing home for postacute care, finding significant but small market share changes in response to better scores in some postacute quality measures. The rationale was that postacute care patients, covered by Medicare, are more able to choose nursing homes. Complementing these studies, survey studies of family members of newly admitted nursing home residents found that only a small percentage of respondents (12%) reported using NHC, which in part explains the small response observed.

The release of the new composite five-star ratings resulted in several studies evaluating the impact of simplified ratings, with more consistent findings showing consumer response to the simplified ratings. Since the composite ratings were applied to all CMS-certified nursing homes, no comparison group was available for evaluation. However, Perraillon, Konetzka, et al. (2019) used a regression discontinuity approach to evaluate if nursing homes with better ratings increased their admissions 6 months after the release of the ratings, taking advantage of the mechanism used to assign stars that relied on a cutoff point to assign stars to compare facilities. The study found that nursing homes receiving higher ratings (5, 4, and 3) increased the number of admissions by 2% to 5%. However, nursing homes that gained two stars compared to one did not increase admissions. The study emphasized that consumers of better-rated nursing homes have different characteristics than consumers of lower-rated nursing homes. These findings were corroborated in qualitative interviews with nursing home administrators (Perraillon, Brauner, & Konetzka, 2019). Administrators of better-rated nursing homes stressed that their clients, and in some cases, referring hospitals, do pay close attention to ratings, while administrators of lower-rated nursing homes stated that their clients, who are more likely to be covered by Medicaid, in general, did not extensively use ratings in part because of lack of choices in their areas. These findings reflect the tiered structure of nursing homes in the United States (Mor et al., 2004).

Other studies of the launch of NHC showed similar findings. For example, Konetzka, Grabowski, et al. (2015) found a significant decline in the number of residents being served in one-star nursing homes and a significant increase in the number being served in five-star nursing homes. Although this study could not establish causality, it highlighted that better-rated nursing homes experienced gains in admissions (Werner et al., 2016). Another study found that one-star facilities lost market share while five-star facilities gained market share after the release of the ratings (Werner et al., 2016).

The empirical evidence more consistently shows that composite ratings shifted admissions to higher-rated facilities, a premise of public reporting. One possible mechanism is that composite ratings are easier to use and understand since consumers are familiar with five-star ratings as they are used by popular websites like Amazon and Yelp.

NURSING HOME RESPONSE

Since the ultimate goal of public reporting is to motivate nursing homes to improve their quality of care, several studies evaluated whether nursing homes improved quality as a result of public reporting. In general, studies found that nursing homes increased *measured* quality in response to ratings. For example, descriptive studies found improvements, albeit small, in some of the long-stay quality measures, with more consistent improvements in the short-stay measures (Castle et al., 2007, 2008). Using surveys of nursing home administrators, a study also found improvements in some measures (Mukamel et al., 2008). Two studies used the pilot program in six states to compare pilot states with nonpilot states, with findings suggesting that only nursing homes facing greater competition improved their quality or that nursing homes only improved quality along the reported dimension (Grabowski & Town, 2011; Lu, 2016).

A few studies evaluated nursing home responses to the five-star ratings. Some found that nursing homes improved quality scores after the release of the ratings (Konetzka, Grabowski, et al., 2015; Werner et al., 2016), including a CMS report that found large improvements in reported quality (2014). Other studies found price responses to ratings. The rationale is that better-rated nursing homes could respond to ratings by increasing private-payer prices. Huang and Hirth (2016) found that star ratings increased the price differential between high- and low-ranked facilities. They reported that high-ranked nursing homes increased prices by 4.8% to 6.0% more than the increase in prices by low-rated facilities. In the same way, a study found that nursing homes with higher ratings experienced higher profit margins due in part to increasing occupancy and the share of Medicare days (Park & Werner, 2011).

In summary, both consumers and nursing homes appear to respond to public reporting of information, especially to the simplified five-star ratings (Konetzka et al., 2021). The response is heterogeneous, with better-rated nursing homes and nursing homes in more competitive areas experiencing larger changes. In the same way, not all patients appear to use ratings when making decisions related to nursing homes. These findings highlight the possible unintended consequences of public reporting.

UNINTENDED CONSEQUENCES

Although the rationale of public reporting suggests that consumers benefit from more information, studies of report cards in other healthcare sectors prompted concerns about unintended consequences. For example, evidence from report cards of cardiac surgery outcomes in New York and Pennsylvania in the 1990s suggested that report cards led to the selection of healthier patients to improve ratings (Dranove et al., 2003). Following Konetzka et al. (2021), we group unintended consequences into four categories: increasing access disparities, selection of patients to improve ratings, improving only measured quality, and manipulating or gaming ratings.

If consumers can choose nursing homes based on quality ratings, public reporting could lead to better outcomes for most patients. However, higher-rated nursing homes are restricted by the availability of beds, especially for Medicaid-covered patients, and these facilities may not be available in all geographic areas (He & Konetzka, 2015). Furthermore, a possible outcome of public reporting is that patients who are more affluent, educated, not racial and ethnic minorities, and living in areas with more choices will benefit more from public reporting, possibly "crowding out" other patients (He & Konetzka, 2015). Thus, public reporting has the potential to exacerbate disparities in the access to higher-quality nursing homes. These concerns have been corroborated by studies showing that comprehension of ratings is lower by racial and ethnic minorities. Furthermore, a larger concentration of Medicare and Medicaid (duals) patients receive care in lower-rated nursing homes, with distance to higher-rated facilities, income, and education explaining a large portion of the difference (Castle, 2009a, 2009b; Konetzka, Brauner, et al., 2015; Sharma et al., 2020).

Another concern is that nursing homes may increase their ratings by selecting patients who are healthier and less likely to hurt ratings since some of the information reported does not have extensive risk adjustment. However, this strategy may be difficult to implement, and its legal validity is questionable. Evidence suggests that most nursing homes do not consider ratings when admitting patients, with concerns about litigation and the match of patient and nursing home being more salient (Perraillon, Brauner, & Konetzka, 2019). At the same time, it is challenging to evaluate this strategy using observational data because there is no information available to determine the precise reason for admission to a nursing home or to detect patients who were not admitted to a facility. Nonetheless, a study found that postacute patients were more likely to be hospitalized just before reaching the number of days required for inclusion in the reported quality measures. This was likely done to avoid negatively affecting the nursing home's ratings (Konetzka et al., 2013). However, this strategy is no longer effective because hospital readmission rates are now included in public report cards (Table 6.1). Additionally, another study found changes in the admission of patients with pain or memory limitations following the 2002 launch of NHC, further supporting concerns about selective admissions (Mukamel et al., 2009). Overall, evidence on patient selection remains limited, possibly due to the difficulty in empirically evaluating this practice.

Nursing homes seeking to improve their ratings to attract more patients may need to make trade-offs to efficiently use resources. One way to do this is by concentrating efforts on the areas that are measured by ratings. This response is often called "teaching to test" in allusion to the response by educators to standardized testing: teaching what is tested to the detriment of other relevant content. Considerable research supports this concern, in part because it is possible to evaluate empirically by comparing the evolution of quality metrics that are reported to those that are not reported by the CMS (Feng, 2012; Werner, Konetzka, & Kruse, 2009; Werner, Konetzka, Stuart, et al., 2009). Surveys of nursing home administrators also found that after the initial release of NHCC, nursing homes prioritize their efforts into areas that would improve reported quality metrics (Mukamel et al., 2007). Another study found that nursing homes changed the ratio of clinical to "hotel" expenditures (increased by 5% following the 2002 report cards publication), especially among nursing homes with initial lower quality that faced more competition. Hotel expenditures refer to services such as room and board, social services, and other services that affect life in nursing homes and are important considerations when choosing a nursing home (Mukamel et al., 2010).

Finally, given the potential financial benefit of high ratings, there have always been concerns about facilities manipulating or "gaming" the system by falsifying data or using strategies that improve ratings without improving quality (Perraillon, Brauner, & Konetzka, 2019). Two developments supported this concern. First, two press reports published by the *New York Times* in 2014 and 2015 argued that nursing homes were manipulating their ratings by providing false self-reported data (Thomas, 2014, 2015). In the initial release of the five-star system, only the health inspection domain relied on more objective data from nursing home inspections, while the staffing and quality measures were largely based on unverified self-reported information. The articles highlighted cases in which consumers felt deceived by the ratings, receiving care in highly rated facilities that nonetheless had previous violations and other quality problems.

The second development was that over time most nursing homes in the country ended up receiving a high number of stars in the staffing and quality domains. As we discussed in the section detailing the construction of ratings, cutoff points in the staffing and quality domains were held constant for many years, which meant that there was no mechanism to prevent most nursing homes in a state from receiving four or five stars. In the health inspection domain, only the top 10% of nursing homes could receive five stars. Either by deception or by making real improvements in measured quality, most nursing homes in the country became top-rated in two of the three rating domains (Thomas, 2014). Therefore, at least in the staffing and quality measures domain, the star system lost its information value. Consumers were not able to separate nursing homes by quality as measured by those two domains.

As with other unintended consequences, it has been difficult to ascertain the extent to which nursing homes engage in gaming of the ratings. Most of the evidence is indirect. For example, a study found that despite dramatic improvements in the staffing ratings there were no corresponding improvements in the staffing expenditures (as captured in cost reports) after the release of the five-star ratings (Sharma et al., 2019). Other studies found weak associations between process measures and health outcomes captured by public reporting (Han et al., 2016), and weak associations between preventable hospitalizations for postacute patients after the five-star ratings were published (Werner et al., 2013). Qualitative evidence also supports the gaming of the ratings. One study found that strategies to improve ratings included timing assessments that are part of ratings in such a way that they would not be counted because of rules about look-back windows or asking about pain levels only after administering pain medications (Perraillon, Brauner, & Konetzka, 2019). Although it is not possible to evaluate how widespread the use of these strategies may be, some nursing homes deem ratings as a key metric of success, which highlights the incentives to improve ratings (Perraillon, Brauner, & Konetzka, 2019).

The press reports and other evidence prompted the CMS to change the design of ratings. In 2018, the CMS replaced self-reported staffing data with data collected electronically through the Payroll-Based Journal, which can help ensure that staffing information is more objective. It also changed the staffing thresholds, with the consequence that fewer nursing homes could receive high ratings in the staffing domain. Similar changes were subsequently applied to quality measures (Figure 6.1).

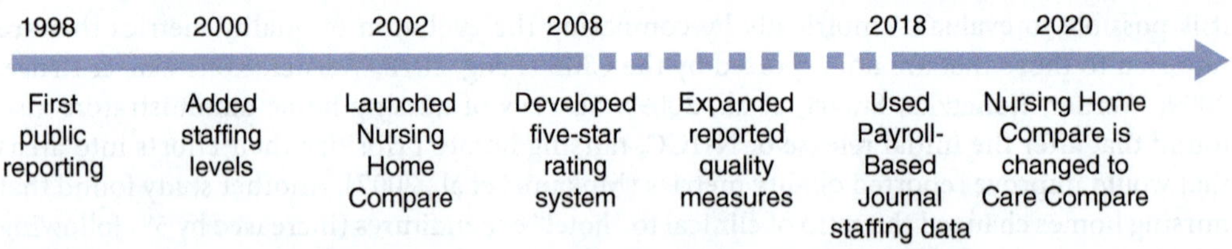

FIGURE 6.1. Timeline of major changes to Nursing Home Care Compare.

Note: From 2009 to 2023, the algorithm to construct the five-star ratings has been constantly revised. The figure depicts the most significant changes.

DO RATINGS REFLECT QUALITY?

When discussing consumer and nursing home responses to the publication of quality measures and five-star composite ratings, it is not necessary to evaluate if report cards accurately reflected care quality. Determining if consumers and nursing homes react to ratings only evaluates the premises underlying public reporting. However, as the discussion of unintended consequences emphasizes, it is consequential to ascertain whether reported information does reflect in some way quality, even if imperfectly. Since evidence suggests that nursing homes attempt to improve measured quality, it follows that a rating system that accurately measures quality would accomplish the stated goals of public reporting, notwithstanding other unintended consequences.

There is circumstantial evidence that the five-star system does reflect some aspects of quality, at least initially. For example, the characteristics of nursing homes that are lower-rated are correlated with other factors known to affect the quality of care, like the proportion of Medicaid patients in a nursing home (indicating lower resources given low Medicaid reimbursements), the location of the nursing home, the size of the nursing home, profit status, and chain status, among others (Perraillon, Konetzka, et al., 2019). On the other hand, studies have found a low correlation between reported measures and quality of life and family satisfaction (Çalıkoğlu et al., 2012; Kim et al., 2014; A. Williams et al., 2016). Another area of inquiry has been the limited risk adjustment in some of the measures, which emphasize a problematic aspect of nursing home ratings and a common complaint of administrators (Perraillon, Brauner, & Konetzka, 2019). Nursing homes that accept the most challenging patients to care for could be nursing homes that receive poor ratings.

Concerns about nursing home ratings not accurately reflecting the quality of care has prompted the CMS to continuously revise the methodology to construct the ratings. Most of the research has concentrated on examining problems and limitations of the current ratings, but more research is needed to devise novel ways of evaluating the quality of care in the medical sector, not just the nursing home sector.

SUMMARY

This chapter has described the evolution of public reporting in nursing homes, from a website that published information on individual quality measures to a website that publishes composite five-star ratings. The intent of nursing home ratings is to allow consumers to evaluate the quality of nursing home care before choosing a facility. Research evaluating the initial release of NHC was somewhat inconclusive, possibly because the information provided was difficult for consumers to understand, and evidence suggested that NHC was not extensively used. However, more recent evidence on the five-star ratings indicates that some consumers do rely on these ratings to select high-quality nursing homes, and some facilities have indeed invested in quality improvement.

Despite the progress made in public reporting, several unintended consequences limit its effectiveness, particularly regarding equitable access to high-quality nursing homes. For instance, public reporting may unintentionally widen disparities because some facilities manipulate their ratings, making it harder for consumers to distinguish between genuinely high-quality homes and those that appear so due to inflated scores. Additionally, the high number of facilities with top ratings dilutes the meaning of staffing and quality metrics, as most nursing homes receive high ratings even without substantial improvements. This trend can mislead families and patients, making it difficult to assess true quality. These issues underscore the need for ongoing evaluation and refinement of the rating system. Future research should focus on creating measurement tools that accurately reflect quality, particularly those that account for patient case-mix and residents' experiences in nursing homes (Bär et al., 2022). As the population ages, accurate and meaningful nursing home ratings will become increasingly essential.

Take-Home Points

- Quality of care concerns have always been a salient problem in nursing homes.
- Data collection in nursing homes related to patients' initial status and changes made it possible to create public reporting measures related to quality in nursing homes (NHCC).
- To facilitate comprehension of report cards, simplified, compositive five-star ratings were created.
- Not all residents and families use NHCC, and there are concerns about unintended consequences and manipulation of ratings.
- The ratings continue to evolve, with several changes made to ensure more objective information is being used in the ratings, but more research is needed on better ways to measure quality.

END-OF-CHAPTER RESOURCES

DISCUSSION QUESTIONS

1. Is it fair for nursing homes to be evaluated using some metrics that are not adjusted for resident mix?
2. Are nursing home ratings useful if many patients do not have a choice given that poorer areas tend to not have highly rated nursing homes and patients relying on Medicaid have fewer opportunities to choose a nursing home?
3. Should NHCC restrict the number of nursing homes that can achieve a high rating in the overall number of stars?
4. Should the ratings be updated regularly to prevent manipulation of ratings?
5. Should the CMS promote the use of ratings and design ratings that permit a causal evaluation of their impact?
6. How could NHCC be redesigned to better reflect the quality of care?

SPRINGER PUBLISHING CONNECT™ A robust set of instructor resources designed to supplement this text is located at http://connect.springerpub.com/content/book/978-0-8261-4935-0. Qualifying instructors may request access by emailing textbook@springerpub.com.

REFERENCES

Bär, M., Bakx, P., Wouterse, B., & van Doorslaer, E. (2022). Estimating the health value added by nursing homes. *Journal of Economic Behavior & Organization*, *203*, 1–23. https://doi.org/10.1016/j.jebo.2022.08.028

Çalıkoğlu, Ş., Christmyer, C. S., & Kozlowski, B. U. (2012). My eyes, your eyes—The relationship between CMS five-star rating of nursing homes and family rating of experience of care in Maryland. *Journal for Healthcare Quality*, *34*(6), 5–12. https://doi.org/10.1111/j.1945-1474.2011.00159.x

Castle, N. G. (2009a). Consumers' use of internet-based nursing home report cards. *The Joint Commission Journal on Quality and Patient Safety, 35*(6), 316–323. https://doi.org/10.1016/s1553-7250(09)35045-x

Castle, N. G. (2009b). The Nursing Home Compare report card: Consumers' use and understanding. *Journal of Aging & Social Policy, 21*(2), 187–208. https://doi.org/10.1080/08959420902733272

Castle, N. G., & Engberg, J. (2010). An examination of special focus facility nursing homes. *The Gerontologist, 50*(3), 400–407. https://doi.org/10.1093/geront/gnq008

Castle, N. G., Engberg, J., & Liu, D. (2007). Have Nursing Home Compare quality measure scores changed over time in response to competition? *BMJ Quality & Safety, 16*(3), 185–191. https://doi.org/10.1136/qshc.2005.016923

Castle, N. G., & Ferguson, J. C. (2010). What is nursing home quality and how is it measured? *The Gerontologist, 50*(4), 426–442. https://doi.org/10.1093/geront/gnq052

Castle, N. G., Liu, D., & Engberg, J. (2008). The association of Nursing Home Compare quality measures with market competition and occupancy rates. *Journal for Healthcare Quality, 30*(2), 4–14. https://doi.org/10.1111/j.1945-1474.2008.tb01129.x

Centers for Medicare & Medicaid Services. (2008, December 18). *Improving the Nursing Home Compare web site: The Five-Star nursing home quality rating system* (Vol. I). https://www.cms.gov/files/document/qsandasfinalpdf

Centers for Medicare & Medicaid Services. (2014, June 16). *Nursing Home Compare five-star quality rating system: Year five report*. https://www.cms.gov/Medicare/Provider-Enrollment-and-Certification/CertificationandComplianc/Downloads/NHC-Year-Five-Report.pdf

Centers for Medicare & Medicaid Services. (2024). *Design for Care Compare nursing home five-star quality rating system: Technical users' guide*. http://www.cms.gov/Medicare/Provider-Enrollment-and-Certification/CertificationandComplianc/downloads/usersguide.pdf

Chen, Z., Gleason, L. J., Konetzka, R. T., & Sanghavi, P. (2023). Accuracy of infection reporting in US nursing home ratings. *Health Services Research, 58*(5), 1109–1118. https://doi.org/10.1111/1475-6773.14195

Dranove, D., Kessler, D., McClellan, M., & Satterthwaite, M. (2003). Is more information better? The effects of "report cards" on health care providers. *Journal of Political Economy, 111*(3), 555–588. https://doi.org/10.1086/374180

Feng, L. S. (2012). Multitasking, information disclosure, and product quality: Evidence from nursing homes. *Journal of Economics & Management Strategy, 21*(3), 673–705. https://doi.org/10.1111/j.1530-9134.2012.00341.x

Grabowski, D. C., & Town, R. J. (2011). Does information matter? Competition, quality, and the impact of nursing home report cards. *Health Services Research, 46*(6 Pt. 1), 1698–1719. https://doi.org/10.1111/j.1475-6773.2011.01298.x

Han, X., Yaraghi, N., & Gopal, R. (2016). *Five-star ratings for sub-par service: Evidence of inflation in nursing home ratings* [Report]. Governance Studies at Brookings. https://www.brookings.edu/wp-content/uploads/2016/12/gs_20161213_nursing-homes.pdf

He, D., & Konetzka, R. T. (2015). Public reporting and demand rationing: Evidence from the nursing home industry. *Health Economics, 24*(11), 1437–1451. https://doi.org/10.1002/hec.3097

Huang, S. S., & Hirth, R. A. (2016). Quality rating and private-prices: Evidence from the nursing home industry. *Journal of Health Economics, 50*, 59–70. https://doi.org/10.1016/j.jhealeco.2016.08.007

Institute of Medicine. (1986). *Improving the quality of care in nursing homes*. National Academies Press. https://www.ncbi.nlm.nih.gov/books/NBK217556

Kim, S. J., Park, E.-C., Kim, S., Nakagawa, S., Lung, J., Choi, J. B., Ryu, W. S., Min, T. J., Shin, H. P., Kim, K., & Yoo, J. W. (2014). The association between quality of care and quality of life in long-stay nursing home residents with preserved cognition. *Journal of the American Medical Directors Association, 15*(3), 220–225. https://doi.org/10.1016/j.jamda.2013.10.012

Kissam, S., Gifford, D., Parks, P., Patry, G., Palmer, L., Wilkes, L., Fitzgerald, M., Petrulis, A. S., & Barnette, L. (2003). Approaches to quality improvement in nursing homes: lessons learned from the six-state pilot of CMS's Nursing Home Quality Initiative. *BMC Geriatrics, 3*, 2. https://doi.org/10.1186/1471-2318-3-2

Konetzka, R. T., Brauner, D. J., Coca Perraillon, M., & Werner, R. M. (2015). The role of severe dementia in nursing home report cards. *Medical Care Research and Review, 72*(5), 562–579. https://doi.org/10.1177/1077558715588436

Konetzka, R. T., Grabowski, D. C., Perraillon, M. C., & Werner, R. M. (2015). Nursing home 5-star rating system exacerbates disparities in quality, by payer source. *Health Affairs*, *34*(5), 819–827. https://doi.org/10.1377/hlthaff.2014.1084

Konetzka, R. T., Polsky, D., & Werner, R. M. (2013). Shipping out instead of shaping up: Rehospitalization from nursing homes as an unintended effect of public reporting. *Journal of Health Economics*, *32*(2), 341–352. https://doi.org/10.1016/j.jhealeco.2012.11.008

Konetzka, R. T., Yan, K., & Werner, R. M. (2021). Two decades of Nursing Home Compare: What have we learned? Review. *Medical Care Research and Review*, *78*(4), 295–310. https://doi.org/10.1177/1077558720931652

Kramer, A. F. (2001). Appropriateness of minimum nurse staffing ratios in nursing homes report. *The Relationship Between Nurse Staffing Levels and the Quality of Nursing Home Care, Report to Congress, Phase 2*. 1–26. https://www.phinational.org/wp-content/uploads/2017/07/Phase_I_VOL_I-1.pdf

Lu, S. F. (2016). The role of donations in quality disclosure: Evidence from nonprofit nursing homes. *American Journal of Health Economics*, *2*(4), 431–462. https://doi.org/10.2139/ssrn.1956689

Mor, V. (2005). Improving the quality of long-term care with better information. *The Milbank Quarterly*, *83*(3), 333–364. https://doi.org/10.1111/j.1468-0009.2005.00405.x

Mor, V., Zinn, J., Angelelli, J., Teno, J. M., & Miller, S. C. (2004). Driven to tiers: Socioeconomic and racial disparities in the quality of nursing home care. *Milbank Quarterly*, *82*(2), 227–256. https://doi.org/10.1111/j.0887-378X.2004.00309.x

Mukamel, D. B., Ladd, H., Weimer, D. L., Spector, W. D, & Zinn, J. S. (2009). Is there evidence of cream skimming among nursing homes following the publication of the Nursing Home Compare report card? *The Gerontologist*, *49*(6), 793–802. https://doi.org/10.1093/geront/gnp062

Mukamel, D. B., Spector, W. D., Zinn, J. S., Huang, L., Weimer, D. L., & Dozier, A. (2007). Nursing homes' response to the Nursing Home Compare report card. *The Journals of Gerontology. Series B, Psychological Sciences and Social Sciences*, *62*(4), S218–S225. https://doi.org/10.1093/geronb/62.4.s218

Mukamel, D. B., Spector, W. D., Zinn, J. S., Weimer, D. L., & Ahn, R. (2010). Changes in clinical and hotel expenditures following publication of the Nursing Home Compare report card. *Medical Care*, *48*(10), 869–874. https://doi.org/10.1097/MLR.0b013e3181eaf6e1

Mukamel, D. B., Weimer, D. L., Spector, W. D., Ladd, H., & Zinn, J. S. (2008). Publication of quality report cards and trends in reported quality measures in nursing homes. *Health Services Research*, *43*(4), 1244–1262. https://doi.org/10.1111/j.1475-6773.2007.00829.x

National Center for Health Statistics. (2004). *National Nursing Home Survey*. https://www.cdc.gov/nchs/nnhs/index.htm

Park, J., & Werner, R. M. (2011). Changes in the relationship between nursing home financial performance and quality of care under public reporting. *Health Economics*, *20*(7), 783–801. https://doi.org/10.1002/hec.1632

Perraillon, M. C., Brauner, D. J., & Konetzka, R. T. (2019). Nursing home response to Nursing Home Compare: The provider perspective. *Medical Care Research and Review*, *76*(4), 425–443. https://doi.org/10.1177/1077558717725165

Perraillon, M. C., Konetzka, R. T., He, D., & Werner, R. M. (2019). Consumer response to composite ratings of nursing home quality. *American Journal of Health Economics*, *5*(2), 165–190. https://doi.org/10.1162/ajhe_a_00115

Sanghavi, P., & Chen, Z. (2023). Underreporting of quality measures and associated facility characteristics and racial cisparities in US nursing home ratings. *JAMA Network Open*, *6*(5), e2314822. https://doi.org/10.1001/jamanetworkopen.2023.14822

Sharma, H., Konetzka, R. T., & Smieliauskas, F. (2019). The relationship between reported staffing and expenditures in nursing homes. *Medical Care Research and Review*, *76*(6), 758–783. https://doi.org/10.1177/1077558717739214

Sharma, H., Perraillon, M. C., Werner, R. M., Grabowski, D. C., & Konetzka, R. T. (2020). Medicaid and nursing home choice: Why do duals end up in low-quality facilities? *Journal of Applied Gerontology*, *39*(9), 981–990. https://doi.org/10.1177/0733464819838447

Thomas, K. (2014, August 24). Medicare star ratings allow nursing homes to game the system. *New York Times*. https://www.nytimes.com/2014/08/25/business/medicare-star-ratings-allow-nursing-homes-to-game-the-system.html

Thomas, K. (2015, April 14). In race for Medicare dollars, nursing home care may lag. *New York Times*. https://www.nytimes.com/2015/04/15/business/as-nursing-homes-chase-lucrative-patients-quality-of-care-is-said-to-lag.html

Werner, R. M., Konetzka, R. T., & Kim, M. M. (2013). Quality improvement under Nursing Home Compare: The association between changes in process and outcome measures. *Medical Care*, *51*(7), 582–588. https://doi.org/10.1097/MLR.0b013e31828dbae4

Werner, R. M., Konetzka, R. T., & Kruse, G. B. (2009). Impact of public reporting on unreported quality of care. *Health Services Research*, *4*(2 Pt. 1), 379–398. https://doi.org/10.1111/j.1475-6773.2008.00915.x

Werner, R. M., Konetzka, R. T., & Polsky, D. (2016). Changes in consumer demand following public reporting of summary quality ratings: An evaluation in nursing homes. *Health Services Research*, *51*(Suppl. 2), 1291–1309. https://doi.org/10.1111/1475-6773.12459

Werner, R. M., Konetzka, R. T., Stuart, E. A., Norton, E. C., Polsky, D., & Park, J. (2009). Impact of public reporting on quality of postacute care. *Health Services Research*, *44*(4), 1169–1187. https://doi.org/10.1111/j.1475-6773.2009.00967.x

Werner, R. M., Norton, E. C., Konetzka, R. T., & Polsky, D. (2012). Do consumers respond to publicly reported quality information? Evidence from nursing homes. *Journal of Health Economics*, *31*(1), 50–61. https://doi.org/10.1016/j.jhealeco.2012.01.001

Williams, A., Straker, J. K., & Applebaum, R. (2016). The nursing home five star rating: How does it compare to resident and family views of care? *The Gerontologist*, *56*(2), 234–242. https://doi.org/10.1093/geront/gnu043

Williams, C., Hadden, L., Mortimore, E., Nagy, F., Plotzke, M., & White, A. (2010). *Measuring nursing home quality—The five-star rating system*. http://support.sas.com/resources/papers/proceedings10/161-2010.pdf

Winter, J. D., Kerns, J. W., Winter, K. M., & Etz, R. (2022). Public Quality Reporting and Nursing Home Admission Decisions. *Journal of the American Medical Directors Association, 23*(12), 2035–2037. https://doi.org/10.1016/j.jamda.2022.08.017

Xu, H., Intrator, O., Culakova, E., & Bowblis, J. R. (2022). Changing landscape of nursing homes serving residents with dementia and mental illnesses. *Health Services Research*, *57*(3), 505–514. https://doi.org/10.1111/1475-6773.13908

CHAPTER 7

MANAGING RECRUITMENT, RETENTION, AND TURNOVER IN LONG-TERM CARE FOR IMPROVED QUALITY AND SUSTAINABILITY

April Temple

Learning Objectives

After completing this chapter, each learner will be able to:

- Understand the critical importance of a stable, qualified workforce to provide high-quality care in long-term care (LTC).
- Review the current state of the LTC workforce.
- Describe the relationship between nursing staff turnover and quality of care in LTC facilities.
- Identify factors that impact recruitment and retention in LTC.
- Discuss policy and practice recommendations to improve staff recruitment and retention in LTC.

INTRODUCTION

Demand for long-term care (LTC) across the continuum of care is increasing rapidly with the aging of the U.S. population. The number of older adults needing LTC is expected to more than double from 6.3 million in 2015 to 15 million by 2050 (National Academy of Social Insurance, n.d.). At the same time, the availability of and reliance on family caregivers to meet this need is projected to decline (Schulz & Eden, 2016). Consequently, there will be a greater reliance than ever before on the LTC industry to fill this gap.

LTC providers rely primarily on nurses and other direct care staff to fulfill their mission to provide quality care to those they serve. Yet, the LTC sector faces persistent staffing challenges compared to other healthcare sectors. The industry has a long-standing history of staffing shortages and high turnover rates, issues that have been further exacerbated by the COVID-19 pandemic. Why is this the case, and what can be done about it? To answer these questions, a growing body of evidence yields recommendations for both policy and practice.

With the increasing demand for LTC coupled with a looming workforce crisis, immediate attention must be given to the critical role of qualified and sufficient staffing in the delivery of high-quality LTC. This chapter will provide an overview of the LTC workforce and its role in the provision of quality care, current and future challenges related to staffing, and evidence-based strategies to improve recruitment and retention. Although a large focus of this chapter will be on staffing in nursing homes, a broad overview of LTC workforce issues will be presented with application across the LTC continuum. This chapter is of particular relevance to all who will lead and manage staff in LTC settings.

LONG-TERM CARE WORKFORCE OVERVIEW

Distribution and Characteristics of the Workforce

The provision of quality care in LTC settings is highly dependent on a well-qualified, stable workforce. The LTC workforce includes a variety of professionals and paraprofessionals who provide for the daily care needs of individuals across a variety of settings including home and community-based services, residential care/assisted living facilities, and skilled nursing facilities (SNFs). As presented in Figure 7.1, a majority of the LTC workforce members in the United States are employed in institutional settings such as SNFs (42%) and assisted living (25%). The remainder (33%) work in the home health sector.

The industry heavily relies on nursing staff, including RNs, LPNs, and licensed vocational nurses (LVNs), as well as direct care workers. Direct care workers assist older adults and individuals with disabilities with personal care and tasks of daily living; job titles vary by setting and include certified nursing assistants (CNAs) or nurse aides, personal care aides, and home health aides. As seen in Figure 7.1, the majority (53%) of the LTC workforce members are comprised of these direct care workers. This is followed by direct contact support workers (16%) in nonclinical areas such as housekeeping, laundry, and food service, and healthcare providers (14%) including licensed nurses, physicians or

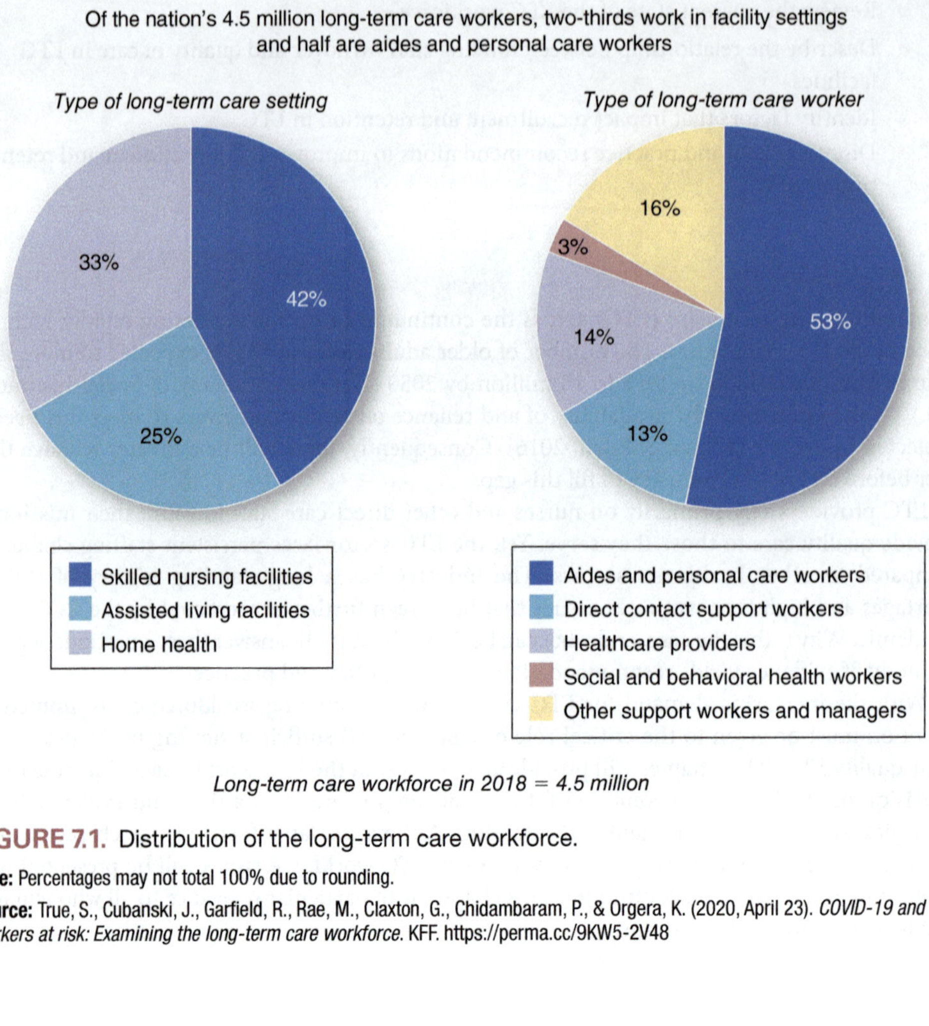

FIGURE 7.1. Distribution of the long-term care workforce.

Note: Percentages may not total 100% due to rounding.

Source: True, S., Cubanski, J., Garfield, R., Rae, M., Claxton, G., Chidambaram, P., & Orgera, K. (2020, April 23). *COVID-19 and workers at risk: Examining the long-term care workforce.* KFF. https://perma.cc/9KW5-2V48

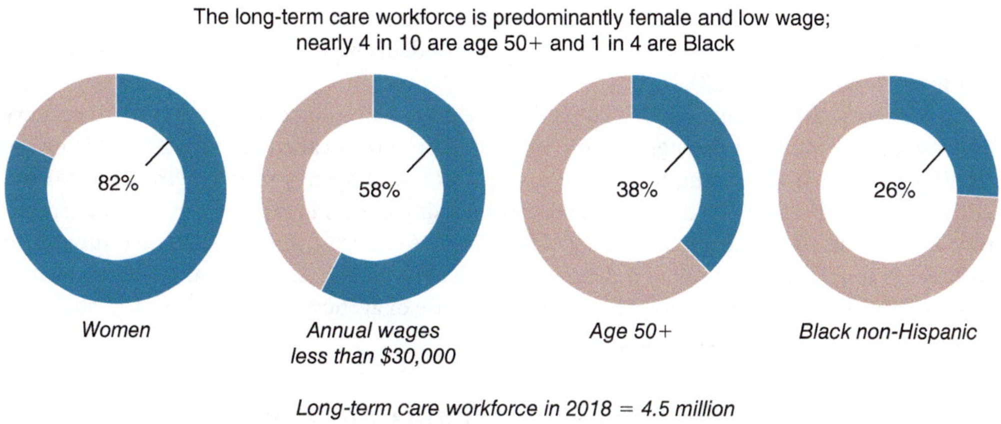

FIGURE 7.2. Characteristics of the long-term care workforce.

Source: True, S., Cubanski, J., Garfield, R., Rae, M., Claxton, G., Chidambaram, P., & Orgera, K. (2020, April 23). *COVID-19 and workers at risk: Examining the long-term care workforce.* KFF. https://perma.cc/9KW5-2V48

nonphysician practitioners, and therapists. Across all staff categories, aides provide the most "hands-on" direct hours of care on a daily basis (Centers for Disease Control and Prevention [CDC], 2018).

Figure 7.2 presents a snapshot of key characteristics of the LTC workforce. Overall, this workforce is predominantly female, racially diverse, and low paid. The majority (58%) earn annual wages below $30,000, and nearly one-third live in low-income families. The workforce itself is aging, with 38% of workers over the age of 50. Data from this source also indicates a large share of both aides (48%) and personal care workers (60%) have a high school education or less (True et al., 2020). Additionally, immigrant workers born outside the United States comprise one in four direct care workers in LTC (Campbell et al., 2021).

A Workforce in Demand

According to the U.S. Bureau of Labor Statistics (Dubina et al., 2022), there is a growing demand across job categories in LTC created by the aging of the population, the resulting increase in chronic conditions and disabilities, and the declining availability of family caregivers. The greatest job growth, however, is occurring in the direct care workforce. In particular, consumer preference and policies supporting home- and community-based services is contributing to the fastest growth among home health and personal aides. Home health and personal aides are projected to increase by 25%, from 3.6 million jobs in 2021 to 4.6 million in 2031 (Dubina et al., 2022). Although the overall demand for nursing home care is declining, an estimated 38% of all nursing home job openings will be for nursing assistants in the next decade (Paraprofessional Health Institute, 2022).

Despite these projections, meeting the demand for LTC workers will be difficult in light of persistent staffing challenges that have plagued the LTC sector and have continued to worsen since the start of the COVID-19 pandemic. Nursing homes face unprecedented labor supply shortages, particularly for nurses and aides (McGarry et al., 2020; Ochieng et al., 2022). During the height of the pandemic, the nursing home industry lost 15% of its total workforce and still has not fully recovered to prepandemic levels (American Health Care Association [AHCA] & National Center for Assisted Living [NCAL], 2022). In a survey of more than 500 nursing home providers in early 2023, the vast majority (84%) reported they are facing significant staffing shortages and difficulty in hiring (AHCA & NCAL, 2023). A similar story is found in assisted living, where a recent poll by LeadingAge found 70% of assisted living respondents report significant or severe staffing shortages (LeadingAge, 2023).

To address staffing shortages, LTC organizations have had to increasingly rely on temporary or contract staff obtained through staffing agencies (commonly called agency staff). During the COVID-19 pandemic, nursing homes increased their use of agency staff by 24% from 2019 to 2020 (Porter et al., 2022). To date, the majority of nursing homes in 2023 reported using temporary agency staff to adjust for shortages (AHCA & NCAL, 2023). Agency staff are estimated to cost two to four times as much as a direct hire (AHCA & NCAL, 2021), contributing to a labor and economic crisis for providers. Moreover, greater use of agency staff has been correlated with poorer quality of care (Porter et al., 2022).

Turnover and Retention of the Long-Term Care Workforce

The discrepancy between the demand and supply of LTC workers is further compounded by high rates of turnover. *Turnover* refers to the number of staff who leave employment, either voluntarily or involuntarily, during a given period of time. Turnover rates across the LTC industry are consistently high but vary widely by occupation and setting. Most recently, the median annual turnover rate for total nursing staff was 94% across U.S. nursing homes, with some facilities experiencing turnover rates as high as 300% (Gandhi et al., 2021). Similarly, recent national surveys report the average annual turnover rate among home care, home health, and hospice workers at 77.1% (Home Care Pulse, 2023) and for assisted living staff at 42% (Hospital & Healthcare Compensation Service, 2023). These high turnover rates further add to the difficulty of achieving adequate staffing in LTC.

While most of the reported data focuses on turnover, staff retention is also a challenge in LTC. *Retention* refers to the number of employees who remain in their position during a given time period and is an additional measure of workforce stability. Retention does not necessarily have an inverse relationship with turnover; for example, LTC providers can experience both high rates of retention and high rates of turnover if turnover repeatedly occurs in select positions. Retention among direct care workers is often most challenging within the first few months of hire (Drake, 2020). Across U.S. nursing homes, one recent study found just above 50% of nurse aides were retained after 1 year (Castle et al., 2020). Similarly, another study of direct care workers across nursing homes and assisted living facilities found retention rates at the end of 1 year at 61% and 66%, respectively (Kennedy et al., 2021).

TURNOVER, RETENTION, AND QUALITY OF LONG-TERM CARE

High turnover and low staff retention have both direct and indirect costs for LTC organizations. It drives up operational costs for providers to recruit, hire, and train new employees as well as to pay overtime or agency staff in the interim. It also contributes to lower morale, lost productivity, and heightened stress and burnout among remaining staff to fill the vacancies. Furthermore, the presence of high LTC staff turnover threatens quality of care as it disrupts continuity of care when residents are regularly receiving care from staff who lack the experience and knowledge of their needs.

A large body of research has supported the link between nursing staff turnover and quality of care in nursing homes. For example, high nursing staff turnover has been associated with poorer performance on several quality measures in nursing homes such as physical restraint use and pressure ulcers (Castle & Engberg, 2005; Castle et al., 2007) as well as more deficiencies given during annual surveys (Lerner et al., 2014; Loomer et al., 2022). Nursing staff turnover has also been associated with higher rates of hospitalizations, hospital readmissions, and emergency department use among nursing home residents (Thomas et al., 2013; Zheng et al., 2022).

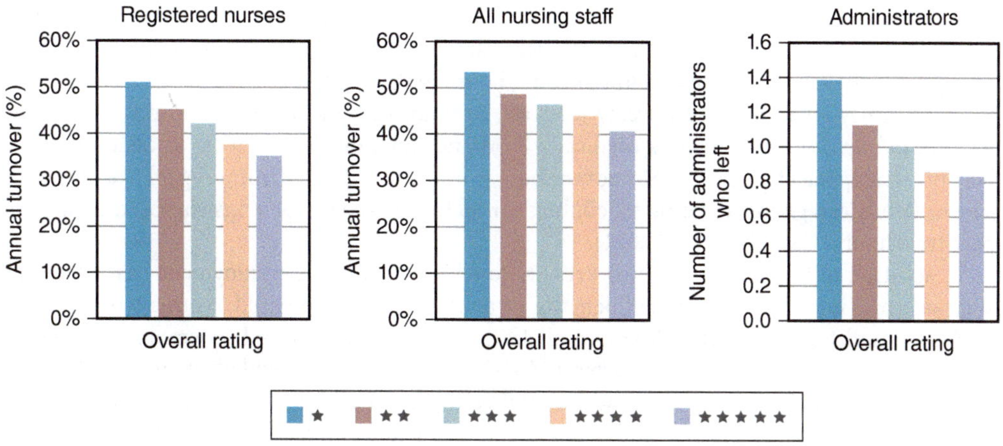

FIGURE 7.3. Nursing home staff turnover by the CMS Nursing Home Five-Star Quality Rating System.

CMS. Centers for Medicare & Medicaid Services

Source: Centers for Medicare & Medicaid Services. (2022, January 7). *Nursing home staff turnover and weekend staffing levels.* [Memorandum]. https://www.cms.gov/files/document/qso-22-08-nh.pdf

Staff retention is also important, as nursing homes with higher retention rates of nurse aides were found to have fewer deficiency citations (Castle et al., 2020).

Moreover, studies have found facilities with high staff turnover consistently receive lower star ratings on the quality metrics in the Nursing Home Five-Star Quality Rating System (Gandhi et al., 2021; Zheng et al., 2022). Given this evidence, the Centers for Medicare & Medicaid Services (CMS) recently began reporting staff turnover measures for the first time on its Care Compare website beginning in January 2022. These measures include percent of all nursing staff (RNs, LPNs, and nurse aides) and percent of RN staff who left as well as the number of administrators who left the nursing facility over the past 12-month period. Initial analyses by the CMS found nursing home staff turnover rates decrease as star ratings increase, suggesting that lower turnover is associated with higher quality of care (Figure 7.3; CMS, 2022). These turnover measures supplement existing staffing data in the Nursing Home Five-Star Quality Rating System and are intended to encourage providers to strengthen staffing and to inform consumer decision-making.

FACTORS IMPACTING RECRUITMENT AND RETENTION IN LONG-TERM CARE

Inadequate Wages and Benefits

The challenge of meeting both current and future demand for LTC workers begins with inadequate compensation. LTC workers at all skill levels earn significantly lower wages compared to their counterparts in other healthcare sectors (Muench et al., 2021). National estimates indicate RNs in nursing homes earn over $10,000 less than the mean annual wage for all RNs (U.S. Bureau of Labor Statistics, 2023). Compensation for direct care workers is particularly low, often around the minimum wage. For example, the median hourly wage in 2021 for all direct care workers was only $14.27 (Paraprofessional Health Institute, 2022). A recent analysis also found that direct care workers in most states earn less than workers in other entry-level jobs such as retail and hospitality (Khavjou et al., 2023).

Furthermore, these low wages contribute to higher poverty rates among LTC workers. One study found the poverty rate for direct care workers to be 10.4%, which is almost twice the average for all U.S. workers (Hickey et al., 2022). Similarly, the Paraprofessional Health Institute (Campbell et al., 2021) found that 15% of direct care workers live below the federal poverty level while 44% are estimated to live in low-income households, defined as living below 200% of the federal poverty level. Because poverty rates are so high, 42% of direct care workers use some form of public assistance such as Medicaid, food and nutritional assistance, or cash assistance benefits (Campbell et al., 2021). Moreover, these workers face difficulty finding affordable child-care or family caregiving, creating scheduling conflicts that impact earnings via absenteeism and part-time hours (Campbell et al., 2021).

In addition to low wages, LTC workers are less likely to receive employment-based benefits such as health insurance, retirement benefits, or paid sick leave compared to other workers. One analysis found less than half (45.4%) of all LTC workers were covered by employer-provided health insurance and only one-quarter (24.7%) had employer-provided retirement benefits (Hickey et al., 2022). Coverage rates were significantly lower among direct care workers (38.9% and 18.9%, respectively; Hickey et al., 2022). A national survey from 2020, during the height of the pandemic, found that 65% of nursing home workers indicated they did not have paid sick days (Service Employees International Union [SEIU], 2020). Additionally, many of these workers lack paid family and medical leave (Campbell et al., 2021).

Limited Training and Career Advancement

The amount of education and training currently required of direct care workers is often cited as inadequate preparation to meet the responsibilities of caring for residents with increasingly complex needs (Institute of Medicine [IOM], 2008). In nursing homes, federal regulations dating back to the Omnibus Budget Reconciliation Act of 1987 require CNAs to have a minimum of 75 hours of training, pass a competency exam, and complete 12 hours of continuing education annually (Requirements for Long Term Care Facilities, 2024). Although some states require more training, most fall short of a national recommendation of at least 120 hours of training for CNAs (IOM, 2008). Standards of training of personal care and home health aides vary by state but are generally even less than that required of CNAs (Campbell et al., 2021; Stone & Bryant, 2019).

Moreover, limited opportunities for career advancement for direct care workers contributes to poor job quality and limits earning potential. Formal career advancement opportunities have been limited to attaining additional certification (e.g., medication aide) or nursing licensure (e.g., LPN or RN). These options are often not accessible due to the time and expense of additional education. Direct care workers consistently express the need for additional training and desire to gain new skills, and there is a need to develop meaningful growth opportunities within the direct care field that are accessible to these workers (Campbell et al., 2021).

Difficult Working Conditions

LTC workers face heavy workloads and difficult working conditions that contribute to high levels of stress, burnout, and job dissatisfaction. Nursing assistants, who provide the most hours of direct care, have an average staff-to-resident ratio of one nursing assistant per 13 nursing home residents (Paraprofessional Health Institute, 2022). Their care tasks are both physically and emotionally demanding. Due to the physical nature of the work, nursing assistants are eight times more likely to experience workplace-related injuries including back injuries, overexertion, slips or falls, and workplace illness such as COVID-19 (Paraprofessional Health Institute, 2022). They also experience higher rates of workplace assaults involving physical and verbal abuse, as well as racially charged abuse such as racial slurs and insults, particularly when caring for residents with dementia (Tak et al., 2010; Xiao et al., 2021). Furthermore, developing meaningful relationships and sustained engagement with individuals experiencing significant physical or cognitive impairments requires additional emotional labor that can contribute to stress and burnout over time (Campbell et al., 2021).

Lack of Recognition

The LTC industry is undervalued and underappreciated and this limits the attractiveness of working in LTC. In today's competitive healthcare environment, workers' perception of organizational attractiveness, or the perceived benefit or value that makes a place of employment desirable, has been shown to be important for recruitment and retention of nurses (Slatten et al., 2019; Van Hoye, 2008). Yet, there is a long-standing negative stigma and poor reputation surrounding LTC, which has been further diminished due to the demoralizing effects of the COVID-19 pandemic. Stigma contributes to recruitment challenges as healthcare professionals with negative perceptions of aged-care work are less willing to work in LTC institutions (Manchha et al., 2022). Further, the occupational stigma attributed to aged-care work has been shown to negatively impact worker outcomes including psychologic distress, job dissatisfaction, and intention to leave (Manchha et al., 2023).

Direct care workers, who are at the bottom of a typical organizational chart, often perceive their work is not valued or respected by the rest of the care team. Aides are often labeled as unskilled, which does not accurately reflect the important and complex tasks they perform (Osterman, 2018). They are also referred to as "just" a nursing assistant and often excluded from decision-making involving patient care. Moreover, since this workforce is primarily comprised of women and people of color, systemic racism and sexism in the United States compounds the undervaluing of this work (Campbell et al., 2021).

The Impact of COVID-19

The COVID-19 pandemic further exacerbated existing LTC workforce challenges and prominently highlighted long-standing issues related to staffing and quality of care (Case Study 7.1). As widely known, the pandemic took a substantial toll on those living and working in LTC institutions. Nursing home residents and staff had disproportionally higher rates of both COVID-19 infections and deaths (Ochieng et al., 2022), and nursing home workers had one of the highest death rates among all occupations during the pandemic (Lewis, 2021). Staff had to take on additional, and evolving, caregiving and infection control practices and often lacked adequate personal protective equipment and resources to provide quality care (McGarry et al., 2020). Staff experienced significant burnout due to staffing shortages, increased workloads, and the emotional burden of caring for their residents in pandemic conditions, adding to an already strained workforce (E. M. White et al., 2021).

Case Study 7.1 The Lesser of Two Evils

Carson is the executive director at Shady Maple, a nonprofit life plan community that includes a 60-bed SNF. Shady Maple has a strong reputation in the community for providing high-quality care and consistently maintains a high occupancy rate. It is also a reputable employer in the community, offering competitive wages and benefits for the local market, and as such has experienced relatively low nursing staff turnover.

Carson has been at Shady Maple for the past 7 years and led the organization through the COVID-19 pandemic. As with other LTC communities, Shady Maple struggled to maintain nurse staffing during the height of the pandemic. Initially, many front-line employees quit out of fear of contracting COVID-19 when little was known about the disease. Staffing shortages were further exacerbated when existing staff had to quarantine for exposure or tested positive for COVID-19. Several staff members also faced new demands at home, such as a lack of childcare, which impacted their availability to work.

(continued)

Case Study 7.1 The Lesser of Two Evils (*continued*)

To ensure adequate staffing to care for the residents, Carson and his department directors became increasingly flexible with staff scheduling policies to retain employees during the height of the pandemic. They worked diligently with staff members who needed to adjust the hours of their workday or reduce the number of their shifts to ensure staff continued to show up for work. Carson and his nurse scheduler began spending more time than ever before on the schedule. Nevertheless, Shady Maple's use of agency staff increased throughout the pandemic to meet staffing needs.

Now 3 years later, some normalcy has finally returned to operations. Carson is facing increasing pressure from the board to lessen the use of agency staff to reduce operating costs. Furthermore, nursing staff are growing increasingly frustrated with agency staff who aren't familiar with the building, organizational culture, or residents. Nurses complain they spend too much time orienting agency staff and lament agency staff don't have the same commitment to the residents or the rest of the team.

Carson sits down to review the nursing staff schedule to see where he can cut back on agency staffing. He finds that agency staff are regularly being used to fill shifts that are not being covered due to the flexible scheduling policies implemented during the pandemic. He has several staff who dropped from a 40-hour to 32-hour work week, leaving a hodgepodge of open 8-hour shifts to fill with agency staff.

One example is Maggie, a full-time CNA who has been at Shady Maple for 5 years and worked throughout the COVID-19 pandemic. She is a valued team member and is beloved by the residents. She has two school age children who were home for virtual schooling during the early days of the pandemic, so flexibility was granted to allow Maggie to drop down to four, 8-hour shifts per week so that she could cover gaps in childcare at home. She has since continued this schedule and has expressed she does not want to return to five shifts per week.

Carson is torn on what to do next. He really needs Maggie to return to the full-time schedule she agreed upon when hired so that he doesn't have to rely on agency staff to fill her shifts. However, he worries if he mandates it, the organization will risk losing a dedicated employee. In this competitive labor market, Carson recognizes it would not be easy to fill a vacant CNA position. Alternatively, he could continue using agency staff for the foreseeable future to fill Maggie's shifts despite concerns from the board and team members. Carson is left pondering, which is the lesser of two evils?

Case Study Discussion Questions

1. What is the main issue(s) in this case?
2. Using information from this chapter, discuss the advantages and disadvantages of the two options Carson is considering to fill Maggie's shifts.
3. Are there any other alternatives Carson could consider in this case to meet staffing needs?
4. The mandate to return to full-time has been given. Maggie knows CNAs are in high demand and that she could easily find a job somewhere else. What should Maggie consider in her decision?
5. Carson expresses concern over being able to hire a new CNA if Maggie were to leave. From what you have learned in the chapter, why is it difficult to recruit and retain direct care workers in LTC?

Source: Courtesy of April Temple, PhD, and Matt Dameron, LNHA.

EVIDENCE-BASED RECOMMENDATIONS TO IMPROVE RECRUITMENT AND RETENTION

The aforementioned workforce challenges and their resulting impact on the quality of LTC are garnering renewed attention following the COVID-19 pandemic. A recent landmark report by the National Academies of Sciences, Engineering, and Medicine (NASEM, 2022) highlighted the essential role of staffing to improve quality of care in our nation's nursing homes. Specifically, high-quality nursing home care requires empowered, knowledgeable staff in sufficient numbers who have adequate supervision and training. It also advocates the importance of consistent staff with low turnover to be able to best meet residents' individual needs. Findings from this report conclude the number, qualifications, and compensation of nursing home staff are currently inadequate, and a major transformation and investment in the LTC workforce is needed to achieve high-quality nursing home care (NASEM, 2022).

On an international level, the Organisation for Economic Co-operation and Development (OECD, 2023) is also calling attention to the need to improve the LTC workforce as worldwide aging is contributing to an increasing demand for LTC and exacerbating shortages of LTC workers. This report included findings that LTC workers across countries are among the lowest paid, face difficult working conditions, and lack social recognition (OECD, 2023). To address LTC workforce challenges, the OECD (2023, p. 5) recommends countries focus efforts on the following areas, summarized as RESPECT for the caring profession in Box 7.1.

Given the staffing challenges in LTC are multifaceted, it will take a multipronged approach to make strides in improving recruitment and retention. These efforts will require sustained support and investment from both LTC providers and policymakers. The following section will highlight select evidence-based strategies to improve LTC staff recruitment and retention.

Provide Competitive Wages and Benefits

Successful recruitment and retention of a high-quality LTC workforce begins with providing competitive wages and benefits (Campbell et al., 2021; NASEM, 2022; OECD, 2023). Competition for staff both from other healthcare settings such as hospitals as well as other industries including retail and food service has intensified following the COVID-19 pandemic. The pandemic prompted many LTC organizations to increase hourly wages, use bonuses, and/or offer hazard pay to recruit and retain staff (Musumeci et al., 2022). Nonetheless, providers have voiced difficulty retaining skilled staff when they can't compete with the wages paid by hospitals or staffing agencies or when direct care workers earn higher wages in other entry-level jobs (Khavjou et al., 2023; Porter et al., 2022).

BOX 7.1 RESPECT for the Caring Profession

Recognize, both economically and socially, care workers.

Enforce (effective regulations) governing the LTC sector.

Sustainably fund the LTC sector.

Pay better salaries.

Equip workers with new technologies.

Collectively bargain for better work conditions.

Train to retain LTC workers

LTC, long-term care.

Source: Organisation for Economic Co-operation and Development. (2023). *Beyond applause? Improving working conditions in long-term care* (p. 5). OECD Publishing. https://doi.org/10.1787/27d33ab3-en

Mechanisms to address compensation will require policy support from federal and state governments. State policy approaches include the recent trend toward increasing the minimum wage or establishing a wage floor for direct care workers (Abbasi, 2022). A number of states have successfully used Medicaid wage-pass through provisions that designate a portion of Medicaid rate increases with the explicit purpose of increasing direct care wages or benefits as one way to ensure improved compensation for workers (Abbasi, 2022; Block et al., 2022). LTC workers also need improved access to employer-based benefits such as affordable health insurance, paid sick leave, and retirement savings. Importantly, LTC providers need policymakers' support through increased Medicaid funding and reimbursement rates to help fund wage and benefit increases (Campbell et al., 2021).

Increase Minimum Staffing Requirements

Until as recently as 2024, federal regulations of nursing home staffing had remained unchanged since the Omnibus Budget Reconciliation Act of 1987 (OBRA-87) despite the increasing complexity and acuity of nursing home residents since then. Historically, federal regulations did not specify specific staffing hours or levels but rather required "sufficient" staff to meet the needs of residents, 24-hour licensed nursing, and RN coverage of 8-hours each day (Wiener et al., 2017). The relationship between higher staffing levels, especially RNs, and improved quality of care in nursing homes has been well documented (Castle, 2008; CMS, 2001; Harrington et al., 2016, 2020; A. White & Olsho, 2023). For decades, increasing overall nurse staffing has been a consistent recommendation for improving the quality of care in nursing homes (CMS, 2001; Harrington et al., 2016; IOM, 2008; NASEM, 2022). A salient report by the CMS (2001) recommended a minimum of 4.1 nursing hours per resident day to provide optimal care. Additionally, experts have recommended 24-hour RN coverage with additional coverage by RNs as needed to reflect acuity and case-mix (IOM, 2008; NASEM, 2022).

Moreover, higher staffing levels have been associated with lower nursing home staff turnover (Castle & Engberg, 2006; Donoghue & Castle, 2007; Temple et al., 2009). Higher staffing levels may alleviate workload and allow nursing staff to provide more high-quality, person-centered care when they support fewer residents (A. White & Olsho, 2023). Among direct care workers, increased staffing is frequently identified as a necessary change to improve their jobs (Kemper et al., 2008).

A majority of states have established minimum staffing standards that exceed federal requirements under OBRA-87, but these vary widely and are often still below recommended staffing levels (Musumeci et al., 2022; Figure 7.4). In addition to staffing standards, states have also used other policy levers including wage pass-through or other payment policies that tie Medicaid reimbursement to direct care wage costs to increase staffing (Medicaid and CHIP Payment and Access Commission, 2022). Previous studies have found that state Medicaid rate increases to nursing home providers were also associated with improved staffing levels, particularly for RNs and LPNs (Bowblis & Applebaum, 2017; Hackmann, 2019).

Notably, for the first time in decades, there is policy action at the federal level related to nursing home staffing. In response to the Biden administration's Action Plan for Nursing Home Reform, the CMS issued a proposed rule in September 2023 to establish minimum staffing standards that would raise staffing levels for more than three-quarters of nursing homes at a cost to providers of $4 billion annually (Burns et al., 2023; CMS, 2023). Despite opposition and concerns raised by the nursing home industry, the CMS issued a final rule in April 2024 with staggered implementation of staffing requirements over the next 3 years (CMS, 2024). The new rule will require a total nurse staffing standard of 3.48 hours of care per resident day, which must include 0.55 hours by an RN and 2.45 hours of direct nurse aide care. It will also increase RN coverage from 8-hours to 24-hours per day, 7 days per week. Additionally, the CMS is launching a $75 million national nursing home staffing campaign with financial incentives to improve nurse recruitment and nurse aide training (CMS, 2024).

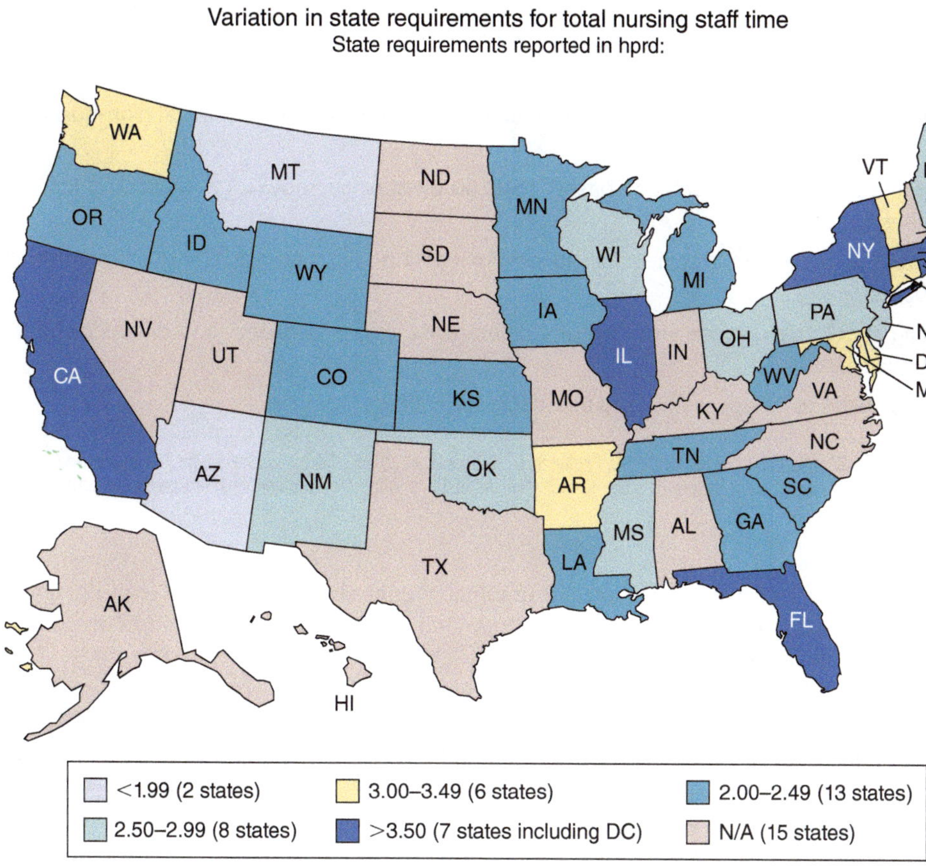

FIGURE 7.4. Nursing home staffing requirements by state.

Note: Hprd = hours per resident per day include total nurse staffing hours by licensed nurses and certified nursing assistants.

Source: Musumeci, M. B., Childress, E., & Harris, B. (2022). *State actions to address nursing home staffing during COVID-19* [Issue brief]. KFF. https://www.kff.org/medicaid/issue-brief/state-actions-to-address-nursing-home-staffing-during-covid-19

Enhance Education and Training Requirements

Across occupations and settings, enhanced education and training requirements are needed in LTC to contribute to the professionalization of this workforce, and, in turn, improvements in quality of care. National recommendations have called for increasing the qualifications and enhancing the education and training of almost all types of nursing home staff (NASEM, 2022), as well as requiring all healthcare workers to receive coursework or training in gerontology and geriatrics (IOM, 2008).

The amount and/or quality of training has also been shown to have an impact on LTC staff recruitment and retention. Prior research has demonstrated that training of nursing assistants is associated with improved job satisfaction (Han et al., 2014) and lower turnover (Temkin-Greener et al., 2020) as well as better nursing home resident outcomes (Trinkoff et al., 2016). Direct care workers consistently report they also desire more training to effectively do their jobs (Campbell et al., 2021).

Among direct care workers, training requirements differ between settings of care and across states. Federal standards for training exist only for nursing assistants and home health aides, and these standards have routinely been criticized as being insufficient to meet the demands of caring for a population with increasing acuity. Several bodies have recommended minimum training requirements of nursing assistants and home health aides should be increased from the current standard of 75 hours to 120 hours (IOM, 2008; NASEM, 2022). Some states have expanded

BOX 7.2 Best Practices for Training of Direct Care Workers

Training should include both relational and technical skills necessary to provide high-quality care.

Programs should be competency-based, focused on specific knowledge, skills, and abilities needed in the job.

It should provide opportunities for hands-on learning and use adult learner-centered instruction.

Training should be responsive to cultural differences, language needs, and differences in learning styles.

Training needs to be accessible and affordable for workers.

Source: Data from Campbell, S., Del Rio Drake, A., Espinoza, R., & Scales, K. (2021). *Caring for the future: The power and potential of America's direct care workforce.* Paraprofessional Health Institute. https://www.phinational.org/caringforthefuture

training requirements beyond the federal minimum, but only a handful require at least 120 hours for nursing assistants (13 states and Washington, DC) and home health aides (six states and Washington, DC; Campbell et al., 2021).

More can also be done so that training is relevant, accessible, and affordable for direct care workers. Since the time and expense of training can be a barrier, some options include offering free or low-cost training and paying workers for the time spent in training (NASEM, 2022). There is also a need to improve the quality of training to ensure direct care workers are equipped to succeed in their roles. For example, competency-based training for CNAs that includes topics such as dementia, infection prevention, behavioral health, chronic diseases, use of assistive devices, and cultural sensitivity is recommended (NASEM, 2022). Best practices for training of direct care workers are outlined in Box 7.2.

Offer Career Advancement Opportunities

In addition to inadequate training, a lack of career growth opportunities has been identified as a barrier to attracting and retaining the direct care workforce (Drake, 2020; NASEM, 2022). There is a need to offer accessible career advancement opportunities for upward mobility for these workers that represent an elevation in title, role, and compensation. Examples of these advanced roles that have been used with success include peer mentorship programs, which train experienced direct care workers to orient and support new workers; care coordination roles to improve care transitions; or condition-specific care such as a dementia care specialist (Drake, 2020; Hostetter & Klein, 2021). LTC providers can also promote direct care workers from within to administrative roles, such as trainer or clinical coordinator roles (Campbell et al., 2021). These advanced roles show promise for improving staff retention (Hegeman et al., 2007) and increasing the efficiency and quality of care delivered to consumers (Drake, 2020).

States can also play a role in formalizing meaningful career pathways, and some states have been innovative in developing advanced training programs for direct care workers that are linked to career advancement and wage increases (Hostetter & Klein, 2021). For example, Washington state created an advanced home care aide specialist program that offers additional training and pay for home care workers to support consumers with complex needs (Drake, 2020). The state of New York designed an advanced home health aide role with additional training and responsibilities to provide tasks such as routine medication administration under the delegation of RNs (National Conference of State Legislatures, 2023). More public investment is needed to scale these types of programs to strengthen the direct care workforce for the future.

Foster a Supportive Work Environment

The last recommendation includes greater focus on the importance of creating a supportive, positive work environment to recruit and retain LTC staff. Although pay is frequently a top concern, direct care workers routinely call for improved working relationships, especially supervisory, and the need to feel appreciated, listened to, and treated with respect (Bishop et al., 2008; Creapeau et al., 2022; Kemper et al., 2008; Krein et al., 2022). Effective supervision is particularly important, as nursing assistants who perceived their supervisors to be respectful, helpful, and to provide positive feedback were found in one study to be more likely to remain in their jobs (Bishop et al., 2008). An additional suggestion is to move to a supportive model of supervision that is focused on coaching, mentoring, and empowering self-managed work teams (McDonald, 2007).

Staffing practices that focus on empowerment of staff also show promise to enhance job satisfaction and improve retention among LTC workers (Berridge et al., 2018, 2020). Empowerment refers to granting staff the autonomy to make decisions, collaborate effectively, and provide person-centered care to residents. Among direct care staff, empowerment includes activities such as involvement in resident care planning teams, shared decision-making, consistent resident assignments, and ongoing training. Moreover, staff empowerment is a guiding principle across culture change initiatives occurring in LTC.

SUMMARY

In summary, this chapter described the current state of workforce challenges in LTC that will likely continue for the foreseeable future. Addressing these challenges will require a multifaceted approach that includes competitive compensation, enhanced training and career advancement opportunities, and improved working conditions. These actions will require collaboration and investment by both policymakers and providers and cannot be overlooked as part of the overall equation to improving quality and patient safety in LTC. If we are to ensure LTC residents receive high quality of care, we must be able to attract and retain qualified workers in this industry by giving them the resources, support, and respect they need.

Take-Home Points

- The provision of quality care in LTC settings is dependent on a well-qualified, stable workforce.
- The LTC industry faces persistent staffing shortages and high turnover rates, which have been further exacerbated since the start of the COVID-19 pandemic.
- Nurse staffing levels and turnover impact quality of care in nursing homes.
- Inadequate compensation, limited training and career advancement opportunities, difficult working conditions, and lack of recognition impact staff recruitment and retention in LTC.
- Both policy and practice approaches are needed to improve staff recruitment and retention in LTC.

END-OF-CHAPTER RESOURCES

DISCUSSION QUESTIONS

1. Discuss the unique characteristics of the LTC workforce.
2. What are the current staffing challenges facing the field of LTC?
3. In what ways did the COVID-19 pandemic exacerbate existing staffing challenges?
4. Discuss the relationship between turnover and quality of care in nursing homes.

5. What factors contribute to the difficulty with recruiting and retaining staff in LTC?
6. What are the evidence-based strategies LTC providers could use to improve nursing staff retention?
7. Where can policy efforts be directed to address staffing concerns in the LTC workforce?

TOOLS FOR FURTHER LEARNING

- CMS Care Compare for Nursing Homes. https://www.medicare.gov/care-compare
- National Academies of Sciences, Engineering, and Medicine. (2022). *The national imperative to improve nursing home quality: Honoring our commitment to residents, families, and staff*. National Academies Press. https://nap.nationalacademies.org/catalog/26526/the-national-imperative-to-improve-nursing-home-quality-honoring-our
- Organisation for Economic Co-operation and Development. (2023). *Beyond applause? Improving working conditions in long-term care*. https://www.oecd.org/publications/beyond-applause-improving-working-conditions-in-long-term-care-27d33ab3-en.htm
- Paraprofessional Health Institute. (2022). *Direct care workers in the United States: Key facts*. https://www.phinational.org/resource/direct-care-workers-in-the-united-states-key-facts-3

REFERENCES

Abbasi, E. (2022, October 12). *States legislatures taking steps to address direct care wages*. LeadingAge. https://leadingage.org/states-legislatures-taking-steps-to-address-direct-care-wages

American Health Care Association & National Center for Assisted Living. (2021, November 3). *Long term care sector continues to battle worsening workforce crisis*. https://www.ahcancal.org/News-and-Communications/Press-Releases/Pages/Long-Term-Care-Sector-Continues-To-Battle-Worsening-Workforce-Crisis.aspx

American Health Care Association & National Center for Assisted Living. (2022). *BLS January jobs report*. https://www.ahcancal.org/News-and-Communications/Fact-Sheets/FactSheets/BLS-JAN2022-JOBS-REPORT.pdf

American Health Care Association & National Center for Assisted Living. (2023, January 10). *Survey: Nursing home providers say workforce and economic challenges persist*. https://www.ahcancal.org/News-and-Communications/Press-Releases/Pages/Survey-Nursing-Home-Providers-Say-Workforce-and-Economic-Challenges-Persist.aspx

Berridge, C., Lima, J., Schwartz, M., Bishop, C., & Miller, S. C. (2020). Leadership, staff empowerment, and the retention of nursing assistants: Findings from a survey of U.S. nursing homes. *Journal of the American Medical Directors Association*, *21*(9), 1254–1259.e2. https://doi.org/10.1016/j.jamda.2020.01.109

Berridge, C., Tyler, D. A., & Miller, S. C. (2018). Staff empowerment practices and CNA retention: Findings from a nationally representative nursing home culture change survey. *Journal of Applied Gerontology*, *37*(4), 419–434. https://doi.org/10.1177/0733464816665204

Bishop, C. E., Weinberg, D. B., Leutz, W., Dossa, A., Pfefferle, S. G., & Zincavage, R. M. (2008). Nursing assistants' job commitment: Effect of nursing home organizational factors and impact on resident well-being. *The Gerontologist*, *48*(Suppl. 1), 36–45. https://doi.org/10.1093/geront/48.Supplement_1.36

Block, L., Maxey, H., Medlock, C., Johnson, K., & Nielson, B. (2022). *Addressing wages of the direct care workforce through Medicaid policies*. National Governors Association. https://www.nga.org/publications/addressing-wages-of-the-direct-care-workforce-through-medicaid-policies

Bowblis, J. R., & Applebaum, R. (2017). How does Medicaid reimbursement impact nursing home quality? The effects of small anticipatory changes. *Health Services Research, 52*(5), 1729–1748. https://doi.org/10.1111/1475-6773.12553

Burns, A., Chidambaram, P., Neuman, T., & Rudowitz, R. (2023). *What share of nursing facilities might meet proposed new requirements for nursing staff hours?* [Issue brief]. KFF. https://www.kff.org/medicaid/issue-brief/what-share-of-nursing-facilities-might-meet-proposed-new-requirements-for-nursing-staff-hours

Campbell, S., Del Rio Drake, A., Espinoza, R., & Scales, K. (2021). *Caring for the future: The power and potential of America's direct care workforce*. Paraprofessional Health Institute. https://www.phinational.org/caringforthefuture

Castle, N. G. (2008). Nursing home caregiver staffing levels and quality of care: A literature review. *Journal of Applied Gerontology, 27*(4), 375–405. https://doi.org/10.1177/0733464808321596

Castle, N. G., & Engberg, J. (2005). Staff turnover and quality of care in nursing homes. *Medical Care, 43*(6), 616–626. https://doi.org/10.1097/01.mlr.0000163661.67170.b9

Castle, N. G., & Engberg, J. (2006). Organizational characteristics associated with staff turnover in nursing homes. *The Gerontologist, 46*(1), 62–73. https://doi.org/10.1093/geront/46.1.62

Castle, N. G., Engberg, J., & Men, A. (2007). Nursing home staff turnover: Impact on nursing home compare quality measures. *The Gerontologist, 47*(5), 650–661. https://doi.org/10.1093/geront/47.5.650

Castle, N. G., Hyer, K., Harris, J. A., & Engberg, J. (2020). Nurse aide retention in nursing homes. *The Gerontologist, 60*(5), 885–895. https://doi.org/10.1093/geront/gnz168

Centers for Disease Control and Prevention. (2018). *QuickStats:* Percentage distribution of long-term care staffing hours, by staff member type and sector—United States, 2016. *Morbidity and Mortality Weekly Report, 67*(17), 506. https://www.cdc.gov/mmwr/volumes/67/wr/mm6717a6.htm

Centers for Medicare & Medicaid Services. (2001). Report to Congress: Appropriateness of minimum nurse staffing ratios in nursing homes phase II final report. *Centers for Medicare and Medicaid Services, I*, 1–12. https://theconsumervoice.org/uploads/files/issues/CMS-Staffing-Study-Phase-II.pdf

Centers for Medicare & Medicaid Services. (2022, July 27). *CMS enhances nursing home rating system with staffing and turnover data*. https://www.cms.gov/newsroom/press-releases/cms-enhances-nursing-home-rating-system-staffing-and-turnover-data

Centers for Medicare & Medicaid Services. (2023, September 1). *HHS proposes minimum staffing standards to enhance safety and quality in nursing homes*. https://www.cms.gov/newsroom/press-releases/hhs-proposes-minimum-staffing-standards-enhance-safety-and-quality-nursing-homes

Centers for Medicare & Medicaid Services. (2024, April 22). *Medicare and Medicaid programs: Minimum staffing standards for long-term care facilities and Medicaid institutional payment transparency reporting final rule* (CMS 3442-F) [Fact sheet]. https://www.cms.gov/newsroom/fact-sheets/medicare-and-medicaid-programs-minimum-staffing-standards-long-term-care-facilities-and-medicaid-0

Creapeau, L. J. G., Johs-Artisensi, J. L., & Lauver, K. J. (2022). Leadership and staff perceptions on long-term care staffing challenges related to certified nursing assistant retention. *The Journal of Nursing Administration, 52*(3), 146–153. https://doi.org/10.1097/NNA.0000000000001122

Donoghue, C., & Castle, N. G. (2007). Organizational and environmental effects on voluntary and involuntary turnover. *Health Care Management Review, 32*(4), 360–369. https://doi.org/10.1097/01.HMR.0000296791.16257.44

Drake, A. (2020). *Direct care work is real work: Elevating the role of the direct care worker*. Paraprofessional Health Institute. https://www.phinational.org/wp-content/uploads/2020/07/Direct-Care-Work-Is-Real-Work-2020-PHI.pdf

Dubina, K. S., Kim, J.-L., Colato, J., & Rieley, M. J. (2022). Projections overview and highlights, 2021–31. *Monthly Labor Review*. U.S. Bureau of Labor Statistics. https://www.bls.gov/opub/mlr/2022/article/projections-overview-and-highlights-2021-31.htm

Gandhi, A., Yu, H., & Grabowski, D. C. (2021). High nursing staff turnover in nursing homes offers important quality information: Study examines high turnover of nursing staff at US nursing homes. *Health Affairs, 40*(3), 384–391. https://doi.org/10.1377/hlthaff.2020.00957

Hackmann, M. B. (2019). Incentivizing better quality of care: The role of Medicaid and competition in the nursing home industry. *American Economic Review, 109*(5), 1684–1716. https://doi.org/10.1257/aer.20151057

Han, K., Trinkoff, A. M., Storr, C. L., Lerner, N., Johantgen, M., & Gartrell, K. (2014). Associations between state regulations, training length, perceived quality and job satisfaction among certified nursing assistants: Cross-sectional secondary data analysis. *International Journal of Nursing Studies, 51*(8), 1135–1141. https://doi.org/10.1016/j.ijnurstu.2013.12.008

Harrington, C., Dellefield, M. E., Halifax, E., Fleming, M. L., & Bakerjian, D. (2020). Appropriate nurse staffing levels for U.S. nursing homes. *Health Services Insights, 13*, 1–14. https://doi.org/10.1177/1178632920934785

Harrington, C., Schnelle, J. F., McGregor, M., & Simmons, S. F. (2016). The need for higher minimum staffing standards in U.S. nursing homes. *Health Services Insights, 9*, 13–19. https://doi.org/10.4137/HSI.S38994

Hegeman, C., Hoskinson, D., Munro, H., Maiden, P., & Pillemer, K. (2007). Peer mentoring in long-term care: Rationale, design, and retention. *Gerontology & Geriatrics Education, 28*(2), 77–90. https://doi.org/10.1300/J021v28n02_06

Hickey, S. M., Sawo, M., & Wolfe, J. (2022, July 27). *The state of the residential long-term care industry: A comprehensive look at employment levels, demographics, wages, benefits, and poverty rates of workers in the industry*. Economic Policy Institute. https://www.epi.org/publication/residential-long-term-care-workers

Home Care Pulse. (2023). *HCP benchmarking report for home care, home health, and hospice*.

Hospital & Healthcare Compensation Service. (2023). *Assisted living salary & benefits report*.

Hostetter, M., & Klein, S. (2021). *Placing a higher value on direct care workers*. The Commonwealth Fund. https://www.commonwealthfund.org/publications/2021/jul/placing-higher-value-direct-care-workers

Institute of Medicine. (2008). *Retooling for an aging America: Building the health care workforce*. National Academies Press. https://www.ncbi.nlm.nih.gov/books/NBK215401

Kemper, P., Heier, B., Barry, T., Brannon, D., Angelelli, J., Vasey, J., & Anderson-Knott, M. (2008). What do direct care workers say would improve their jobs? Differences across settings. *The Gerontologist, 48*(Suppl. 1), 17–25. https://doi.org/10.1093/geront/48.Supplement_1.17

Kennedy, K. A., Applebaum, R., Bowblis, J. R., & Straker, J. K. (2021). Organizational factors associated with retention of direct care workers: A comparison of nursing homes and assisted living facilities. *The Gerontologist, 61*(4), 530–539. https://doi.org/10.1093/geront/gnaa130

Khavjou, O., Suarez, G., Tyler, D., Squillace, M., Dey, J., & Oliveira, I. (2023). *Wages of direct care workers lower than other entry-level jobs in most states*. Office of the Assistant Secretary for Planning and Evaluation, U.S. Department of Health and Human Services. https://aspe.hhs.gov/sites/default/files/documents/7a611d901c615e5611ea095b1dcf8d08/wages-dcw-lower-ib.pdf

Krein, S. L., Turnwald, M., Anderson, B., & Maust, D. T. (2022). "Sometimes it's not about the money . . . it's the way you treat people . . .": A qualitative study of nursing home staff turnover. *Journal of the American Medical Directors Association, 23*(7), 1178–1184. https://doi.org/10.1016/j.jamda.2021.11.036

LeadingAge. (2023). *LeadingAge workforce informal snap poll: Toplines*. https://leadingage.org/wp-content/uploads/2023/03/Workforce-Snap-Poll-Toplines-2023-1.pdf

Lerner, N. B., Johantgen, M., Trinkoff, A. M., Storr, C. L., & Han, K. (2014). Are nursing home survey deficiencies higher in facilities with greater staff turnover. *Journal of the American Medical Directors Association, 15*(2), 102–107. https://doi.org/10.1016/j.jamda.2013.09.003

Lewis, T. (2021, February 18). Nursing home workers had one of the deadliest jobs of 2020. *Scientific American*. https://www.scientificamerican.com/article/nursing-home-workers-had-one-of-the-deadliest-jobs-of-2020

Loomer, L., Grabowski, D. C., Yu, H., & Gandhi, A. (2022). Association between nursing home staff turnover and infection control citations. *Health Services Research, 57*(2), 322–332. https://doi.org/10.1111/1475-6773.13877

Manchha, A. V., Way, K. A., Tann, K., & Thai, M. (2022). The social construction of stigma in aged-care work: Implications for health professionals' work intentions. *The Gerontologist, 62*(7), 994–1005. https://doi.org/10.1093/geront/gnac002

Manchha, A. V., Way, K. A., Thai, M., & Tann, K. (2023). "The stigma is what you do": Examining the relationship between occupational stigma and worker outcomes in the aged care context. *Journal of Applied Gerontology, 42*(2), 221–230. https://doi.org/10.1177/07334648221129849

McDonald, I. J. (2007). *Respectful relationships: The heart of Better Jobs Better Care* [Issue brief]. Institute for the Future of Aging Services. https://leadingage.org/wp-content/uploads/drupal/Respectful_Relationships.pdf

McGarry, B. E., Grabowski, D. C., & Barnett, M. L. (2020). Severe staffing and personal protective equipment shortages faced by nursing homes during the COVID-19 pandemic. *Health Affairs, 39*(10), 1812–1821. https://doi.org/10.1377/hlthaff.2020.01269

Medicaid and CHIP Payment and Access Commission. (2022). *State policy levers to address nursing facility staffing issues* [Issue brief]. https://www.macpac.gov/wp-content/uploads/2022/03/State-Policy-Levers-to-Address-Nursing-Facility-Staffing-Issues.pdf

Muench, U., Jura, M., Spetz, J., Mathison, R., & Herrington, C. (2021). Financial vulnerability and worker well-being: A comparison of long-term services and supports workers with other health workers. *Medical Care Research and Review, 78*(5), 607–615. https://doi.org/10.1177/1077558720930131

Musumeci, M. B., Childress, E., & Harris, B. (2022). *State actions to address nursing home staffing during COVID-19* [Issue brief]. KFF. https://www.kff.org/medicaid/issue-brief/state-actions-to-address-nursing-home-staffing-during-covid-19

National Academies of Sciences, Engineering, and Medicine. (2022). *The national imperative to improve nursing home quality: Honoring our commitment to residents, families, and staff.* The National Academies Press. https://nap.nationalacademies.org/catalog/26526/the-national-imperative-to-improve-nursing-home-quality-honoring-our

National Academy of Social Insurance. (n.d.). *Demand for long-term services and supports will rise.* Retrieved May 10, 2024, from https://www.nasi.org/learn/long-term-services-and-supports/demand-for-long-term-services-and-supports-will-rise

National Conference of State Legislatures. (2023, March 10). *Strengthening the direct care workforce.* https://www.ncsl.org/health/strengthening-the-direct-care-workforce

Ochieng, N., Chidambaram, P., & Musumeci, M. (2022, April 4). *Nursing facility staffing shortages during the COVID-19 pandemic* [Issue Brief]. KFF. https://www.kff.org/coronavirus-covid-19/issue-brief/nursing-facility-staffing-shortages-during-the-covid-19-pandemic

Organisation for Economic Co-operation and Development. (2023). *Beyond applause? Improving working conditions in long-term care.* OECD Publishing. https://doi.org/10.1787/27d33ab3-en

Osterman, P. (2018). Improving long-term care by finally respecting home-care aides. *Hastings Center Report, 48*(S3), S67–S70. https://doi.org/10.1002/hast.917

Paraprofessional Health Institute. (2022). *Direct care workers in the United States: Key facts.* https://www.phinational.org/resource/direct-care-workers-in-the-united-states-key-facts-3

Porter, K. A., Tyler, D. A., Gasdaska, A., Segelman, M., Khatutsky, G., Squillace, M., Dey, J., & Oliveira, I. (2022). *COVID-19 pandemic increased nursing homes' reliance on contract staff to address staffing shortages in 2020* [Issue brief]. U.S. Department of Health and Human Services, Office of the Assistant Secretary for Planning and Evaluation. https://www.aspe.hhs.gov/sites/default/files/documents/67e96aa09cd62304787c331ea6c2c6a6/nh-reliance-contract-staff-brief.pdf

Requirements for Long Term Care Facilities, 42 C.F.R. 483 Subpart B (2024). https://www.ecfr.gov/current/title-42/chapter-IV/subchapter-G/part-483/subpart-B

Schulz, R., & Eden, J. (Eds.). (2016). *Families caring for an aging America*. National Academies Press. https://doi.org/10.17226/23606

Service Employees International Union. (2020, June 9). *National survey shows government, employers are failing to protect nursing home workers and residents.* https://www.seiu.org/2020/06/national-survey-shows-government-employers-are-failing-to-protect-nursing-home-workers-and-residents

Slatten, T., Lien, G., & Svenkerud, J. (2019). The role of organizational attractiveness in an internal market-oriented culture (IMOC): A study of hospital frontline employees. *BMC Health Services Research, 19*, 307. https://doi.org/10.1186/s12913-019-4144-8

Stone, R. I., & Bryant, N. S. (2019). The future of the home care workforce: Training and supporting aides as members of home-based care teams. *Journal of the American Geriatrics Society*, *67*(S2), S444–S448. https://doi.org/10.1111/jgs.15846

Tak, S., Sweeney, M. H., Alterman, T., Baron, S., & Calvert, G. M. (2010). Workplace assaults on nursing assistants in US nursing homes: A multilevel analysis. *American Journal of Public Health*, *100*(10), 1938–1945. https://doi.org/10.2105/AJPH.2009.185421

Temkin-Greener, H., Cen, X., & Li, Y. (2020). Nursing home staff turnover and perceived patient safety culture: Results from a national survey. *The Gerontologist*, *60*(7), 1303–1311. https://doi.org/10.1093/geront/gnaa015

Temple, A., Dobbs, D., & Andel, R. (2009). Exploring correlates of turnover among nursing assistants in the National Nursing Home Survey. *Health Care Management Review*, *34*(2), 182–190. https://doi.org/10.1097/HMR.0b013e31819c8b11

Thomas, K. S., Mor, V., Tyler, D. A., & Hyer, K. (2013). The relationships among licensed nurse turnover, retention, and rehospitalization of nursing home residents. *The Gerontologist*, *53*(2), 211–221. https://doi.org/10.1093/geront/gns082

Trinkoff, A. M., Storr, C. L., Lerner, N. B., Yang, B. K., & Han, K. (2016). CNA training requirements and resident care outcomes in nursing homes. *The Gerontologist*, *57*(3), 501–508. https://doi.org/10.1093/geront/gnw049

True, S., Garfield, R., Rae, M., Claxton, G., Chidambaram, P., & Orgera, K. (2020, April 23). *COVID-19 and workers at risk: Examining the long-term care workforce* [Issue brief]. KFF. https://perma.cc/9KW5-2V48

U.S. Bureau of Labor Statistics. (2023, May). *Occupational employment and wages, May 2023: 29–1141 registered nurses*. https://www.bls.gov/oes/current/oes291141.htm#nat

Van Hoye, G. (2008). Nursing recruitment: Relationship between perceived employer image and nursing employees' recommendations. *Journal of Advanced Nursing*, *63*(4), 366–375. https://doi.org/10.1111/j.1365-2648.2008.04710.x

White, A., & Olsho, L. E. W. (2023, June). *Nursing home staffing study: Comprehensive report*. Centers for Medicare & Medicaid Services. https://kffhealthnews.org/wp-content/uploads/sites/2/2023/08/Abt-Associates-CMS-NH-Staffing-Study_Final-Report_-Apndx_June_2023.pdf

White, E. M., Wetle, T. F., Reddy, A., & Baier, R. R. (2021). Front-line nursing home staff experiences during the COVID-19 pandemic. *Journal of the American Medical Directors Association*, *22*(1), 199–203. https://doi.org/10.1016/j.jamda.2020.11.022

Wiener, J. M., Freiman, M. P., & Brown, D. (2007, December). *Nursing home care quality: Twenty years after the Omnibus Budget Reconciliation Act of 1987*. Kaiser Family Foundation. https://www.kff.org/wp-content/uploads/2013/01/7717.pdf

Xiao, C., Winstead, V., & Jablonski, R. (2021). Certified nursing assistants' perceived workplace violence in long-term care facilities: A qualitative analysis. *Workplace Health & Safety*, *69*(8), 366–374. https://doi.org/10.1177/2165079920986159

Zheng, Q., Williams, C. S., Shulman, E. T., & White, A. J. (2022). Association between staff turnover and nursing home quality—evidence from payroll-based journal data. *Journal of the American Geriatrics Society*, *70*(9), 2508–2516. https://doi.org/10.1111/jgs.17843

CHAPTER 8

NAVIGATING THE UNEXPECTED: PREPARING FOR CHALLENGES IN LONG-TERM CARE QUALITY AND SAFETY

Lindsay J. Peterson

Learning Objectives

After completing this chapter, each learner will be able to:

- Understand the effects of a changing climate on the older adult population, including how vulnerability varies depending on the older adults' health conditions and types of disaster.
- Describe the varied risks that disasters pose to residents of long-term care (LTC) facilities and the features of the facility or its response that affect the potential level of harm to the resident.
- Describe existing disaster preparedness regulations and how these regulations have evolved in recent years.
- Analyze the challenges of an all-hazards approach to disaster preparedness in LTC and to examine the role and limits of using regulations to ensure disaster preparedness in LTC.
- Assess multiple approaches to ensuring the safety of LTC facilities in emergencies and disasters and why some approaches may be more effective than others.

INTRODUCTION

Much is written about the people and processes required to ensure nursing home and assisted living residents receive the care needed to recuperate after a hospitalization or live safely and comfortably despite their illnesses. We hear less about what to do when usual routines are upended by serious threats, such as a hurricane or a deadly virus—the times when long-term care (LTC) residents are at greatest risk.

Consider the LTC nurse who had come to her nursing home after years of caring for acutely ill patients in hospitals. She was proud of her experience and professionalism and felt confident that the needed systems were in place to keep her residents safe when Hurricane Irma approached Florida in 2017. It all started to go wrong when one of a group of buildings she oversaw began to evacuate its residents and she realized that the beds did not fit in the elevator. Taking the beds apart and putting them back together turned the evacuation into an all-day task, but she and her staff got it done, and though she was already exhausted, she made plans to stay at one of the other nursing homes where residents and staff would be sheltering in place because it was not at risk of flooding. The nursing home fared well in the storm but lost electrical power, as did most of Florida. A generator was available, but only for essential resident care functions, not for air conditioning. With temperatures rising, residents became anxious.

The nurse had some help from administrative staff, but a number of direct care workers did not show up as expected, possibly because they evacuated with their families based on the state's widespread and dire warnings about the danger Irma posed. For more than two full days, the lone nurse cared for about 60 high-need residents with her skeleton crew, many of whom were not licensed to give nursing care. Medications ran out, as residents' needs grew, with too few hands available to clean, turn, and provide other care they needed. Finally, help arrived to relieve the nurse and the others, but it left her with emotional scars and hard-won knowledge of the price that both staff and residents pay when a healthcare facility lacks adequate power, critical supplies such as medication, and back up direct care staff.

Research going back to Hurricane Katrina, in 2005, has shown that disaster exposure is associated with increased hospitalization and ED visits for older adults with diabetes, congestive heart failure, and other chronic conditions (Bell et al., 2022; Malik et al., 2018). The risks are even greater for LTC residents living with multiple chronic conditions, mobility impairments, and medication needs. This is based on studies finding they are more likely to die, require hospitalization, or decline in function (Dosa et al., 2010) and are particularly vulnerable to harm if they experience an evacuation (Castle & Engberg, 2011; Dosa et al., 2012; Thomas et al., 2012). After Hurricanes Katrina and Rita, also in 2005, researchers, policy makers, and administrative leaders in LTC worked together to persuade and help nursing homes to improve their disaster preparedness (Hyer et al., 2010).

The John A. Hartford Foundation helped fund a series of workshops and publications (Florida Health Care Association [FHCA], 2008), including sessions that led to the development of an evacuation decision framework (Figure 8.1). This framework presents the decision as an analysis of specific external factors (e.g., the nature of the event, the location of the facility related to flooding risk) and internal factors (e.g., resident acuity, staff availability, transportation, and supply needs) to guide an LTC facility in deciding whether to evacuate or shelter in place.

A decade later, Hurricane Irma struck Florida. Research that followed showed that despite the preparedness work of so many years earlier, the risks persisted. Long-stay nursing home residents—who are considered to be permanent residents and are generally frailer than those

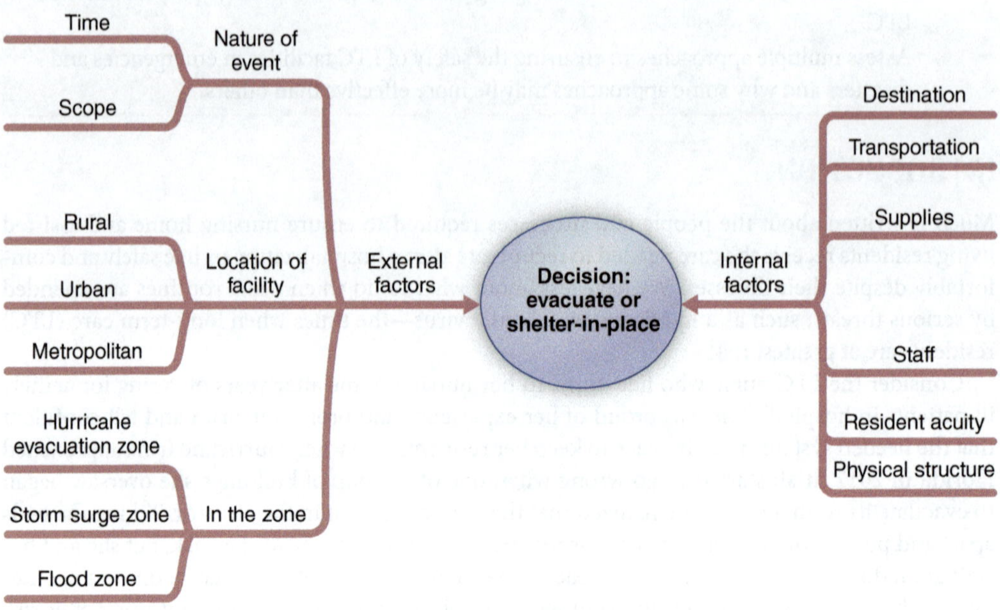

FIGURE 8.1. A decision model of key factors to consider when assessing whether to evacuate or shelter in place for a hurricane.

Source: Florida Health Care Association. (2008). *National criteria for evacuation decision-making in nursing homes*. https://www.fhca.org/images/uploads/NationalCriteriaforEvacuationDecision-Making2008.pdf

receiving short-term rehabilitation services—were found to be at greater risk of death or hospitalization in the weeks after the storm (Dosa et al., 2020). Risks were also higher for residents in facilities that lost power during the hurricane and may have suffered from exposure to extreme heat (Skarha et al., 2021). Assisted living community residents exposed to Hurricane Irma had higher rates of ED use in the weeks after the storm (Hua et al., 2021); injury-related visits were 13% higher 30 days after Irma, compared to 2016. Additionally, assisted living residents who were evacuated had higher rates of ED use and nursing home placement within 30 days of the storm, compared to counterparts who sheltered in place (Hua et al., 2024). Looking at the effects of Hurricane Harvey, in Texas, also in 2017, Hua et al. (2023) found that the risk of death for long-stay nursing home residents was higher, with 196 excess deaths within the sample of 15,111 residents in the 3 months after the storm. Compared to the year before when there was no hurricane, death rates after Harvey were higher for those with chronic-obstructive pulmonary disease (Hua et al., 2023).

Several of these studies have provided a critical perspective on the effect of disasters on this population, finding the harm is not always immediately evident. The resident may survive the event but experience a shock to the system—from the trauma of a sudden relocation or the lack of needed medication or a fall in a disrupted environment—leading to a serious or fatal decline several weeks afterward. Because of this, the number of disaster-related casualties in nursing homes and assisted living communities is likely to be much higher than the usual postemergency estimates, which typically count only casualties that occur during or immediately after an event (Dosa et al., 2020).

The COVID-19 pandemic also provided a stark view of the vulnerability of older adults, with U.S. data showing that nearly a fourth of the deaths related to COVID-19 occurred in LTC settings (Chidambaram, 2022). What these events have in common is that they created severe disruption in living environments that older adults depended on for stability and safety. Today, rising numbers of older adults require care for diabetes, heart and lung diseases, dementia, and other serious chronic illnesses. Also on the rise are a range of events affecting LTC facilities across the United States, from intensifying heat spells to winter storms, wildfires, and floods that threaten human health and disrupt healthcare operations on a massive scale (Smith, 2021). The convergence of these trends increases the urgency of ensuring that nursing homes and assisted living communities are well prepared (Harper, 2023).

DISASTER PREPAREDNESS REGULATIONS FOR LONG-TERM CARE

The National Response Framework (NRF) has long guided the response to disasters and emergencies in the United States through a system created to coordinate the many organizational entities needed to maintain critical functions at these times. These entities include hospital systems and public health organizations. The NRF relies on each one to develop procedures to protect those who rely on their care and services, and to work in coordination with other critical organizations and service providers (Federal Emergency Management Agency, 2019). The U.S. Gulf Coast hurricanes of 2004 and 2005, including Hurricane Katrina, drew new attention to nursing home preparedness. In 2006, the U.S. Office of the Inspector General (OIG) documented numerous gaps in the preparedness that the OIG inspectors viewed as essential, even though 94% of nursing homes nationwide were technically in compliance with the Centers for Medicare & Medicaid Services (CMS) preparedness standards at the time, based on their state inspection survey results (OIG, 2006). In the U.S. Gulf Coast nursing homes examined, several plans lacked essential elements, including:

- criteria on how to decide whether to evacuate or shelter in place;
- information on the specific characteristics of residents that would enable staff to modify plans based on the need for oxygen, for instance, or mobility assistance;
- formal agreements with host sites in the event of an evacuation; and
- the need to supply water for an evacuation (Case Study 8.1).

Case Study 8.1 Unprecedented Flooding After Hurricane Ian Delivers Hard Lessons

Nursing home and assisted living administrators in Florida know from experience what to do when they learn a hurricane is approaching. And if experience is not enough, state rules require them to create detailed plans for annual review and approval by their county emergency management officials. So, in late September, 2022, when the staff of Avante at Orlando got word that Hurricane Ian was headed for the state, "we prepped as usual," said company CEO Kimberly Biegasiewicz. That meant organizing the staff; contacting families; readying generators in case power went out; checking food, water, and medical supplies; and preparing to either shelter in place or evacuate, depending on what emergency officials directed them to do. Hurricane Ian made a devastating landfall, with 150 mph winds, along Florida's southeastern coast, 140 miles from Orlando.

By the time it crossed central Florida, it had powered down to a tropical storm. The staff of Avante, which is not in a flood zone, had been advised to shelter in place, and thought they had escaped the worst of it. That is, until about 12 hours after Ian's afternoon landfall. At home on a video call with staff members, Biegasiewicz saw a scene that she later likened to something from the movie *Titanic*. Water was pouring into the facility, down the hallways, and toward residents' rooms. And it wasn't just rainwater. What no one had imagined was that the wastewater lift station nearby would fail. Wastewater that typically flowed away from Avante was rushing into it.

Biegasiewicz and her staff were responsible for the safety of 106 people with varied chronic and acute care needs, many of whom were unable to walk. It was the middle of the night. Where could they go? How would they get there? Her calls for help were answered by staff from the county emergency management office. Over the next few hours, working together with the help of emergency medical workers, they used mattresses and stretchers to float and roll the residents out of their rooms. A staff member used her own boat to get residents through the flooded parking lot to higher ground and buses, including a public bus, that took them to public special needs shelters opened for the storm. Hospitals took in some with higher needs. But the management's job was far from over. For the next several hours, they worked the phones to find beds in sister facilities for their residents and rent vans and other vehicles to transport them. The residents were safely in other facilities by the next day, but still, their losses were great. The waters that flooded into Avante or Orlando destroyed most of their possessions, clothes, documents, photos, and mementos. The damage caused by the water—and related issues, such as mold—was so extensive, the building was closed for extensive renovations.

Biegasiewicz came away from the experience with several tips and recommendations:

- Call your contact with your state regulatory office ASAP, and have a cell phone number.
- Be sure to have a system to identify where all residents are being taken, especially if they are going to different locations.
- Check for skin tears on every resident before they go out.
- Have a staff member at the receiving location to supervise residents' arrival at the new location.
- Concerning communication with families, she said, "Be transparent. Communication is huge!"
- Concerning insurance, be able to account for every item in the facility, down to each paperclip. Here again, constant communication with the insurance company is critical.
- Don't store documents, or other precious items, on the floor.
- Look out for staff members and their needs. All vehicles in the parking lot were inundated in the flood, and Avante established a "Go Fund Me" page, raising $12,000 to help with vehicle repairs.
- Finally, "Expect the unexpected," she emphasized. "Even if you are not in a flood zone, you could get it. You need an evacuation plan."

(*continued*)

Case Study 8.1 Unprecedented Flooding After Hurricane Ian Delivers Hard Lessons (*continued*)

Case Study Discussion Questions

1. What can LTC facilities do differently to enhance their preparedness for more extreme forms of natural disasters?
2. From this case study, which factors contributed to the magnitude of damage caused by Hurricane Ian, and how can these factors be mitigated in future natural disasters?
3. Based on the lessons learned from the case study, what improvements would you recommend in emergency management and response strategies for nursing homes and assisted living facilities?

Concerted efforts followed to bolster nursing home emergency and disaster regulations and included nursing homes as healthcare facilities within the National Incident Management System, as part of the NRF (Hyer et al., 2010). Today, all nursing homes that receive Medicare and Medicaid funds are expected to meet a range of emergency preparedness requirements, as set by the CMS. The preparedness of each nursing home is assessed with all other federal requirements during the CMS recertification surveys that are supposed to occur every 9 to 15 months. Plans are expected to address hazards "most likely to occur in the surrounding area," including natural disasters, man-made disasters, and facility-based disasters, such as equipment and utility failures, interruptions to the normal supply of needed resources (e.g., water, food, fuel), and emerging infectious diseases, including hazardous waste, bioterrorism, pandemic flu, and highly communicable diseases, such as COVID-19 (CMS, 2021). See Table 8.1 for the broad categories nursing homes are expected to address. The events of the past several years, including the COVID-19 pandemic and multiple climate disasters, however, have raised new questions about disaster preparedness in LTC, while also highlighting the extraordinary challenges posed by these events.

TABLE 8.1 CMS Emergency Preparedness Requirements

CATEGORY	REQUIREMENT
Emergency Plan	Develop and maintain an emergency preparedness program; update annually. Plan should be based on documented facility- and community-based risk assessment, considering all risks that could disrupt operations, categorized by likelihood of occurrence. Risk assessments and plan should include the potential for an emerging infectious disease outbreak.
	Address resident needs and ability to meet needs during a disaster; develop plan to ensure continuity of operations.
	Have a process for cooperation and collaboration with local, state, and federal officials.
Policies and Procedures	Create and maintain emergency preparedness policies and procedures based on emergency plan, risk assessment, and communication plan; have procedures to review and update annually or more frequently if necessary, such as during a pandemic when guidance is in flux.
	Plan for residents' basic needs, including food, water, power, lighting, and waste disposal, whether evacuating or sheltering in place.
	Create systems to track staff and residents during and after emergency.
	Evacuation plans should consider residents' needs, staff responsibilities, transportation, and identification of evacuation location, as well as means of communication with outside sources of assistance.

(*continued*)

TABLE 8.1 CMS Emergency Preparedness Requirements (*continued*)

CATEGORY	REQUIREMENT
	Include staff and volunteers in plans involving sheltering in place.
	Ensure resident records are available, maintained, and kept confidential.
	Address the use of volunteers or other emergency staffing strategies.
	Arrange for other providers to receive patients to maintain continuity of services.
	Address how to request a 1,135 waiver and allow services to be temporarily provided at an alternate site.
Communication Plan	Include contact information for staff, physicians, service providers, volunteers, government emergency preparedness staff (e.g., local, state), state regulatory agency, LTC ombudsmen, and other sources of assistance; include primary and alternate ways to communicate with staff and emergency officials.
	Have ways to share resident medical information to maintain continuity of care, provide information about the facility's needs and ability to provide services, and share emergency plan information with residents and their families.
Training and Testing	Develop and maintain an emergency preparedness training and testing program based on preparedness plan; review and update annually.
	Train all new and existing staff on disaster plan at least annually; document training; demonstrate staff knowledge of emergency procedures.
	Conduct exercises to test emergency plan at least twice a year, including unannounced staff drills using emergency plan procedures. At least one of the two should be a full-scale community-based exercise or facility-based functional exercise.
Emergency Power Systems	Must follow applicable healthcare facilities' code in location, inspection, testing, and maintenance of emergency power system; if using onsite fuel, must plan for how to keep systems functioning during emergency, except if evacuating.
Integrated Health Systems	If the facility is part of a larger system with an integrated emergency plan, the facility may choose to be part of this plan but must show it participated in the plan's development, that the plan accounts for unique circumstances and resident populations, and was based on documented community-based and facility-based risk assessments; it must also include all other required elements (e.g., communication plan, testing and training programs).

CMS, Centers for Medicare & Medicaid Services; LTC, long-term care.

Source: Data from Centers for Medicare & Medicaid Services. (2021, April 16). *State operations manual: Appendix Z—Emergency preparedness for all provider and certified supplier types Interpretive guidance.* https://www.cms.gov/Regulations-and-Guidance/Guidance/Manuals/Downloads/som107ap_z_emergprep.pdf

Federal regulations apply only to federally funded nursing homes. Though assisted living communities are subject to many of the same challenges as nursing homes (Peterson et al., 2021), they are subject only to regulation at the state level, which may or may not address disaster preparedness.

"WE DID NOT KNOW THE FOREIGN TERRITORY WE WERE EMBARKING ON"

Dozens of informal and formal assessments have attempted to explain the high COVID-19 mortality rate in LTC facilities across the country. They varied from media reports blaming feckless nursing home management (Fraser & Penzenstadler, 2023) to academic studies showing the connection between high infection rates and the characteristics of a nursing home's neighborhood—factors beyond a facility's control (Abrams et al., 2020). However, LTC administrators who were interviewed during the pandemic for qualitative research studies did not hesitate to say they were not prepared (Hackett et al., 2023). They were prepared for the threats of the past, they said, but COVID-19 was both deadlier and more infectious than anything they had encountered before. One nursing home administrator's comment exemplified the views of many:

When we create our policies and our procedures, we base it off of the likelihood of something happening in our area, and there was no history of a pandemic in a very, very long time. So we didn't actually have a plan besides just our infection control plan. (Interviewee #1, personal communication, November 4, 2020)

Another administrator described the challenge of knowing what to expect:

We're located within an hour of (an industrial) plant . . . . I mean, honestly you would plan more for a train derailment that had a chemical than, honestly, a pandemic. (Interviewee #2, personal communication, November 4, 2020)

The difficulty of organizing a response extended beyond the nursing homes to statewide health and emergency management officials, as one nursing home operator explained:

The pandemic response plan was to coordinate with local and state level DOH and emergency response teams. Unfortunately, at the beginning of the pandemic, those agencies were not able to provide comprehensive guidance. In addition, the guidance provided often conflicted with other agencies. (Interviewee #3, personal communication, November 4, 2020)

As another administrator put it:

COVID was and has so many variables that all contingencies could not be addressed . . . . We did not know the foreign territory we were embarking on. (Interviewee #4, personal communication, November 4, 2020)

At the beginning of the pandemic, in early 2020, few facilities had the personal protective equipment (PPE) they needed. An advance practice clinician interviewed noted, "When everything first hit, nothing was in place. There was no COVID unit, there [were] no COVID swabs available" (as cited in White et al., 2021, p. 200). And in the words of a certified nursing aide, staff were "reusing . . . gowns and going in and out of rooms with the same gown. The face masks [are] being reused for a week" (as cited in White et al., 2021, p. 200).

The COVID-19 emergency was unique in many ways, but one characteristic that magnified its severity was its long duration. While critical supply shortages abated over time, and treatments and processes were developed to help manage the disease, the virus evolved and continued to spread in waves across the United States, and the world. Research during the pandemic provided evidence that COVID-19 vaccinations helped to prevent cases and deaths and enabled nursing homes to reopen to visitors (Sinha & Konetzka, 2022), but uptake of at least two doses of the vaccine among nursing home staff was inconsistent, very low in some areas, mirroring the varying rates among the general public (Chidambaram & Musumeci, 2022). Reports on COVID-19 vaccination highlighted critical staffing issues, such as how to retain staff members while also compelling them to do something, get a vaccination, they feared or considered to be unfair (Gadbois et al., 2023). Nursing home and assisted living personnel grappled with other vexing issues in that time, including frequently changing, sometimes conflicting guidance from the multiple government agencies, in particular requirements that limited visits from family members and friends. Every day, administrators and staff faced the arguably impossible task of shielding residents from the virus while also minimizing the damage to residents of being isolated from their family members and other residents (Hackett et al., 2023; White et al., 2021).

One frequent complaint from both nursing home and assisted living administrators was that public health and regulatory officials provided little to no guidance on how to manage COVID-19 in a facility with high proportions of residents with dementia.

Our guidance was to shut down! And to 'go to your room' and 'shut the door' and 'go to your room' and 'stay in your room' and 'put your mask on' and 'don't come out of your room!' And for someone with dementia, it was horrible! (Hackett et al., 2023, p. 1571)

Administrators acknowledged a certain level of success with virtual options (e.g., Zoom calls), but as one said, "It was very difficult for dementia residents to understand what a Zoom phone call and seeing a family member (on Zoom) was. I'm not sure it helped as much as we thought it was going to help" (Hackett et al., 2023, p. 1569).

Said another: "(Seeing a family member) on a computer monitor was not enough, especially if they had poor eyesight. How do they know that's their daughter?" (Hackett et al., 2023, p. 1569).

THE UNPREDICTABILITY OF TODAY'S CLIMATE DISASTERS

As COVID-19 redefined the concept of a pandemic in healthcare, climate disasters of the past decade also have challenged providers. Hurricane Harvey caused days of unexpected rain and catastrophic flooding in Texas in 2017. Nursing homes and assisted living communities in counties that received no evacuation orders wound up evacuating residents through rising waters—in one case after an administrator was physically assaulted by volunteers who converged on his facility, insisting on taking the residents away in fishing boats (Pearce, 2017). The unprecedented rainfall and flooding forced the release of pollutants from oil refineries into the air in the Houston area, which may explain the increased mortality found among nursing home residents in the area with chronic obstructive pulmonary disease (Hua et al., 2023).

Soon after Hurricane Harvey, Hurricane Irma made landfall on Florida's west coast as a category 4 storm that was originally forecast to strike the east coast. Many nursing home and assisted living communities that had planned to shelter in place, not expecting to be affected, were forced to quickly evacuate. In qualitative research, one administrator described receiving the evacuation order from a county emergency management official after several staff and the transportation contractor had been told their services were not needed (Peterson et al., 2021). She turned to social media in desperate need of buses and people to gather supplies and help the residents out of their rooms for a trip across the state.

> *We sent out a request on Facebook to our community and our local forestry department, our sheriff's office, and local community members came and helped me load all the residents. . . . Only one of the buses had a wheelchair accessible ramp, so we had to carry the rest of them up the stairs. That's all we had available. (Interviewee #5, personal communication, November 4, 2020)*

Another administrator in a different county described her plans to shelter in place being countermanded by emergency managers. She was in a multistory building, and the management had made plans to move residents to higher floors if necessary. Instead, the residents wound up in a crowded public shelter for 3 days. "We had 90–100 residents that were in frail condition lying on mats" on the floor, she told researchers (Peterson et al., 2021, p. 9).

In both cases, the evacuations turned out to be unnecessary when the storm made landfall well to the south of their locations. However, sheltering in place was also a hazard for residents in facilities that overheated when utility power was lost nearly statewide. At least 12 residents died from extreme heat exposure at a nursing home in South Florida when its generator-powered air conditioning system failed. Several staff members and the owner were charged in the case but acquitted when prosecutors failed to prove they were negligent, partly because they had made documented calls to their power utility and the governor's office asking for help (Berklan, 2023).

After Hurricane Irma, Florida passed a law requiring nursing homes and assisted living communities to have sources of back-up power (e.g., generators) and fuel for at least 4 days to maintain internal temperatures of 81 degrees or below. This law, however, would not have helped residents at another Florida nursing home whose primary generator failed after being in use for 10 days, as regional power outages continued after Hurricane Irma. The administrator called on local friends, family members, and other contacts to bring ice, cold drinks, and anything else to protect their residents from succumbing to the heat, again highlighting the critical need for relationships with people who can provide needed help in a disaster (Peterson et al., 2021).

Rising temperatures and sea levels dominate concerns about how to keep long-term residents safe. However, freezing temperatures threatened nursing home and assisted living residents in Texas in 2021 when an upper-level polar vortex of frigid air descended from Canada to encompass the entire state. During the ensuing Winter Storm Uri, Texas experienced a near-catastrophic power grid failure amid record low temperatures, ice storms, and snowstorms. Indoor temperatures remained at or below freezing as the outages continued for days in some parts of the state (City of Austin, 2021). Loss of power exposed nursing homes and assisted living residents to profound cold for extended periods of time (West, 2021). More than 570 of the 1,200 nursing homes in Texas reported emergencies to the Texas Health & Human Services Commission, with more than 400 nursing homes losing power or access to potable water (U.S. Senate Finance Committee & U.S. Senate Special Committee on Aging, 2023). Some were able to provide adequate care only because they had staff members with all-terrain vehicles who could navigate the snow- and ice-covered roads to get to other staff members' homes and bring them to work.

Climate extremes result as well in drought conditions and worsening wildfire threats. Among California's largest wildfires, 10 have occurred in the past 2 decades—half of those in 2020 alone (Turco et al., 2023). In 2018, fast-moving wildfires destroyed three nursing homes in the community of Paradise, California (Stempniak, 2018). The so-called "Camp Fire" started around 6:30 a.m., giving nursing home administrators in Paradise only a few hours to activate staff members and transportation contractors to move residents before being overtaken by smoke and flames. In the case of at least one nursing home in Paradise, staff members hurriedly loaded residents into their own vehicles, which they filled as well with equipment, medications, food, water, and residents' "go" bags as the fire raced toward them (LaGanga, 2018).

CAN REGULATIONS ENSURE PREPAREDNESS?

This compressed time to react makes preparedness for wildfires and other suddenly occurring events especially critical. Administrators and others in charge of the response must be ready to move their residents at a moment's notice. These critical concerns add to the importance of research on wildfire risks, which found (see Figure 8.2) that more than half of nursing homes in the continental western United States were within 5 km of areas with elevated wildfire risk (Festa, Throgmorton, et al., 2023).

Furthermore, those at higher risk in the Mountain West and Pacific Northwest were less likely to have adequately prepared, compared to nursing homes at lower risk. And despite the higher risk, facilities in the Mountain West region were reinspected, on average, 91 days later than lower-risk facilities. This study and others have raised questions about the effectiveness of nursing home regulation and the involvement of nursing homes in the preparedness system envisioned by the NRF (Bell et al., 2023; Dosa et al., 2020; Festa, Heaphy, et al., 2023). After the CMS updated regulations for Medicare providers in 2017, the OIG conducted audits focused on emergency preparedness in eight states (OIG, 2022). In 150 of 154 nursing homes visited, the auditors found 1,139 areas of noncompliance with federal rules requiring emergency supplies and power, plans for evacuation or sheltering in place and tracking residents and staff, emergency communications plans, and emergency plan training and testing (see Table 8.2 for details). As a general conclusion, the OIG stated that management and staff turnover contributed to the emergency preparedness deficiencies. It recommended that the CMS and state survey agencies develop plans to more frequently survey nursing homes with repeat deficiencies but conceded that this might not be possible given the limited resources of some state survey agencies.

FURTHER REGULATORY UPDATES AMID COMPLEXITIES

Following the COVID-19 pandemic and further climate emergencies (e.g., Hurricane Ida in Louisiana, wildfires in California), the CMS again updated its emergency preparedness requirements in 2021. Before this, pandemic threats were only briefly mentioned in LTC. However, post-COVID-19 revisions call for greater focus on emerging infectious diseases, requiring more robust measures. These updates mandate processes to ensure adequate supplies of PPE, as well as resident and visitor screening protocols when necessary. They also emphasize the critical importance of coordination with public health emergency officials and other precautions that experience has proven critical (CMS, 2021). In addition, the new guidelines place greater focus on preparedness

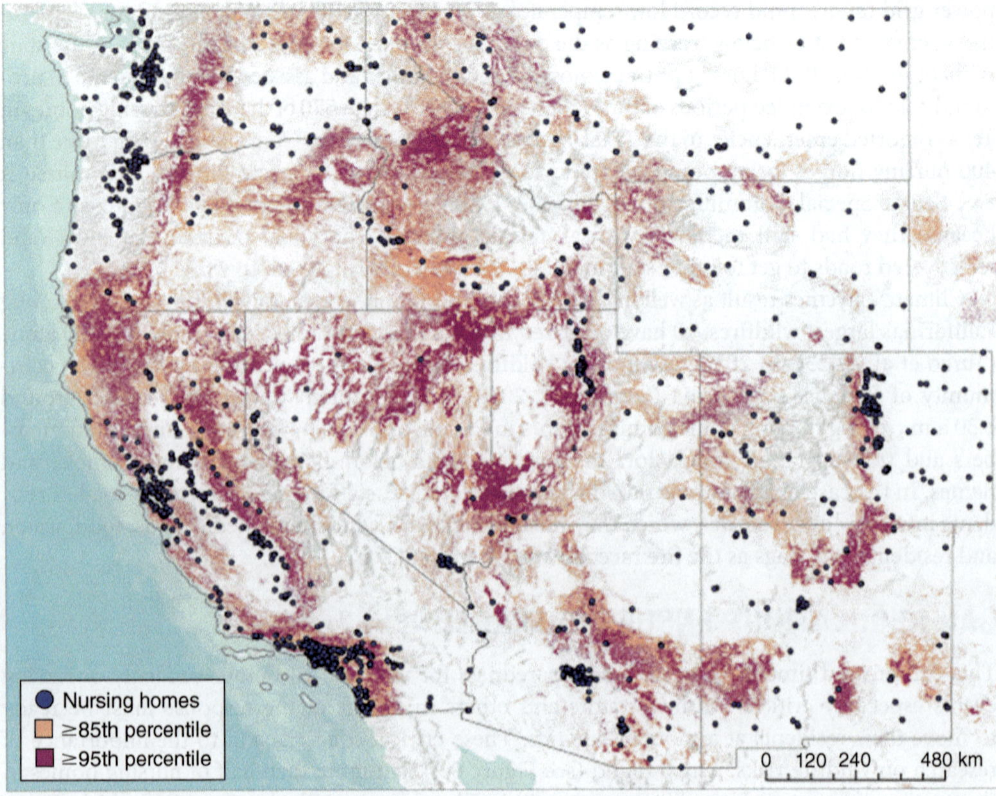

FIGURE 8.2. Nursing homes in high-risk areas of the western United States.

Note: The map displays geocoded locations of Centers for Medicare & Medicaid Services-certified nursing homes as of December 1, 2017. These nursing home locations are overlaid on a visual representation of the U.S. Wildfire Hazard Potential Index, which illustrates national wildfire risk at a 270-meter resolution. Two risk thresholds are highlighted, representing areas at or above the 85th and 95th percentiles of national wildfire potential. Dots indicate the proximity of nursing homes to areas of elevated wildfire risk. Of the nursing homes shown, 1,219 (55.0%) are situated within 5 kilometers of areas at or above the 85th percentile of wildfire risk.

Source: Festa, N., Throgmorton, K. F., Davis-Plourde, K., Dosa, D. M., Chen, K., Zang, E., Kelly, J., & Gill, T. M. (2023). Assessment of regional nursing home preparedness for and regulatory responsiveness to wildfire risk in the Western US. *JAMA Network Open*, *6*(6), e2320207. https://doi.org/10.1001/jamanetworkopen.2023.20207

for climate-related disasters. The CMS reinforced the need for regular training and testing exercises, and stressed the importance of building community partnerships and collaborating with local emergency preparedness officials for effective disaster planning and response.

Notably, CMS regulations outlined in 2019 had stated that nursing homes should document their efforts to contact their local emergency managers to integrate themselves into local disaster planning. However, in the 2021 revisions, the CMS reworded this section of the regulations, stating only that nursing homes "must have a process" to engage in collaborative disaster planning. They softened this requirement despite government oversight reports calling for more communication and collaboration between nursing homes and state and local emergency officials (OIG, 2006, 2012) and research showing that relationships and collaboration with local health and safety officials, as well as community contacts, can be critical to the safety of nursing home residents in a disaster (Hackett et al., 2023; Peterson et al., 2021).

Florida's experience provides an example of why such collaboration often fails to occur. In addition to the CMS regulations, Florida law requires nursing homes to have their emergency management plans reviewed and approved by county-level emergency management officials each year.

TABLE 8.2 Summary of Emergency Preparedness Deficiencies in Eight States

	NEW YORK	CALIFORNIA	TEXAS	FLORIDA	MISSOURI	ILLINOIS	NORTH CAROLINA	IOWA	TOTAL
Number of Nursing Homes Audited	20	19	20	20	20	15	20	20	154
Number of Nursing Homes With Deficiencies	20	19	18	20	20	15	18	20	150
Deficiencies									
Emergency Plans	40	31	13	20	38	37	17	33	229
Emergency Supplies and Power	59	11	4	9	37	5	4	11	140
Plans for Evacuations, Sheltering in Place	40	30	0	17	7	47	29	24	194
Emergency Communications Plans	56	88	10	21	21	66	39	30	331
Emergency Plan Training and Testing	24	28	28	20	46	29	35	35	245
Total—Emergency Preparedness Deficiencies	219	188	55	87	149	184	124	133	1,139

Source: Office of Inspector General. (2022). *Audits of nursing home life safety and emergency preparedness in eight states identified noncompliance with federal requirements and opportunities for the Centers for Medicare & Medicaid Services to improve resident, visitor, and staff safety.* U.S. Department of Health & Human Services. https://oig.hhs.gov/oas/reports/region2/22101010.pdf

However, during an audit of Florida nursing homes after Hurricane Irma (OIG, 2022), a sample of emergency managers described several challenges, including insufficient resources to complete nursing home plan reviews and a lack of knowledge about how to assess the nursing homes' plans. The OIG recommended that the Florida Agency for Health Care Administration, which is the state survey agency, work with county emergency managers to explain nursing homes' roles and responsibilities and provide them with more details about the results of nursing home surveys concerning disaster preparedness. The state's response was that it already provided multiple training opportunities each year to educate local officials.

In other work, researchers who interviewed Florida nursing home and assisted living administrators after Hurricane Irma found evidence of strained relationships between nursing homes and local emergency managers in many counties (Peterson et al., 2021). Indeed, some administrators reported strong connections with their local emergency managers and other community-based contacts, but others described multiple challenges, such as emergency managers who were new to their jobs or had several overlapping job tasks and knew little about nursing homes. Gaps were evident on the part of nursing homes, as well, with some having little to no knowledge of community-level planning resources, such as the regional healthcare coalitions that the CMS has urged them to work with.

MOVING FORWARD

It is important to recognize the disaster preparedness work of the past two decades in LTC; residents are likely safer than they were before Hurricane Katrina. The stories that emerged from research on COVID-19 and varied climate disasters speak to the ingenuity and leadership of some nursing home and assisted living administrative and direct care personnel. Several described the standard processes and impromptu workarounds they established to get through the crises. These included systems to track and manage the constantly changing COVID-19 emergency orders and more efficient ways to communicate with family members of residents, using automation, for instance, to issue text alerts about infection rates or evacuation status during a blackout. And many have adapted the systems for daily use, to message family members about care plan changes, for instance.

Evidence suggests, however, that significant safety gaps continue to exist in LTC. A substantial number of nursing homes have been found to be deficient in their planning, as targeted audits have found (OIG, 2022). But even larger questions loom. Will any nursing home, even those without past deficiencies, be ready for the next disaster, given that preparedness regulations and practices tend to address the demands of past occurrences rather than the unimagined event on the horizon? For instance, the new pandemic preparedness language focuses on the specific issues that arose during the COVID-19 emergency (e.g., supplies of PPE and procedures to screen visitors), as though the next pandemic will pose the same challenges. And while the requirement for "all-hazards" risk assessment does encourage facilities to think beyond the expected occurrences, providers are instructed throughout the regulations to plan for hazards and disasters that are "likely to occur" in their regions. What appears to be missing in the current framework of nursing home preparedness is explicit consideration of the unexpected crisis (e.g., a weather system that brings arctic air thousands of miles south [Winter Storm Uri]) or the expected event that is unexpected in its scope or severity (e.g., a hurricane that knocks out power to an entire state or region [Hurricane Irma]). The questions also loom for assisted living, with state-by-state and potentially lesser regulation.

Given the changing nature of disasters, prescriptive regulations may not be enough to ensure preparedness, suggesting there is a need for a complementary approach that centers on activities that are more closely linked to the daily functions of a healthcare organization. Researchers have suggested adapting the 4Ms paradigm (What Matters, Medication, Mentation, and Mobility) to disaster preparedness planning (Dosa et al., 2023). This approach focused on nursing home preparedness but relates as well to assisted living. The potential is described as follows:

What Matters involves ensuring that residents and family members have a voice in the development of a disaster plan and that residents' advance care preferences are known and documented in resident records. It could additionally help to ensure residents have all possible comforts (e.g., hot food, comfortable bedding, preferred items, and activities) and minimal disruptions to their daily routines, acknowledging that some disruption may be unavoidable. During a disaster, residents should also be afforded the support of family, friends, and preferred staff members who know what matters to them.

Medications are another consideration. Nursing home residents receive, on average, nine prescribed medications daily (Moore et al., 2014). Timely administration during an emergency is critical for the management of multiple chronic conditions (e.g., congestive heart failure, diabetes). Research following Hurricanes Katrina and Rita noted that one third of all visits to EDs in the days following the hurricane occurred due to chronic medical illness (Miller & Arquilla, 2008). Disasters that involve heat-related exposure are particularly problematic for residents who become dehydrated, which can alter the function of many medications. Access to other medications, such as antibiotics and anxiolytics, is essential but may also interact with residents' prescribed medications.

Mentation deals with identifying, treating, and managing dementia, depression, and delirium. Given research showing that up to half of nursing home residents are living with dementia, it is critical to consider the anxiety that changing residents' schedules or environments can evoke. Transfer trauma from evacuation can erode cognitive and physical functioning (Brown et al., 2012; Dosa et al., 2012). Beyond paying special attention to those with dementia, identifying those with higher levels of cognition can be helpful in a disaster, because they may be willing to provide emotional support to other residents while staff are otherwise occupied.

Mobility addresses the importance of knowing and meeting residents' mobility needs, because disaster preparedness often requires residents to be physically moved. Previous research has revealed that even under optimal circumstances, nursing home residents who are moved in healthcare transitions are at heightened risk of mortality and morbidity from falls (Hoffman et al., 2019). Research specific to disasters has identified functional impairment and mobility as key factors contributing to increased morbidity and mortality following a hurricane (Thomas et al., 2012). Additional research has highlighted mobility as critical in the decision of whether to evacuate or shelter-in-place, and especially critical in disasters requiring a rapid response (e.g., sudden flooding, wildfires; FHCA, 2008). Overall, the success of a nursing home or assisted living disaster plan hinges on how well it assesses all residents' mobility risks and secures the spaces, supplies, equipment, and staff members necessary to provide for their safety and comfort as they are transferred.

Marshaling staff and resources is a fifth M suggested in research (Dosa et al., 2023) to address the organizational factors—having the necessary staff, equipment, and supplies—needed to provide undisrupted care to residents despite the disruptions of an emergency. See Figure 8.3 for a diagram of the 5Ms approach in the context of the steps to developing an age friendly healthcare environment (Dosa et al., 2023). Adequate nursing and support staff are among the core needs of a LTC facility during a disaster. Direct-care nurse staffing levels are strongly associated with the quality of resident care, given their knowledge of resident needs and the resources needed to meet those needs. A higher skill mix (i.e., a greater ratio of RNs to LPNs and certified nursing assistants [CNAs]) is associated with lower avoidable hospitalization rates (Xing et al., 2013) and fewer ED visits

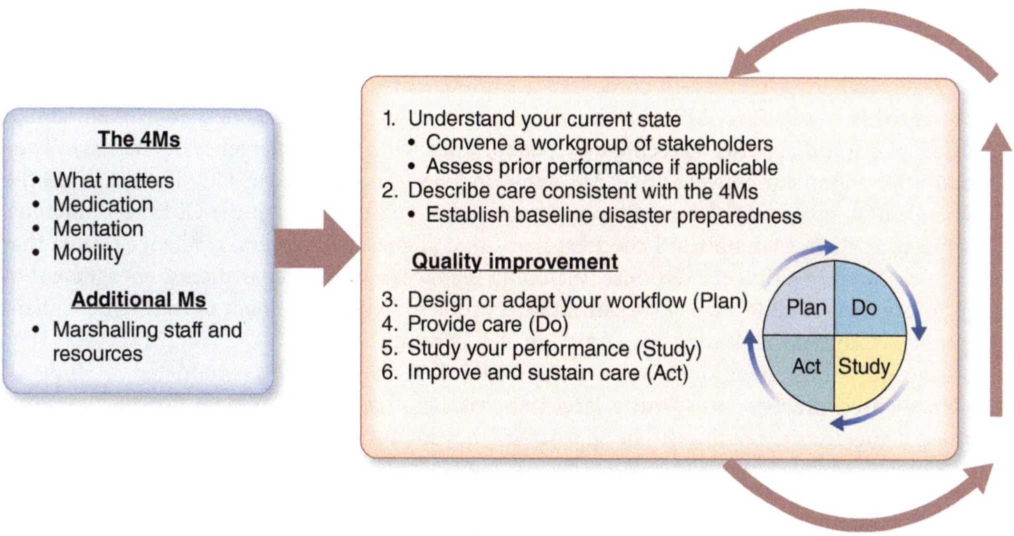

FIGURE 8.3. The Institute for Healthcare Improvement's six steps to developing an age-griendly healthcare environment, in relation to the 5Ms approach to disaster preparedness in long-term care.

Source: Dosa, D. M., Jester, D., Peterson, L., Dobbs, D., Black, K., & Brown, L. (2023). Applying the age-friendly-health system 4M paradigm to reframe climate-related disaster preparedness for nursing home populations. *Health Services Research, 58*, 36–43. https://doi.org/10.1111/1475-6773.14043

(Yang et al., 2021). Prior work from Hurricane Irma suggests that nursing homes increase direct-care nurse staff in preparation for major hurricanes, but that evacuating a facility requires an even greater staffing response (Jester et al., 2021). Full preparedness additionally requires communication and collaboration with outside entities, such as health officials, emergency managers, and first responders, who can communicate the expected severity of a threat and help a nursing home meet unexpected needs. Overall, the value of viewing preparedness through a 4Ms or 5Ms lens is that it brings disaster preparedness to a person-centered level and shows that several key preparedness tasks (e.g., administering medications, attending to residents' mobility needs) are no different from those required every day in a nursing home or assisted living community.

Lane and McGrady (2018) proposed another way of reconceptualizing disaster preparedness, focusing on the idea of building organizational resilience and the use of a resilience benchmark tool. The tool used the following indicators of a facility's ability to adapt (adaptive capacity) to an unexpected circumstance:

- minimization of silos
- internal resources
- staff engagement and involvement
- information and knowledge
- leadership
- innovation and creativity
- decision-making
- situation monitoring and reporting

The tool additionally used these indicators of planning:

- planning strategies
- participation in exercises
- proactive posture
- external resources
- recovery priorities

The researchers systematically compared the resilience tool with a CMS disaster checklist that represented the tasks the CMS considered most important for preparedness (e.g., maintaining staffing plans and supplier agreements, collaborating with local emergency managers). They found poor alignment between the CMS items and several adaptive capacity indicators on the resilience tool, suggesting the need for approaches that go beyond what the CMS recommends. For instance, there were no CMS checklist items that aligned with several resilience factors that can be essential in a disaster response, including teamwork across departments, engagement of staff to use their skills to manage organizational problems, encouragement of staff to be vigilant to problems, and having leaders who function well in crises.

Using an implementation science perspective, Bell et al. (2023) conducted a study of evidence-based practices to identify larger approaches that could improve nursing home or assisted living disaster readiness. The approaches they identified and their benefits are as follows:

- Increasing Staff Engagement in Emergency Preparedness Planning:
  - involves multiple levels of nursing home staff, including direct care workers
  - uses diverse perspectives to identify specific barriers and facilitators of best emergency preparedness practices
  - promotes peer-to-peer dissemination of readiness approaches and initiatives
- Tailoring Emergency Preparedness Plans to Facility Needs:
  - matches strategies to specific barriers and facilitators

- uses facility-specific analyses to adapt emergency preparedness plans to meet the facility's needs
- promotes age-friendly approaches to disaster preparedness, such as the 5Ms
- Improving Integration of LTC Facilities Into Healthcare Readiness Initiatives:
  - facilitates joint planning with emergency management officials
  - broadens emergency preparedness collaborations through network weaving and coalition building
  - promotes information and resource sharing during disasters

SUMMARY

These varied ways of viewing disaster preparedness include multiple overlapping elements, such as engagement of multiple staff members in plan development, and they show the value of using larger frameworks to guide nursing home disaster planning. Qualitative research on nursing home and assisted living community responses to climate disasters and the COVID-19 emergency found that staff frequently confronted emergency situations and challenges they never expected and did not plan for. And many provided examples of creative solutions, such as a nursing home administrator near the beach persuading a nearby resort to lend its spacious beach chairs during a hurricane so family members and residents sheltering in the facility would have places to rest. Others gave examples of leadership, such as cleaning showers side by side with nurse aides when a hurricane left them low on staff (Peterson et al., 2021). Some described being better equipped to manage the COVID-19 emergency because staff members were cross trained. Others discussed the importance of being decisive when regulations were unclear or even harmful to residents, such as allowing in-person visits for residents with dementia who severely missed seeing their loved ones (Hackett et al., 2023). Improving the safety of nursing home and assisted living residents in emergencies and disasters still requires regulatory approaches. However, preparedness can be reframed, not only as a set of procedures outlined in a large binder, but as a set of larger regular practices. These practices include cross training staff, nurturing natural leaders, building relationships with family members and public officials who can be resources in a crisis, integrating technology that facilitates communication everyday as well as during a disaster. Many LTC facilities already do this and can be trained and encouraged to continue these practices and share them with their industry partners.

Take-Home Points

- Federal regulations have evolved since Hurricane Katrina to require nursing homes funded by Medicare and Medicaid to develop and maintain all-hazard disaster plans that address a wide range of needs, including food, water, power supplies, and staffing for sheltering in place and evacuation; communication with families; collaboration with local health and safety officials; and testing a plan's effectiveness.
- Residents of LTC facilities are more likely to die, be hospitalized, or need emergency treatment in the weeks after exposure to a disaster, such as a hurricane, meaning that data that counts only those harmed during or immediately after an event will underestimate the effect on residents of LTC facilities.
- Even with federal regulation, and additional regulation in some states, administrators of both nursing homes and assisted living communities are often confronted with unexpected challenges during a disaster, the management of which requires ingenuity and leadership.
- Plans designed only to adhere to regulations may not be sufficient to provide needed protections to residents of LTC facilities affected by an emergency or disaster. Full preparedness requires the application of more holistic, broadly designed approaches to care.

- Working and communicating with community, public health, and safety organizations during normal times and in the preparation of disaster plans is essential for LTC facilities, given they may need emergency help from individuals and organizations in their communities before, during or after a disaster occurs.

END-OF-CHAPTER RESOURCES

DISCUSSION QUESTIONS

1. Which older adults are more vulnerable to harm in an emergency or disaster and why are LTC residents considered to be at even higher risk? What chronic conditions increase a resident's risk of harm in a disaster and why?
2. Why are statistics on casualties that occur during a disaster unlikely to provide a clear picture of the risks for nursing home residents?
3. What are the critical factors for an LTC administrator to consider before evacuating residents in a disaster, why are these factors important, and how can a long-term facility minimize evacuation risks for residents?
4. How would a 5Ms or resilience-focused approach lead to a higher level of disaster preparedness than an approach that follows only federal regulatory preparedness requirements?
5. Why do LTC facilities continue to struggle with disaster preparedness, despite the availability of multiple tools, reports, and documents to guide the development of emergency and disaster plans?
6. What steps can LTC administrators take to ensure, to the greatest extent possible, that their disaster preparedness plans are adequate to protect their residents?

TOOLS FOR FURTHER LEARNING

- *CMS and Disasters: Resources at Your Fingertips*, ASPR TRACIE: https://files.asprtracie.hhs.gov/documents/cms-ep-rule-resources-at-your-fingertips.pdf
- *2017–2022 Health Care Preparedness and Response Capabilities*, Office of the Assistant Secretary of Preparedness and Response: https://aspr.hhs.gov/HealthCareReadiness/guidance/Documents/Health-Care-Preparedness-and-Response-Capabilities-for-Health-Care-Coalitions.pdf
- *Toolkit on State Actions to Mitigate COVID-19 Prevalence in Nursing Homes*, Centers for Medicare & Medicaid Services: https://www.cms.gov/files/document/covid-toolkit-states-mitigate-covid-19-nursing-homes.pdf
- *Long-Term Care Preparedness Toolkit*, Minnesota Department of Health: https://www.health.state.mn.us/communities/ep/ltc/baseplan.pdf
- *Toolkit: Insights for Health Care Facilities From OIG's Historical Work on Emergency Response*, U.S. Office of Inspector General: https://oig.hhs.gov/reports-and-publications/featured-topics/response/toolkit-healthcare.asp
- *State Health Care Coalitions*, Centers for Medicare & Medicaid Services: https://www.cms.gov/about-cms/what-we-do/emergency-response/providers-states-tribes/state-health-care-coalitions

SPRINGER PUBLISHING CONNECT™

A robust set of instructor resources designed to supplement this text is located at http://connect.springerpub.com/content/book/978-0-8261-4935-0. Qualifying instructors may request access by emailing textbook@springerpub.com.

REFERENCES

Abrams, H. R., Loomer, L., Gandhi, A., & Grabowski, D. C. (2020). Characteristics of U.S. nursing homes with COVID-19 cases. *Journal of the American Geriatrics Society, 68*(8), 1653–1656. https://doi.org/10.1111/jgs.16661

Bell, S. A., Donnelly, J. P., Li, W., & Davis, M. A. (2022). Hospitalizations for chronic conditions following hurricanes among older adults: A self-controlled case series analysis. *Journal of the American Geriatrics Society, 70*(6), 1695–1703. https://doi.org/10.1111/jgs.17702

Bell, S. A., Inloes, J. B., Donnelly, J., Wasserman, M., & Wyte-Lake, T. (2023). Improving nursing home disaster readiness through implementation science. *Journal of the American Medical Directors Association, 25*(4), 617–622. https://doi.org/10.1016/j.jamda.2023.02.004

Berklan, J. M. (2023, February 27). *"No win" scenario in Hollywood Hills manslaughter case leads to nursing home administrators' acquittal.* McKnights. https://www.mcknights.com/news/no-win-scenario-in-hollywood-hills-manslaughter-case-leads-to-nursing-home-administrators-acquittal

Brown, L. M., Dosa, D. M., Thomas, K., Hyer, K., Feng, Z., & Mor, V. (2012). The effects of evacuation on nursing home residents with dementia. *American Journal of Alzheimer's Disease & Other Dementias, 27*(6), 406–412. https:/doi.org/10.1177/1533317512454709

Castle, N. G., & Engberg, J. B. (2011). The health consequences of relocation for nursing home residents following Hurricane Katrina. *Research on Aging, 33*(6), 661–687. https://doi.org/10.1177/0164027511412197

Centers for Medicare & Medicaid Services. (2021). *Updated guidance for emergency preparedness: Appendix Z of the State Operations Manual (SOM).* https://www.cms.gov/medicareprovider-enrollment-and-certificationsurveycertificationgeninfopolicy-and-memos-states-and/updated-guidance-emergency-preparedness-appendix-z-state-operations-manual-som

Chidambaram, P. (2022, February 3). *Over 200,000 residents and staff in long term care facilities have died from COVID-19.* KFF. https:/www.kff.org/policy-watch/over-200000-residents-and-staff-in-long-term-care-facilities-have-died-from-covid-19

Chidambaram, P., & Musumeci, M. B. (2022, February 17). *Nursing home staff vaccination rates vary widely by state as vaccination mandates take effect.* KFF. https://www.kff.org/coronavirus-covid-19/issue-brief/nursing-home-staff-vaccination-rates-vary-widely-by-state-as-vaccination-mandates-take-effect

City of Austin. (2021, October 27). *City of Austin and Travis County Winter Storm Uri after-action report & improvement plan technical report.* https://www.austintexas.gov/sites/default/files/files/HSEM/Winter-Storm-Uri-AAR-and-Improvement-Plan-Technical-Report.pdf

Dosa, D. M., Feng, Z., Hyer, K., Brown, L. M., Thomas, K., & Mor, V. (2010). Effects of Hurricane Katrina on nursing facility resident mortality, hospitalization, and functional decline. *Disaster Medicine and Public Health Preparedness, 4*(S1), S280–S32. https://doi.org/10.1001/dmp.2010.11

Dosa, D. M., Hyer, K., Thomas, K., Swaminathan, S., Feng, Z., Brown, L., & Mor, V. (2012). To evacuate or shelter in place: Implications of universal hurricane evacuation policies on nursing home residents. *Journal of the American Medical Directors Association, 13*(2), 190. E10–190.E7. https://doi.org/10.1016/j.jamda.2011.07.011

Dosa, D. M., Jester, D., Peterson, L., Dobbs, D., Black, K., & Brown, L. (2023). Applying the age-friendly-health system 4M paradigm to reframe climate-related disaster preparedness for nursing home populations. *Health Services Research, 58*, 36–43. https://doi.org/10.1111/1475-6773.14043

Dosa, D. M., Skarha, J., Peterson, L. J., Jester, D. J., Sakib, N., Ogarek, J., Thomas, K. S., Andel, R., & Hyer, K. (2020). Association between exposure to Hurricane Irma and mortality and hospitalization in Florida nursing home residents. *JAMA Network Open, 3*(10), e2019460. https://doi.org/10.1001/jamanetworkopen.2020.19460

Federal Emergency Management Agency. (2019, October 28). *National Response Framework* (4th ed.). U.S. Department of Homeland Security. https://www.fema.gov/sites/default/files/2020-04/NRF_FINALApproved_2011028.pdf

Festa, N., Heaphy, N. M., Throgmorton, K. F., Canavan, M., & Gill, T. M. (2023). Evaluating California nursing homes' emergency preparedness for wildfire exposure. *Journal of the American Geriatrics Society, 71*(3), 895–902. https://doi.org/10.1111/jgs.18142

Festa, N., Throgmorton, K. F., Davis-Plourde, K., Dosa, D. M., Chen, K., Zang, E., Kelly, J., & Gill, T. M. (2023). Assessment of regional nursing home preparedness for and regulatory responsiveness to wildfire risk in the Western US. *JAMA Network Open, 6*(6), e2320207. https://doi.org/10.1001/jamanetworkopen.2023.20207

Florida Health Care Association. (2008). *National criteria for evacuation decision-making in nursing homes.* https://www.fhca.org/images/uploads/NationalCriteriaforEvacuationDecision-Making2008.pdf

Fraser, J., & Penzenstadler, N. (2023, January 5). This nursing home chain reported highest COVID death rate. Then it deleted deaths. *USA Today.* https://www.usatoday.com/story/news/investigations/2022/04/15/trilogy-nursing-home-deletes-covid-deaths-medicare-medicaid-investigate/7319020001. (Original work published April 15, 2022)

Gadbois, E. A., Brazier, J. F., Meehan, A., Madrigal, C., White, E. M., Rafat, A., Grabowski, D., & Shield, R. R. (2023). COVID-19 Vaccination among skilled nursing facility staff: Challenges and strategies identified by administrators. *Medical Care Research and Review, 80*(6), 608–618. https://doi.org/10.1177/10775587231168435

Hackett, S. E., Peterson, L. J., Vogel, C. E., & Dobbs, D. (2023). "We did more damage": How COVID-19 collapsed the care convoys of residents living with dementia. *Journal of Applied Gerontology, 42*(7), 1565–1573. https://doi.org/10.1177/07334648231162360

Harper, S. (2023). The implications of climate change for the health of older adults. *Journal of Population Ageing, 16*(3), 565–568. https://doi.org/10.1007/s12062 023-09425-6

Hoffman, G. J., Liu, H., Alexander, N. B., Tinetti, M., Braun, T. M., & Min, L. C. (2019). Posthospital fall injuries and 30-day readmissions in adults 65 years and older. *JAMA Network Open, 2*(5), e194276. https://doi.org/10.1001/jamanetworkopen.2019.4276

Hua, C. L., Patel, S., Thomas, K. S., Jester, D. J., Kosar, C. M., Peterson, L. J., Dobbs, D., Andel, R., & Dosa, D. M. (2024). Evacuation and health care outcomes among assisted living residents after Hurricane Irma. *JAMA Network Open, 7*(4), e248572. https://doi.org/10.1001/jamanetworkopen.2024.8572

Hua, C. L., Patel, S., Thomas, K. S., Peterson, L. J., Andel, R., Gordon, L., Jester, D. J., & Dosa, D. M. (2023). The relationship between exposure to Hurricane Harvey and mortality among nursing home residents. *Journal of the American Geriatrics Society, 71*(3), 888–894. https://doi.org/10.1111/jgs.18143

Hua, C. L., Thomas, K. S., Peterson, L. J., Hyer, K., & Dosa, D. M. (2021). Emergency department use among assisted living residents after Hurricane Irma. *Journal of the American Medical Directors Association, 22*(4), 918–922. https://doi.org/10.1016/j.jamda.2020.10.010

Hyer, K., Brown, L. M., Polivka-West, L., & Berman, A. (2010). Helping nursing homes prepare for disasters. *Health Affairs, 29*(10), 1961–1965. https://doi.org/10.1377/hlthaff.2010.0665

Jester, D. J., Thomas, K. S., Peterson, L. J., Dosa, D. M., Andel, R., & Hyer, K. (2021). Effect of Hurricane Irma on daily direct-care nurse staffing in nursing homes. *Journal of the American Geriatrics Society, 69*(8), 2298–2305. https://doi.org/10.1111/jgs.17220

LaGanga, M.L. (2018, November 17). California fire: If you stay, you're dead. How a Paradise nursing home evacuated. *Los Angeles Times.* https://www.latimes.com/local/california/la-me-ln-nursing-home-fire-evac-20181117-story.html

Lane, S. J., & McGrady, E. (2018). Measures of emergency preparedness contributing to nursing home resilience. *Journal of Gerontological Social Work, 61*(7), 751–774. https://doi.org/10.1080/01634372.2017.1416720

Malik, S., Lee, D. C., Doran, K. M., Grudzen, C. R., Worthing, J., Portelli, I., Goldfrank, L. R., & Smith, S. W. (2018). Vulnerability of older adults in disasters: Emergency department utilization by geriatric patients after Hurricane Sandy. *Disaster Medicine and Public Health Preparedness, 12*(2), 184–193. https:/doi.org/10.1017/dmp.2017.44

Miller, A. C., & Arquilla, B. (2008). Chronic diseases and natural hazards: Impact of disasters on diabetic, renal, and cardiac patients. *Prehospital and Disaster Medicine, 23*(2), 185–194. https://asprtracie.hhs.gov/technical-resources/resource/2872/chronic-diseases-and-natural-hazards-impact-of-disasters-on-diabetic-renal-and-cardiac-patients

Moore, K. L., Boscardin, W. J., Steinman, M. A., & Schwartz, J. B. (2014). Patterns of chronic co-morbid medical conditions in older residents of US nursing homes: Differences between the sexes and across the agespan. *The Journal of Nutrition, Health & Aging, 18*, 429–436. https://doi.org/10.1007/s12603-014-0001-y

Office of Inspector General. (2006, August). *Nursing home emergency preparedness and response during recent hurricanes* (OEI-06-06-00020). U.S. Department of Health & Human Services. https://oig.hhs.gov/oei/reports/oei-06-06-00020.pdf

Office of Inspector General. (2012, April). *Gaps continue to exist in nursing home emergency preparedness and response during disasters: 2007–2010* (OEI-06-09-00270). U.S. Department of Health & Human Services. https://oig.hhs.gov/documents/evaluation/2956/OEI-06-09-00270-Complete%20Report.pdf

Office of Inspector General. (2020, March). *Florida should improve its oversight of selected nursing homes' compliance with federal requirements for life safety and emergency preparedness* (Report No. A-04-18-08065). U.S. Department of Health & Human Services. https://oig.hhs.gov/documents/audit/7317/A-04-18-08065-Complete%20Report.pdf

Office of Inspector General. (2022, July). *Audits of nursing home life safety and emergency preparedness in eight states identified noncompliance with federal requirements and opportunities for the Center for Medicare & Medicaid Services to Improve Resident, Visitor, and Staff Safety* (A-02-21-01010). U.S. Department of Health & Human Services. https://oig.hhs.gov/documents/audit/6534/A-02-21-01010-Complete%20Report.pdf

Pearce, M. (2017, September 29). After Harvey hit, one Texas nursing home evacuation began with a gun drawn. *Los Angeles Times*. https://www.latimes.com/nation/la-na-texas-harvey-nursing-homes-20170929-story.html

Peterson, L. J., Dobbs, D., June, J., Dosa, D. M., & Hyer, K. (2021). "You just forge ahead": The continuing challenges of disaster preparedness and response in long-term care. *Innovation in Aging*, *5*(4), igab038. https://doi.org/10.1093/geroni/igab038

Sinha, S., & Konetzka, R. T. (2022). Association of COVID-19 vaccination rates of staff and COVID-19 illness and death among residents and staff in US nursing homes. *JAMA Network Open*, *5*(12), e2249002. https://doi.org/10.1001/jamanetworkopen.2022.49002

Skarha, J., Gordon, L., Sakib, N., June, J., Jester, D. J., Peterson, L. J., Andel, R., & Dosa, D. M. (2021). Association of power outage with mortality and hospitalizations among Florida nursing home residents after Hurricane Irma. *JAMA Health Forum*, *2*(11), e213900. https://doi.org/10.1001/jamahealthforum.2021.3900

Smith, A. B. (2021, January 8). *2020 U.S. billion-dollar weather and climate disastersin historical context*. https://www.climate.gov/disasters2020

Stempniak, M. (2018). *Wildfire destroys three skilled nursing facilities*. McKnights. https://www.mcknights.com/news/camp-fire-destroys-three-skilled-nursing-facilities

Thomas, K. S., Dosa, D., Hyer, K., Brown, L. M., Swaminathan, S., Feng, Z., & Mor, V. (2012). Effect of forced transitions on the most functionally impaired nursing home residents. *Journal of the American Geriatrics Society*, *60*(10), 1895–1900. https://doi.org/10.1111/j.1532-5415.2012.04146.x

Turco, M., Abatzoglou, J. T., Herrera, S., Zhuang, Y., Jerez, S., Lucas, D. D., AghaKouchak, A., & Cvijanovic, I. (2023). Anthropogenic climate change impacts exacerbate summer forest fires in California. *Proceedings of the National Academy of Sciences*, *120*(25), e2213815120. https://doi.org/10.1073/pnas.2213815120

U.S. Senate Finance Committee, & U.S. Senate Special Committee on Aging. (2023). *Left in the dark: The impact of the 2021 Texas blackout on long-term care residents and the need to improve emergency preparedness*. https://www.finance.senate.gov/imo/media/doc/02222023%20Left%20in%20the%20Dark%20-%20Wyden-Casey%20final.pdf

West, S. (2021, March 10). *Texas winter storm exposes gaps in senior living oversight*. KFF Health News. https://khn.org/news/article/texas-winter-storm-exposes-gaps-in-senior-living-oversight

White, E. M., Wetle, T. F., Reddy, A., & Baier, R. R. (2021). Front-line nursing home staff experiences during the COVID-19 pandemic. *Journal of the American Medical Directors Association*, *22*(1), 199–203. https://doi.org/10.1016/j.jamda.2020.11.022

Xing, J., Mukamel, D. B., & Temkin-Greener, H. (2013). Hospitalizations of nursing home residents in the last year of life: Nursing home characteristics and variation in potentially avoidable hospitalizations. *Journal of the American Geriatrics Society*, *61*(11), 1900–1908. https://doi.org/10.1111/jgs.12517

Yang, B. K., Carter, M. W., Trinkoff, A. M., & Nelson, H. W. (2021). Nurse staffing and skill mix patterns in relation to resident care outcomes in US nursing homes. *Journal of the American Medical Directors Association*, *22*(5), 1081–1087. https://doi.org/10.1016/j.jamda.2020.09.009

PART III

STRATEGIES FOR CONTINUOUS IMPROVEMENT OF QUALITY AND SAFETY

CHAPTER 9

NAVIGATING HEALTHCARE DISPARITIES IN LONG-TERM CARE

Darren Liu and Betty Burston

Learning Objectives

After completing this chapter, each learner will be able to:

- Identify the objectives of the National Healthcare Quality and Disparities Report and the long-term care (LTC) facilities it covers.
- Explain how healthcare disparities influence LTC options and the quality and safety of care.
- Evaluate the potential role of public report cards in exacerbating disparities in access to higher-quality nursing homes.
- Critically evaluate the effectiveness of different strategies for reducing healthcare disparities, such as increasing staffing levels, improving training and education for LTC workers, implementing cultural competency training, involving family caregivers more actively, and using technology to improve communication and care coordination.

INTRODUCTION

Persistent disparities within the realm of long-term care (LTC) have resulted in unequal access to essential services, variable adherence to care plans, and distinct health outcomes across demographic groups, directly impacting the overall quality of care within these facilities (Shippee, Akosionu, et al., 2020). Discrepancies in factors such as medication adherence or safety incidents disproportionately affect certain ethnic or socioeconomic groups, posing risks to consumers' safety, well-being, and overall satisfaction with care services. Adding to the complexity, the substantial expenses associated with LTC significantly contribute to unequal access, particularly affecting individuals from marginalized communities who often find themselves compelled toward lower-quality care options. These disparities extend beyond financial considerations, intricately intertwining with factors such as socioeconomic status, ethnicity, cultural nuances, and resource availability.

A recent report by the National Academies of Sciences, Engineering, and Medicine (NASEM; 2022) highlights the fact that disparities in quality of life and care in the nursing home sector are influenced by a range of factors. For instance, disparities among racial and ethnic minorities are often linked to the facility's racial composition and staffing levels, which can increase the risk of poor-quality care. Moreover, long-standing systemic issues such as neighborhood segregation, racism, and ageism have deeply affected healthcare practices and policies, contributing to the ongoing failures in LTC, including nursing home care. These ingrained inequalities have shaped the structure and delivery of care, resulting in persistent shortcomings that disproportionately affect vulnerable populations. The report also highlights data constraints, privacy-related issues, and the lack of robust data specific to race and ethnicity as challenges that make it difficult to fully understand the extent and impact of disparities in care (NASEM, 2022, p. 12).

Understanding the root causes of these disparities through data analysis is crucial, given the staggering costs of LTC which now exceeds $467.1 billion (about $1,400 per person in the United States) annually (Colello, 2023). The resultant financial burdens disproportionately affect specific demographic groups, leading to varying levels of access and care quality for those reliant on Medicaid or Medicare programs, and thereby perpetuating a cycle of financial and health-related challenges (Gorges et al., 2019).

This chapter seeks to offer a comprehensive examination of healthcare disparities within LTC settings by emphasizing their impact on the quality and safety of care delivery. Through an exploration of the multifaceted influences of disparities, we aim to elucidate their correlation with various concerns pertinent to LTC. Furthermore, the chapter introduces strategies for addressing and analyzing healthcare outcomes, and provides valuable insights to inform the design of interventions. By illuminating pathways to enhance care quality and safety, this chapter endeavors to contribute to the mitigation of healthcare disparities in LTC.

DEFINITIONS AND CONCEPTS: HEALTH INEQUALITIES

The study of *health inequalities* has a rich history that spans several decades. Exploring health inequalities involves examining differences in health status and outcomes among diverse populations, particularly regarding social, economic, and environmental factors. The origins of the term *health inequalities* can be traced back to the 1960s in the United Kingdom when researchers and social reformers explored the link between social class and health. This research revealed a clear *gradient*, demonstrating that individuals in higher social classes tended to have better health outcomes, even with uniform access to healthcare (Marmot et al., 1991).

Subsequent research has highlighted systematic differences across social groups or classes in the distribution of health outcomes, such as morbidity, mortality, and life expectancy (Scambler & Higgs, 1999). These variations can be categorized as avoidable or unavoidable factors. Avoidable factors, such as challenges associated with healthcare accessibility, socioeconomic disparities, and specific environmental conditions, can be mitigated through targeted interventions and policies. Unavoidable factors, which may not be entirely preventable, include genetic predispositions, age, and sex.

While the initial discussion primarily addresses disparities in health outcomes and their underlying causes, it is crucial to recognize that these inequalities extend beyond mere differences in health status or outcomes. They encompass a wide array of influences, including the prevalence of diseases such as diabetes, genetic predispositions, socioeconomic status, access to education, and access to care. This broader perspective offers a more comprehensive understanding of the complex factors contributing to healthcare disparities within diverse populations.

In recent years, interdisciplinary approaches have gained prominence in the study of health inequalities, incorporating the fields of social epidemiology, medicine, anthropology, and population health management (D. Liu et al., 2018, pp. 31–51). Scholars in these disciplines extensively explore the unequal distribution of health risks and resources by considering factors such as socioeconomic status, race/ethnicity, gender, age, geographical location, and other determinants. This holistic examination allows for a comprehensive understanding of the social, cultural, and structural determinants contributing to health disparities (Krieger et al., 1997).

Contemporary research often uses the term *health disparities*, thereby inheriting the definition of health inequalities, but focusing primarily on avoidable (remediable) differences and unjust inequalities in health and healthcare among distinct population groups. *Healthcare disparities*, on the other hand, target inequities in processes and outcomes related to access to and use of care, health insurance coverage, and quality of healthcare services (Agency for Healthcare Research and Quality [AHRQ], 2023; D. Liu et al., 2018)

While the terms *health inequality*, *health disparities*, and *healthcare disparities* are often used interchangeably, they differ slightly in emphasis and scope. This chapter establishes a framework in which healthcare disparities focus on inequalities in both access to and the quality of medical services within long-term services and supports (LTSS). The overarching goal is to achieve *health equity*, characterized by the fair distribution of health determinants, outcomes, and resources among various segments of the aging population, regardless of their social standing. This goal aligns with the objectives outlined in *The National Institute on Aging: Strategic Directions for 2020–2025* (NIA, 2020).

THE CAUSES OF HEALTHCARE DISPARITIES IN LONG-TERM CARE

In the complex realm of LTC, healthcare disparities arise from diverse factors that impact access, care quality, and health outcomes. This section disentangles the causes of these disparities by encompassing geographic, racial, language, cultural, and age-related dimensions. Understanding these complexities is crucial for crafting interventions that meet the diverse needs of the population.

Geographic Disparities

Geographic disparities are influenced by neighborhood socioeconomic disadvantage and urban–rural distinctions, both of which play a pivotal role in shaping care outcomes (Park & Martin, 2018). In regions marked by socioeconomic disadvantage, LTC consumers face multifaceted challenges in accessing quality care. These challenges manifest as limited facility availability, insufficient staffing, and an overall diminished capacity to deliver comprehensive care, all of which contribute to significant disparities in health outcomes, quality of life, and other areas. Nursing home closures also exhibit a distinct concentration in minority and economically disadvantaged communities (Feng et al., 2011).

Urban settings, with a higher concentration of healthcare facilities, may offer a broader range of services, but challenges such as overcrowding and heightened demand can strain healthcare systems, potentially impacting the overall quality of care. Conversely, rural areas may face shortages in LTC, thereby creating significant accessibility barriers, especially with transportation challenges in remote areas (Coburn et al., 2019; Siconolfi et al., 2019). Addressing these geographic disparities is essential for targeted interventions and policies that meet diverse community needs.

Racial and Ethnic Disparities

The impact of diversity on healthcare service utilization reveals disparities along racial and ethnic lines. Residential care communities (89.4% non-Hispanic White) and hospices (82.3%) show the highest percentages. Adult day services centers emerge as the most diverse, with only 44.8% non-Hispanic White, including 16.8% non-Hispanic Black and 22.2% Hispanic individuals. In specific care settings, nursing homes have 73.3% non-Hispanic White short-stay residents (Sengupta et al., 2022).

Persisting racial and ethnic disparities in healthcare outcomes reveal systemic inequalities that impact access to essential facilities and services. For instance, nursing homes with a larger proportion of non-White consumers often experience insufficient staffing, resulting in neglect and a lower care quality (Shippee, Ng, & Bowblis, 2020). This is evident in the higher average number of deficiency citations and an increased number of complaints related to residents' rights observed in nursing homes with a significant non-White demographic (K. Lee et al., 2021; Li et al., 2015).

Disparities extend to quality-of-life scores, with higher concentrations of minorities displaying lower scores and reduced vaccination rates (Shippee, Ng, & Bowblis, 2020; Travers et al., 2018). The amplification of these disparities is further pronounced by racial segregation within nursing homes. This segregation exacerbates disparities because it can lead to differential access to resources, healthcare services, and staff attention based on residents' race or ethnicity, contributing to divergent outcomes (Smith et al., 2007).

Addressing systemic issues is crucial for promoting equitable healthcare across diverse populations. Efforts to combat racial segregation within nursing homes and other LTC settings and to improve access to resources and care for all consumers are essential steps toward achieving health equity. By dismantling institutional barriers and implementing policies that prioritize inclusivity and fairness, healthcare systems can work toward ensuring that every individual, regardless of race or ethnicity, receives the care and support they need to thrive.

Language and Cultural Disparities

Language and cultural disparities in LTC pose challenges for individuals with limited English proficiency (LEP) and diverse cultural backgrounds. These disparities result in communication barriers and misunderstandings between healthcare providers and LTC consumers. Language disparities, coupled with issues related to health literacy, hinder navigation of the LTC system, highlighting the need for inclusive and culturally competent environments (Batista et al., 2021).

For instance, consider a scenario where an older individual who primarily speaks a language other than English enters a LTC setting. The healthcare providers, predominantly English speakers, may encounter difficulties in effectively communicating vital information regarding the individual's medical history, medication instructions, and overall care plan. This language barrier can prevent individuals from fully understanding their treatment, potentially leading to complications or dissatisfaction with the care provided.

Furthermore, *cultural discordances* play a significant role in influencing expectations and preferences related to LTC (Weng & Landes, 2017). Diverse cultural norms, practices, and beliefs between care recipients and providers may impact the individual's comfort level within the care setting. For instance, traditional dietary preferences, religious practices, or specific cultural rituals may not be adequately addressed or respected, which can affect the overall well-being and satisfaction of individuals in LTC.

Addressing language and cultural disparities in LTC is crucial for providing inclusive and culturally competent environments. Healthcare providers and facilities need to implement strategies such as employing multilingual staff, offering interpretation services, and providing cultural sensitivity training to ensure effective communication and understanding between caregivers and care recipients with diverse linguistic and cultural backgrounds. This approach fosters a more inclusive and equitable LTC system.

Sex-Related Disparities

Sex-related disparities play a prominent role in healthcare workforce dynamics. For example, while women make up the majority of healthcare workers, they are often concentrated in lower-paying roles and face barriers to career advancement (Campbell, 2017). Pay inequities persist across gender and racial/ethnic lines, with women and minority healthcare workers frequently earning less than their male and White counterparts. This contributes to financial insecurity and widening socioeconomic disparities (McCall & Scales, 2022).

However, sex-related disparities also stem from other causes. Addressing disparities related to sexual orientation and gender identity requires understanding the unique challenges faced by sexual and gender minorities, particularly LGBTQ individuals. The term *LGBTQ+* represents a spectrum of identities, including those beyond the initial letters, such as asexuality and intersexuality, which are often overlooked in mainstream discourse. Concerns about dependence on healthcare providers, the higher prevalence of dementia, mistreatment, and social isolation can contribute to identity concealment and psychologic distress, including thoughts of suicide (Putney et al., 2018).

Comprehensive efforts are needed to combat discrimination effectively, from interpersonal interventions to policy changes, aiming to enhance the health and well-being of aging LGBTQ+ populations. This requires an intersectional approach, actively engaging underrepresented LGBTQ+ older communities. By fostering inclusive research, we can address the diverse experiences of LGBTQ+ older survivors of sexual violence, LGBTQ+ older adults of color, older LGBTQ+ immigrants, and older bisexual individuals (Lampe et al., 2024).

Age-Related Disparities

Age-related disparities in LTC refer to differences or inequalities in various aspects of life that arise due to age differences among individuals or groups within aging populations. These disparities, stemming from ageism and ableism, significantly impact the well-being of older individuals and those with disabilities within the healthcare system.

Ageism refers to prejudice or discrimination against individuals based on their age, often leading to negative stereotypes, unequal treatment, and limited access to healthcare services (D. Liu, Burston, et al., 2020, pp. 7–10). *Ableism* involves discrimination against individuals with disabilities, devaluing their abilities and creating barriers to full participation in society, including healthcare (D. Liu, Burston, et al., 2020, p. 12). These biases manifest in various forms, such as assumptions about cognitive decline or limited capacity for older adults, and overlooking the healthcare needs and rights of individuals with disabilities. Such systemic prejudices not only undermine the dignity and rights of these populations but also result in disparities in access to healthcare, employment opportunities, education and training, social support and services, and legal and policy issues (Rochon et al., 2021).

Effectively addressing age-related disparities often requires targeted interventions and policies that promote equity, reduce barriers, and improve opportunities for individuals across the lifespan. Key initiatives include promoting age-friendly environments, combating ageism, enhancing healthcare access, and supporting lifelong learning and employment opportunities for people of all ages. A focus on age inclusivity has emerged strongly in higher education, particularly within gerontology programs and healthcare training, where it is recognized as essential for preparing future LTC professionals (Silverstein et al., 2022). Emphasizing age inclusivity in educational settings deepens understanding of age-related issues and fosters practices that support equity throughout life. When applied in healthcare, age-inclusive practices create systems that respect individuals of all ages, ensure equitable access to quality care, and address the unique needs of aging and disabled populations.

Disparities Amplified by Insufficient Community Resources

Insufficient community resources significantly contribute to exacerbating healthcare disparities, particularly preventive care. The absence of support services and educational programs within communities can impede individuals' access to crucial information and interventions, leading to disparities in health outcomes. This challenge is especially pronounced during the COVID-19 pandemic, where shortages of vaccine, masks, testing, and personal protective equipment disproportionately affected those reliant on LTC (Schwartz et al., 2023). Communities with barriers to healthcare access and limited resources may struggle to stay informed and access preventive measures (Chen et al., 2020). This lack of access, including healthcare facilities and transportation services, contributes to the accelerated spread of the virus within these communities, resulting in a higher incidence of cases and worsening health outcomes.

Consider a community with a high proportion of older adults who could benefit from preventive health measures such as regular screenings and wellness programs. However, due to limited resources, there is a lack of easily accessible healthcare facilities, educational materials, and tailored support services. This deficiency can lead to delayed detection of health issues, missed opportunities for early intervention, and a higher likelihood of adverse outcomes. Addressing these resource gaps is crucial for creating a proactive healthcare environment that ensures equitable access to preventive care measures.

Digital Disparities

Digital disparities, characterized by differences in technology access and digital literacy, pose significant challenges in the healthcare landscape, particularly for older adults (D. Liu, Yamashita, et al., 2020). These discrepancies can exacerbate health inequities based on differences in technology access and proficiency levels (Hall et al., 2015).

Imagine an older adult living in an area with limited internet connectivity or lacking access to essential digital devices. In such circumstances, tasks such as utilizing telehealth services or accessing health information online becomes daunting. The digital divide widens existing healthcare disparities, depriving those unable to navigate the digital realm of the advantages offered by telehealth, such as convenience, timely medical consultations, and better management of chronic conditions (D. Liu et al., 2018, pp. 146–157).

Socioeconomic status also plays a role in digital disparities. Individuals with lower income levels may struggle to afford necessary technology or lack resources to develop digital literacy skills. Effectively addressing these disparities involves implementing initiatives to enhance technology access and digital literacy, especially among older adults. Community-based programs, educational workshops, and outreach efforts emerge as crucial components, empowering individuals with the skills and resources needed to navigate the digital landscape confidently.

Disparities Stemming From Cultural Stigma and Mistrust

The intricacies of healthcare disparities are often compounded by cultural stigma and mistrust, particularly affecting communities with diverse cultural backgrounds. These factors act as significant barriers, dissuading individuals from seeking appropriate care and thereby contributing to disparities in health outcomes (Waymouth et al., 2023).

Consider a community where cultural stigma surrounds mental health, fostering fear of societal judgment or exclusion among its members. This stigma poses a formidable obstacle, leading to delayed or avoided mental health interventions and resulting in pronounced disparities in mental health outcomes compared to communities without such cultural phenomena.

In LTC facilities lacking cultural competence, consumers from diverse backgrounds encounter challenges in communication, dietary preferences, and understanding health beliefs (Raj et al., 2023). For example, consider a healthcare facility where staff members lack adequate training to navigate the cultural nuances of the residents they serve. This deficiency may lead to misunderstandings regarding treatment plans, dissatisfaction with care, and potential adverse health outcomes due to the misalignment with cultural phenomena and preferences.

Addressing cultural stigma and enhancing cultural competence within healthcare settings are crucial steps toward fostering an environment of inclusivity and reducing disparities in care outcomes.

COVID-19's Impact on Disparities

The COVID-19 pandemic has heightened the vulnerability of older adults, especially those in senior living communities, who already face disparities in healthcare access (Rozenfeld et al., 2020). Factors such as age, race/ethnicity, income, and living conditions further exacerbate this vulnerability, making LTC facilities a focal point of concern.

Among older adults, particularly people of color, there is a notable increase in emotional distress compared to their White counterparts, largely due to systemic barriers in healthcare access (Bui et al., 2021). This distress, stemming from the loss of loved ones, fear of infection, and challenges in accessing timely and appropriate healthcare, further compounds the mental health impacts of the pandemic.

Addressing the impact of the COVID-19 pandemic on health disparities requires a comprehensive and targeted approach. This involves ensuring the equitable distribution of healthcare resources, enhancing access to testing and vaccination in underserved communities, and addressing the social determinants of health (SDOH) that contribute to existing disparities. Key strategies may include providing support to LTC administrators through robust communication and relationship-building initiatives among staff, families, hospitals, health departments, and community members (Lane et al., 2023). Such efforts are essential in mitigating the disproportionate effects of the pandemic on vulnerable populations and promoting health equity.

Workforce Disparities

Workforce disparities exist within both informal care and the formal healthcare workforce, impacting the composition, experiences, and opportunities of caregivers and healthcare professionals alike. In informal caregiving, which involves approximately 53 million adults in the United States providing support to individuals with disabilities or older adults (AARP and National Alliance for Caregiving, 2020), disparities often arise due to cultural norms and societal expectations (Dilworth-Anderson et al., 2005). These caregivers, often family members or friends, play a critical role in supporting vulnerable populations but frequently face significant challenges.

A significant portion of *informal caregivers* (21%) report fair or poor health, reflecting the toll of caregiving burden on their well-being (Edwards et al., 2020). The concept of *caregiver burden* encapsulates adverse effects on emotional, social, financial, and physical well-being experienced by many caregivers (Cohen et al., 2019; Zarit et al., 1986). Women, for instance, typically assume a larger share of caregiving responsibilities compared to men (27% vs. 20%), while rural caregivers often bear heavier burdens, caring for multiple individuals (34% vs. 23% in suburban or urban areas; AARP and National Alliance for Caregiving, 2020).

The COVID-19 pandemic has exacerbated the strain on caregivers' health and well-being, adding to the challenges they face (Choi et al., 2021; University of Pittsburgh, 2020). Furthermore, experiences of caregiving burden are not uniform and vary significantly across gender and racial/ethnic lines, underscoring the importance of recognizing *intersectionality* in addressing disparities (R. Liu et al., 2022).

In the *formal* healthcare workforce, disparities manifest in various ways, including underrepresentation of minority groups and gender disparities in leadership positions and pay equity. Minority healthcare workers may encounter barriers to entry and advancement, while women face challenges such as wage gaps, limited access to leadership roles, and workplace discrimination (Scales, 2021). These disparities affect not only individual healthcare workers but also have implications for patient care and health outcomes. Thus, incorporating diverse perspectives and experiences is essential for providing high-quality and culturally competent care.

Addressing workforce disparities in both informal care and the formal healthcare workforce requires systemic changes and comprehensive strategies. Efforts should focus on promoting diversity, equity, and inclusion across all levels of the healthcare system (D. Liu, Burston, et al., 2020). This includes increasing representation of underrepresented groups, providing equal opportunities for career advancement and leadership roles, ensuring pay equity, and fostering inclusive workplace cultures.

Supporting caregiver well-being and providing resources and support for informal caregivers are essential steps in addressing disparities in caregiving burden and health outcomes. For example, the Recognize, Assist, Include, Support and Engage (RAISE) Family Caregivers Act (2018) aimed at providing education, health resources, workplace support, and financial stability. The Act's duration was later extended to 2024 under the Supporting Older Americans Act of 2020 (Reinhard et al., 2023). The Balancing Incentives Program (BIP), established under the Affordable Care Act, seeks to shift LTC from institutions to home-based settings, improving access to noninstitutional LTSS.

Through these efforts, we can work toward a more equitable and inclusive healthcare system that meets the diverse needs of both caregivers and patients. While these initiatives have shown promise, policy variations among states underscore the need for more comprehensive and consistent policies to address disparities in informal caregiving (Anastos-Wallen et al., 2020).

UNDERSTANDING THE INFLUENCES OF HEALTHCARE DISPARITIES

In the realm of healthcare inequalities, influences are the multifaceted variables that intricately influence an individual's health outcomes. A comprehensive understanding of these determinants is essential for discerning the root causes of healthcare disparities. These determinants encompass both SDOH and non-SDOH, categorizing factors based on their nature and characteristics (Hahn, 2021).

Non-Social Determinants of Health

Non-SDOH include biological factors (e.g., genetics, age, sex), healthcare system factors (e.g., access to healthcare services), and individual behavior (e.g., personal lifestyle choices, diet). While not directly tied to social and environmental contexts, these factors significantly shape health outcomes.

Social Determinants of Health

SDOH encapsulate conditions and factors in the social, economic, and physical environment that influence individuals across their lifespan. These encompass social (e.g., socioeconomic status, education, employment, social support networks), economic (e.g., income, poverty, wealth distribution), and environmental factors (e.g., housing conditions, neighborhood safety, access to healthy food, exposure to environmental pollutants). Recognizing the significance of socioeconomic status, education, employment, social networks, access to healthcare, and the physical environment is paramount, as highlighted by initiatives such as *Healthy People 2030* (Office of Disease Prevention and Health Promotion [ODPHP], n.d.-c) and the World Health Organization (WHO; n.d.).

THE INTERPLAY OF DETERMINANTS IN LONG-TERM CARE

Disparities in LTC settings manifest across multiple dimensions, shaped by factors such as race/ethnicity, nativity, gender, and disability status, creating a *social stratification* system where access to care varies in both availability and quality of care (D. Liu et al., 2018, pp. 34, 35). This complexity underscores the challenge of addressing healthcare inequalities. The convergence of these factors significantly shapes access to resources, opportunities, and life experiences, consequently affecting health outcomes. This *intersectionality*[1] is clearly evidenced by the unequal distribution of unmet care needs among diverse social groups with the consumer population (Lin & Liu, 2023).

Recognizing and navigating these intersections is crucial in developing comprehensive strategies to ensure equitable and inclusive healthcare services for all individuals, regardless of their social backgrounds. A nuanced understanding of determinants at both individual and systemic (community) levels is essential. This comprehension enables targeted interventions for individuals while addressing broader social, economic, and environmental factors that shape community health (Hatef et al., 2021).

Table 9.1 offers a detailed overview of health determinants, distinguishing between individual and systemic influences. It underscores the significance of aligning personalized healthcare interventions with systemic reforms to establish a more inclusive and equitable LTC system. Through the development of tailored care plans that accommodate financial constraints and the implementation of policy changes aimed at bridging socioeconomic gaps, this dual approach ensures a synergistic and comprehensive strategy for enhancing accessibility and equity in LTC.

[1] *Intersectionality*: A concept that describes how different aspects of an individual's identity (such as race, gender, class, sexual orientation, ability, etc.) intersect and overlap, leading to unique and interconnected forms of discrimination or privilege. Coined by *Kimberlé Crenshaw* (1991), it emphasizes that these various elements of identity don't exist independently but interact to shape experiences and societal treatment. Understanding intersectionality helps recognize how multiple forms of discrimination can compound, affecting individuals or groups differently and influencing social structures and systems.

TABLE 9.1 Mapping Health Determinants: Individual Versus Systemic Influences

DETERMINANTS	INDIVIDUAL LEVEL	SYSTEMIC LEVEL
Scope	Factors specific to an individual's characteristics	Broader societal, economic, and environmental conditions affecting groups
Examples	Health behaviors, access to care, socioeconomic status	SDOH, structural factors, intersectionality
Impact on health	Directly affects an individual's health status	Indirectly shapes health outcomes for communities and populations
Possible data source	EHRs for individual patient data	Census data, community surveys, and public health databases for community-level data
Study focus	Assessment of patient-level social needs (e.g., housing issues)	Examination of community-level SDOH impact on healthcare utilization and outcomes
Intervention strategies	Influenced by personal choices, education, lifestyle changes	Requires systemic changes such as policy reforms, community interventions
Emphasis on equity	Tailoring care to individual needs	Addressing systemic disparities, promoting health equity

EHRs, electronic health records; SDOH, social determinants of health.

Source: Date from Hatef, E., Ma, X., Rouhizadeh, M., Singh, G., Weiner, J. P., & Kharrazi, H. (2021). Assessing the impact of social needs and social determinants of health on health care utilization: Using patient-and community-level data. *Population Health Management*, *24*(2), 222–230. https://doi.org/10.1089/pop.2020.0043

Individual-Level Determinants

Individual-level determinants focus on factors specific to an individual's characteristics, such as health behaviors, access to care, and socioeconomic status. These determinants directly impact an individual's health status and are typically assessed using electronic health records (EHR) for patient-level data. Interventions targeting individual-level determinants are influenced by personal choices, education, and lifestyle changes, with an emphasis on tailoring care to individual needs for promoting health equity.

Systemic Level Determinants

Systemic level determinants pertain to broader societal, economic, and environmental conditions that affect groups rather than individuals. Examples include SDOH, structural factors, and intersectionality. Unlike individual-level determinants, systemic factors indirectly shape health outcomes for communities and populations. Data for systemic determinants are typically gathered from sources such as census data, community surveys, and public health databases, allowing for an examination of their impact on healthcare utilization and outcomes at a community level. Interventions aimed at systemic determinants necessitate systemic changes such as policy reforms and community interventions to address systemic disparities and promote health equity.

ASSESSING INEQUALITIES IN LONG-TERM CARE

Understanding and addressing healthcare disparities in LTC requires a multifaceted approach, starting with robust data sources that provide insights into the complexities of these inequalities. In this section, we explore various data sources and methodological considerations necessary for effectively measuring and analyzing disparities in LTC settings.

Data Sources

Sound, reliable, and accurate data sources are key to continuous improvements in LTC quality and safety. These datasets are essential for evaluating outcomes and assessing disparities in healthcare. They provide crucial information that helps uncover the root causes of healthcare disparities, including SDOH such as income, education, and neighborhood characteristics. By integrating data from these sources, analysts can gain comprehensive insights into the factors influencing healthcare outcomes and use that knowledge to develop strategies that effectively promote equity and address disparities.

Healthy People 2030

Healthy People 2030 provides valuable insights into healthcare disparities among the older population (ODPHP, n.d.-b). This federal initiative includes health disparities data for core objectives, with breakdowns by demographic groups such as age, race, and ethnicity. Researchers can analyze these data (ODPHP, n.d.-a) to identify and understand disparities related to these factors. By tracking changes over time, it helps researchers and policymakers to understand where improvements are needed. This enables them to assess disparities, particularly among older adults, and target interventions more effectively. Key metrics such as the highest rate (R_{max}), lowest rate (R_{min}), maximal rate difference (MRD), and rate ratios (RR) allow for a precise assessment of disparities. Additionally, its data tools summarize disparities while simultaneously highlighting priority populations. This information is crucial for policymakers and healthcare providers to tailor interventions aimed at promoting health equity. By utilizing the comprehensive data and objectives provided, stakeholders can monitor progress, focus on areas such as chronic disease prevention and management, and work toward reducing healthcare disparities among older adults.

Race, Ethnicity and Language Data

The collection and analysis of REaL (**R**ace, **E**thnicity, **a**nd **L**anguage) data play a crucial role in addressing healthcare disparities. These data capture essential information about a patient's REaL preferences. Although not mandatory, hospitals and health systems gather REaL data during patient interactions to better understand the demographics of their communities. By analyzing REaL data, healthcare providers can identify disparities, develop patient-centered strategies, and work toward advancing health equity (Rowen et al., 2022).

Healthcare systems are encouraged to integrate REaL data collection into quality improvement initiatives. Utilizing national, regional, and state resources helps ensure the data's relevance and accuracy. Regularly reviewing, revising, and refining data collection processes and categories is essential for maintaining their effectiveness. By leveraging REaL data, healthcare organizations can (American Hospital Association [AHA], 2020):

1. *Capture patient demographics:* Understand the REaL preferences of patients to gain insights into their unique healthcare needs.
2. *Deliver culturally competent care:* Apply care practices that respect and accommodate patients' cultural backgrounds, ensuring that care quality does not vary based on race, ethnicity, or language.
3. *Stratify quality metrics:* Analyze healthcare quality metrics by different demographic groups to identify and address disparities.

Ultimately, the strategic use of REaL data enables healthcare providers to offer more personalized and equitable care, fostering an inclusive healthcare environment that meets the diverse needs of all patients (W. C. Lee et al., 2016).

Centers for Medicare & Medicaid Services Minimum Data Set

To study healthcare disparities in nursing home care, researchers typically employ various datasets and methodologies. One common approach involves analyzing datasets such as the

Minimum Data Set (MDS), which systematically collects comprehensive data on residents' health, functional abilities, and service needs within nursing homes. By leveraging this data alongside other sources such as hospitalization records, demographic information, and facility characteristics, researchers can assess quality measures and disparities based on factors such as REaL preferences. These analyses can reveal significant disparities in quality measures and star ratings across different racial and ethnic groups, highlighting areas for improvement. Additionally, researchers can investigate how residents of color may receive care in facilities with more substantial regulatory violations or staffing shortages, shedding light on systemic issues within the LTC system (Sanghavi & Chen, 2023). Ultimately, these studies provide valuable insights that can inform policymakers and healthcare providers about the need to address disparities in nursing home care to ensure equitable access and quality of care for all residents.

National Healthcare Quality and Disparities Reports

The National Healthcare Quality and Disparities Reports (NHQDR) website (https://datatools.ahrq.gov/nhqdr), published annually by AHRQ, provides national and state-level data on healthcare topics—such as access, diseases, demographics, and care types—organized into 15 subject areas. It emphasizes healthcare disparities, framing equity as central to quality improvement, and leverages data to support evidence-based solutions. The website provides comprehensive data on patient safety measures across various settings, including hospitals, ambulatory care, nursing homes, home health care, and others.

National and State Surveys

Various national surveys, including the Healthcare Cost and Utilization Program (HCUP), the National Health Interview Survey (NHIS), and the Behavioral Risk Factor Surveillance System (BRFSS), collect data on health behaviors, access to healthcare, and health outcomes (Ver Ploeg & Perrin, 2004). These surveys offer insights into disparities across different demographic groups. Additionally, state health departments often conduct surveys and compile reports on healthcare access, quality, and disparities within their jurisdictions, providing valuable regional insights (Zephyrin, 2021).

Population Health Data

Population health data, sourced from healthcare systems including clinical trials, research studies, and EHRs, are invaluable for dissecting and addressing healthcare disparities, particularly concerning equitable access to cutting-edge treatments and the inclusivity of diverse demographic groups (Zhang et al., 2017). Through meticulously analyzing this data, researchers gain insights into the multifaceted factors influencing healthcare outcomes among diverse populations, spanning socioeconomic status, race/ethnicity, gender, age, geographic location, and cultural background.

This comprehensive examination facilitates the identification of barriers hindering certain groups from accessing novel therapies or participating in clinical trials, empowering stakeholders to implement targeted interventions and policies aimed at fostering greater inclusivity and fairness within healthcare systems. Moreover, such analyses not only unveil disparities but also facilitate the development of tailored approaches to bridge these gaps, ultimately advancing the goal of achieving health equity for all individuals, regardless of their background or circumstances.

Measuring and Analyzing Healthcare Disparities

Addressing healthcare disparities in LTC requires a thorough understanding of the underlying complexities and nuances involved in data collection and analysis. This section navigates through the methodologies and considerations essential for measuring and analyzing these inequalities effectively.

Exploring healthcare disparities in LTC necessitates a methodical approach due to challenges in social class measures and potential biases in self-reported data. Braveman and colleagues (2004) advocate for a systemic method that encompasses three fundamental approaches: selecting health indicators or determinants, identifying social positions, and comparing indicators across social groups. Monitoring changes over time and analyzing higher-risk groups play pivotal roles in effective disparities reduction.

To ensure the robustness of results, it is crucial to adopt alternative outcome measures and control variables. *Sensitivity analysis*, a valuable methodology, involves repeating an analysis with different outcome measures or alternative variables included as controls to examine the robustness of results to these decisions (Lê Cook et al., 2012). One practical application of this approach is the inclusion of diverse experiences of discrimination and sociocultural factors in the data selection process. This involves integrating appropriate socioeconomic measures into public health surveys, aligning them with vital statistics and health data for a more comprehensive perspective (Krieger et al., 1997).

Thorough analysis utilizing various methods is essential for exploring healthcare disparities comprehensively. Table 9.2 outlines various common approaches, including RR, prevalence ratio, regression analysis, and more. These tools aid researchers and practitioners in unraveling disparities in healthcare outcomes, treatment access, and adherence among diverse demographic groups.

Caution in Within- and Across-Group Comparisons

Interpreting study outcomes requires a nuanced exploration of contextual factors. *Within-group disparities* unveil variations in care and outcomes among residents of the same race, emphasizing diversity within racial or ethnic groups. Meanwhile, *across-group disparities* highlight differences among residents of different races, offering insights into systemic issues. Caution is essential in both within- and across-group comparisons, emphasizing the need for predefined criteria to discern genuine differences (Whitfield et al., 2008), since statistically significant race effects might arise from measurement discrepancies rather than authentic variations in the underlying construct. To address this concern, an alternative approach focuses on within-group designs to uncover qualitative differences, assessing the *magnitude* of heterogeneity within a group.

In a study by Fashaw-Walters et al. (2024), the analysis of home health agencies (HHAs) revealed both within- and across-group variations among low-income home health (HH) patients. Through multinomial-logit analyses, the research categorized functional improvement outcomes into several categories, including any functional improvement, no functional improvement, death, transfer to inpatient settings, and continuing HH. The study specifically examines within-group variations, highlighting disparities existing among patients *within* the same bracket (e.g., racial, ethnic, or income), and *between*-group disparities, where differences *across HHAs* may contribute to disparities across various groups. The finding showed that Black, Hispanic, American Indian/Alaska Native (AIAN), and low-income HH patients were more likely to be discharged without functional improvement compared to White and higher-income patients, indicating *within*-group variation. Furthermore, the research underscores across-group variation in income-based disparities persisting within HHAs. By analyzing the impact of HHA fixed effects, researchers concluded that differences across HHAs were the primary drivers of remaining income-based disparities in the study, emphasizing the need for culturally and socioeconomically sensitive HH interventions to address these disparities effectively.

Understanding both within- and across-group variations is crucial for identifying and addressing the root causes of disparities in healthcare settings. Assuming homogeneity within a racial or ethnic group can overlook significant disparities existing within that group. This method identifies factors contributing to disparities at individual, systemic, and institutional levels, enabling the proper design of targeted interventions to address healthcare inequities across diverse racial and ethnic groups in a specific healthcare setting (Grabowski & McGuire, 2009).

TABLE 9.2 Methods for Analyzing Health Disparities

METHOD	DESCRIPTION
Prevalence ratio	Compares the prevalence of a particular condition or disease in different populations
Absolute differences	Calculates the absolute difference in health outcomes between groups
Summary measures	Combines multiple health indicators to create an overall measure of disparity (e.g., the Gini coefficient)
Concentration index	Measures inequalities across the socioeconomic spectrum by considering both the prevalence of a health condition and its distribution across different socioeconomic groups
Regression analysis	Assesses the relationship between demographic factors (race, income, education) and health outcomes, while controlling for other variables
Survival analysis	Analyzes the likelihood of survival after a diagnosis or treatment among different demographic groups
Rate ratio (RR)	Compares rates of a health outcome (e.g., disease incidence, mortality) between two groups
Odds ratio (OR)	Measures the odds of a particular health outcome occurring in one group compared to another group
Risk difference (RD)	Quantifies the difference in risk of a health outcome associated with a particular intervention or exposure

Source: Data from Anand, S., Diderichsen, F., Evans, T., Shkolnikov, V. M., & Wirth, M. (2001). Measuring disparities in health: Methods and indicators. In T. Evans, M. Whitehead, F. Diderichsen, A. Bhuiya, & M. Wirth (Eds.), *Challenging inequities in health: From ethics to action* (pp. 49–67). Oxford University Press; Asada, Y. (2010). Peer reviewed: A summary measure of health inequalities for a pay-for-population health performance system. *Preventing Chronic Disease, 7*(4), A72. https://www.ncbi.nlm.nih.gov/pmc/articles/PMC2901570; Braveman, P. A. (2006). Health disparities and health equity: Concepts and measurement. *Annual Review of Public Health, 27*, 167–194. https://doi.org/10.1146/annurev.publhealth.27.021405.102103; Braveman, P. A., Egerter, S. A., Cubbin, C., & Marchi, K. S. (2004). An approach to studying social disparities in health and health care. *American Journal of Public Health, 94*(12), 2139–2148. https://doi.org/10.2105/ajph.94.12.2139; Chin, M. H., Clarke, A. R., Nocon, R. S., Casey, A. A., Goddu, A. P., Keesecker, N. M., & Cook, S. C. (2012). A roadmap and best practices for organizations to reduce racial and ethnic disparities in health care. *Journal of General Internal Medicine, 27*, 992–1000. https://doi.org/10.1007/s11606-012-2082-9; Keppel, K., Pamuk, E., Lynch, J., Carter-Pokras, O., Kim, I., Mays, V., Pearcy, J., Schoenbach, V., & Weissman, J. S. (2005). Methodological issues in measuring health disparities. *Vital and Health Statistics. Series 2, Data Evaluation and Methods Research*, (141). U.S. Department of Health & Human Services, Centers for Disease Control and Prevention, National Center for Health Statistics. https://www.cdc.gov/nchs/data/series/sr_02/sr02_141.pdf; King, N. B., Harper, S., & Young, M. E. (2012). Use of relative and absolute effect measures in reporting health inequalities: Structured review. *BMJ, 345*, e5774. https://doi.org/10.1136/bmj.e5774; Liu, D., Burston, B., Stewart, S. C., & Mulligan, H. H. (2018). *The challenges of health disparities: Implications and actions for health care professionals* (pp. 83–108). Jones & Bartlett Learning; Scanlan, J. P. (2007, November). *Measurement problems in the national healthcare disparities report* (pp. 3–7). American Public Health Association 135th Annual Meeting & Exposition, Washington, DC.

Roles of Mediators Versus Moderators

Understanding the difference between mediators and moderators is crucial for designing effective interventions to address healthcare disparities. Illustrated in Figure 9.1, the relationship among independent, dependent, and mediator or moderator variables highlights how they interact to shape outcomes. A mediator explains the process or mechanism through which the independent variable influences the dependent variable. In contrast, a moderator affects the strength or direction of this relationship, but does not directly influence the outcome itself. *Mediators*, defined as variables explaining the intricate process through which an intervention influences an outcome,

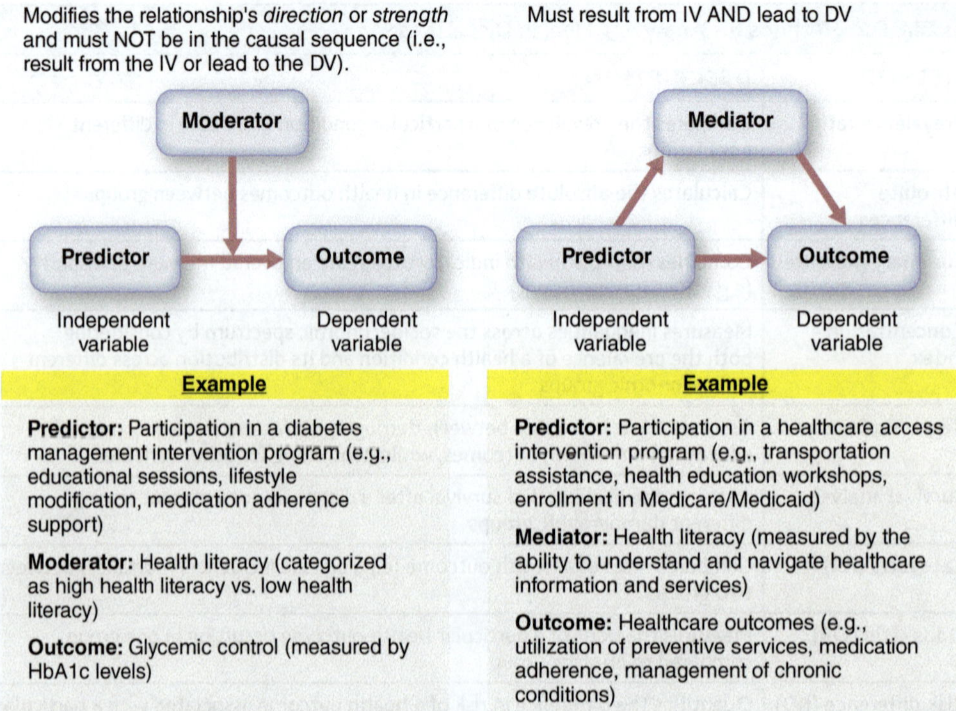

FIGURE 9.1. Moderator versus mediator.
DV, dependent variable; IV, independent variable.

assume a critical role in healthcare disparities research (Naimi et al., 2016). For instance, in interventions targeting improved healthcare access for older adults, variables such as health literacy may account for the relationship between an intervention and its impact on healthcare outcomes, enabling the development of more effective intervention strategies.

In a study by Nkimbeng and colleagues (2022), the duration of residence in the United States emerged as a mediator influencing health risks and outcomes among immigrant populations. Prolonged stays were associated with heightened connections between SDOH and health risks, underscoring the potential efficacy of targeted *acculturation* programs as mediators. These programs support immigrants in adjusting to U.S. cultural and healthcare systems, though this adaptation process is filled with challenges and stress, involving shifts in beliefs, values, attitudes, and behaviors (Lum & Vanderaa, 2010).

Conversely, *moderators* represent variables influencing the strength or direction of the relationship between an intervention and its outcome. For example, in interventions aimed at mitigating disparities in diabetes management, socioeconomic status could serve as a moderator. Individuals with lower socioeconomic status may encounter additional hurdles, such as restricted access to quality healthcare or resources for effective diabetes management. Tailoring support programs specifically for individuals with lower income levels could yield more impactful outcomes.

Encouraging LTC administrators, policymakers, and practitioners to prioritize offering accessible and high-quality home- and community-based services (HCBS) to vulnerable older adults holds promise for improving their overall well-being and promoting aging in place. Both concepts of mediators and moderators are indispensable in devising targeted and effective interventions to address healthcare disparities (MacKinnon, 2011).

SUMMARY

Chapter 9 focuses on the critical issue of healthcare disparities and their profound impact on the quality and safety of LTC, such as medication adherence, patient satisfaction, and safety incidents. It begins by elucidating the definition of healthcare inequalities and their ramifications on LTCservices. Subsequently, it introduces various data sources, including published surveys, clinical trial studies, and research findings, providing insights into healthcare disparities at both national and regional levels.

The chapter emphasizes the importance of targeted interventions, cultural competence training, equitable resource allocation, and community engagement in mitigating these disparities and fostering a care environment that is fair and inclusive, regardless of an individual's background. Through meticulous data analysis, areas for improvement are pinpointed, and the financial implications of addressing healthcare disparities are comprehensively understood.

Ultimately, the chapter advocates for the imperative of addressing healthcare disparities to cultivate an equitable and secure LTC delivery system that transcends the mere improvement of health outcomes, thereby ensuring that every individual receives dignified and unbiased care.

END-OF-CHAPTER RESOURCES

DISCUSSION QUESTIONS

1. What are healthcare disparities, and how do they impact the quality and safety of LTC?
2. How do factors such as distance to higher-rated facilities, income, and education influence the concentration of Medicare and Medicaid consumers in lower-rated nursing homes, and what are the implications of such disparities?
3. What is the difference between mediators and moderators in the context of healthcare disparities, and why is it important to understand these distinctions when designing effective interventions?
4. What are some examples of interventions and programs aimed at promoting equity and patient-centeredness in LTC, and how do they work?
5. What actions can LTC administrators, policymakers, and researchers take to address healthcare disparities and promote an equitable and secure LTC delivery system?

SPRINGER PUBLISHING CONNECT™

A robust set of instructor resources designed to supplement this text is located at http://connect.springerpub.com/content/book/978-0-8261-4935-0. Qualifying instructors may request access by emailing textbook@springerpub.com.

REFERENCES

AARP and National Alliance for Caregiving. (2020, May 14). *Caregiving in the United States 2020*. AARP. https://www.aarp.org/pri/topics/ltss/family-caregiving/caregiving-in-the-united-states

Agency for Healthcare Research and Quality. (2023, December). *National healthcare quality and disparities report* (AHRQ Pub. No. 23(24)-0091-EF). U.S. Department of Health & Human Services. https://www.ncbi.nlm.nih.gov/books/NBK600459/

American Hospital Association. (2020). *Addressing health care disparities through race, ethnicity and language (REaL) data*. https://www.aha.org/system/files/media/file/2020/06/ifdhe_real_data_resource.pdf

Anastos-Wallen, R., Werner, R. M., & Chatterjee, P. (2020). Prevalence of informal caregiving in states participating in the US Patient Protection and Affordable Care Act balancing incentive program, 2011-2018. *JAMA Network Open*, *3*(12), e2025833. https://doi.org/10.1001/jamanetworkopen.2020.25833

Batista, R., Prud'homme, D., Rhodes, E., Hsu, A., Talarico, R., Reaume, M., Guérin, E., Bouchard, L., Desaulniers, J., Manuel, D., & Tanuseputro, P. (2021). Quality and safety in long-term care in Ontario: The impact of language discordance. *Journal of the American Medical Directors Association*, *22*(10), 2147–2153. https://doi.org/10.1016/j.jamda.2020.12.007

Braveman, P. A., Egerter, S. A., Cubbin, C., & Marchi, K. S. (2004). An approach to studying social disparities in health and health care. *American Journal of Public Health*, *94*(12), 2139–2148. https://doi.org/10.2105/AJPH.94.12.2139

Bui, C. N., Peng, C., Mutchler, J. E., & Burr, J. A. (2021). Race and ethnic group disparities in emotional distress among older adults during the COVID-19 pandemic. *The Gerontologist*, *61*(2), 262–272. https://doi.org/10.1093/geront/gnaa217

Campbell, S. (2017). *Racial and gender disparities within the direct care workforce: Five key findings*. PHI. https://www.phinational.org/wp-content/uploads/legacy/research-report/racial_and_gender_disparities_in_dcw_-_phi_2017.pdf

Chen, A. T., Ryskina, K. L., & Jung, H. Y. (2020). Long-term care, residential facilities, and COVID-19: An overview of federal and state policy responses. *Journal of the American Medical Directors Association*, *21*(9), 1186–1190. https://doi.org/10.1016/j.jamda.2020.07.001

Choi, H., Heisler, M., Norton, E. C., Langa, K. M., Cho, T. C., & Connell, C. M. (2021). Family care availability and implications for informal and formal care used by adults with dementia in the US: Study examines family care availability and implications for informal and formal care used by adults with dementia in the United States. *Health Affairs*, *40*(9), 1359–1367. https://doi.org/10.1377/hlthaff.2021.00280

Coburn, A. F., Ziller, E. C., Paluso, N., Thayer, D., & Talbot, J. A. (2019). Long-term services and supports use among older Medicare beneficiaries in rural and urban areas. *Research on Aging*, *41*(3), 241–264. https://doi.org/10.1177/0164027518824117

Cohen, S. A., Sabik, N. J., Cook, S. K., Azzoli, A. B., & Mendez-Luck, C. A. (2019). Differences within differences: Gender inequalities in caregiving intensity vary by race and ethnicity in informal caregivers. *Journal of Cross-Cultural Gerontology*, *34*, 245–263. https://doi.org/10.1007/s10823-019-09381-9

Colello, K. J. (2023). *Who pays for long-term services and supports?* Congressional Research Service. https://crsreports.congress.gov/product/pdf/IF/IF10343

Crenshaw, K. (1991). Mapping the margins: Intersectionality, identity politics, and violence against women of color. *Stanford Law Review*, *43*(6), 1241–1299. https://www.jstor.org/stable/1229039

Dilworth-Anderson, P., Brummett, B. H., Goodwin, P., Williams, S. W., Williams, R. B., & Siegler, I. C. (2005). Effect of race on cultural justifications for caregiving. *The Journals of Gerontology Series B: Psychological Sciences and Social Sciences*, *60*(5), S257–S262. https://doi.org/10.1093/geronb/60.5.S257

Edwards, V. J., Bouldin, E. D., Taylor, C. A., Olivari, B. S., & McGuire, L. C. (2020). Characteristics and health status of informal unpaid caregivers—44 states, District of Columbia, and Puerto Rico, 2015–2017. *Morbidity and Mortality Weekly Report*, *69*(7), 183. https://doi.org/10.15585/mmwr.mm6907a2

Fashaw-Walters, S. A., Rahman, M., Jarrin, O. F., Gee, G., Mor, V., Nkimbeng, M., & Thomas, K. S. (2024). Getting to the root: Examining within and between home health agency inequities in functional improvement. *Health Services Research*, *59*(2), e14194. https://doi.org/10.1111/1475-6773.14194

Feng, Z., Lepore, M., Clark, M. A., Tyler, D., Smith, D. B., Mor, V., & Fennell, M. L. (2011). Geographic concentration and correlates of nursing home closures: 1999-2008. *Archives of Internal Medicine*, *171*(9), 806–813. https://doi.org/10.1001/archinternmed.2010.492

Gorges, R. J., Sanghavi, P., & Konetzka, R. T. (2019). A national examination of long-term care setting, outcomes, and disparities among elderly dual eligibles. *Health Affairs*, *38*(7), 1110–1118. https://doi.org/10.1377/hlthaff.2018.05409

Grabowski, D. C., & McGuire, T. G. (2009). Black-White disparities in care in nursing homes. *Atlantic Economic Journal*, *37*, 299–314. https://doi.org/10.1007/s11293-009-9185-7

Hahn, R. A. (2021). What is a social determinant of health? Back to basics. *Journal of Public Health Research*, *10*(4), 2324. https://doi.org/10.4081/jphr.2021.2324

Hall, A. K., Bernhardt, J. M., Dodd, V., & Vollrath, M. W. (2015). The digital health divide: Evaluating online health information access and use among older adults. *Health Education & Behavior*, *42*(2), 202–209. https://doi.org/10.1177/1090198114547815

Hatef, E., Ma, X., Rouhizadeh, M., Singh, G., Weiner, J. P., & Kharrazi, H. (2021). Assessing the impact of social needs and social determinants of health on health care utilization: Using patient- and community-level data. *Population Health Management*, *24*(2), 222–230. https://doi.org/10.1089/pop.2020.0043

Krieger, N., Williams, D. R., & Moss, N. E. (1997). Measuring social class in US public health research: Concepts, methodologies, and guidelines. *Annual Review of Public Health*, *18*(1), 341–378. https://doi.org/10.1146/annurev.publhealth.18.1.341

Lampe, N. M., Barbee, H., Tran, N. M., Bastow, S., & McKay, T. (2024). Health disparities among lesbian, gay, bisexual, transgender, and queer older adults: A structural competency approach. *The International Journal of Aging and Human Development*, *98*(1), 39–55. https://doi.org/10.1177/00914150231171838

Lane, S. J., Liu, D., & Rados, R. (2023). Post-acute and long-term care leaders' perspectives on leading during COVID-19. *Journal of Applied Gerontology*, *42*(11), 2179–2188. https://doi.org/10.1177/07334648231188282

Lê Cook, B., McGuire, T. G., & Zaslavsky, A. M. (2012). Measuring racial/ethnic disparities in health care: Methods and practical issues. *Health Services Research*, *47*(3pt2), 1232–1254. https://doi.org/10.1111/j.1475-6773.2012.01387.x

Lee, K., Mauldin, R. L., Tang, W., Connolly, J., Harwerth, J., & Magruder, K. (2021). Examining racial and ethnic disparities among older adults in long-term care facilities. *The Gerontologist*, *61*(6), 858–869. https://doi.org/10.1093/geront/gnab035

Lee, W. C., Veeranki, S. P., Serag, H., Eschbach, K., & Smith, K. D. (2016). Improving the collection of race, ethnicity, and language data to reduce healthcare disparities: A case study from an academic medical center. *Perspectives in Health Information Management, 13(*Fall*),* 1g. PMCID: PMC5075235

Li, Y., Harrington, C., Temkin-Greener, H., You, K., Cai, X., Cen, X., & Mukamel, D. B. (2015). Deficiencies in care at nursing homes and racial/ethnic disparities across homes fell, 2006–11. *Health Affairs*, *34*(7), 1139–1146. https://doi.org/10.1377/hlthaff.2015.0094

Lin, Z., & Liu, H. (2023). Race/ethnicity, nativity, and gender disparities in unmet care needs among older adults in the United States. *The Gerontologist*, *64*(4), gnad094. https://doi.org/10.1093/geront/gnad094

Liu, D., Burston, B., Stewart, S. C., & Mulligan, H. H. (2018). *The challenges of health disparities: Implications and actions for health care professionals.* Jones & Bartlett Learning.

Liu, D., Burston, B., Stewart, S. C., & Mulligan, H. H. (2020). *Isms in health care human resources.* Jones & Bartlett Learning.

Liu, D., Yamashita, T., Burston, B., & Keene, J. R. (2020). The use of online health-management tools and health care utilization among older Americans. *The Gerontologist*, *60*(7), 1224–1232. https://doi.org/10.1093/geront/gnaa068

Liu, R., Chi, I., & Wu, S. (2022). Caregiving burden among caregivers of people with dementia through the lens of intersectionality. *The Gerontologist*, *62*(5), 650–661. https://doi.org/10.1093/geront/gnab146

Lum, T. Y., & Vanderaa, J. P. (2010). Health disparities among immigrant and non-immigrant elders: The association of acculturation and education. *Journal of Immigrant and Minority Health*, *12*, 743–753. https://doi.org/10.1007/s10903-008-9225-4

MacKinnon, D. P. (2011). Integrating mediators and moderators in research design. *Research on Social Work Practice*, *21*(6), 675–681. https://doi.org/10.1177/1049731511414148

Marmot, M. G., Smith, G. D., Stansfeld, S., Patel, C., North, F., Head, J., White, I., Brunner, E., & Feeney, A. (1991). Health inequalities among British civil servants: The Whitehall II study. *The Lancet*, *337*(8754), 1387–1393. https://doi.org/10.1016/0140-6736(91)93068-K

McCall, S., & Scales, K. (2022, February). *Direct care worker disparities: Key trends and challenges.* https://www.phinational.org/wp-content/uploads/2022/02/Direct-Care-Worker-Disparities-2022-PHI.pdf

Naimi, A. I., Schnitzer, M. E., Moodie, E. E., & Bodnar, L. M. (2016). Mediation analysis for health disparities research. *American Journal of Epidemiology, 184*(4), 315–324. https://doi.org/10.1093/aje/kwv329

National Academies of Sciences, Engineering, and Medicine. (2022). *The national imperative to improve nursing home quality: Honoring our commitment to residents, families, and staff.* The National Academies Press. https://doi.org/10.17226/26526.

National Institute on Aging. (2020). *The National Institute on Aging: Strategic directions for research, 2020–2025.* https://www.nia.nih.gov/sites/default/files/2020-05/nia-strategic-directions-2020-2025.pdf

Nkimbeng, M., Commodore-Mensah, Y., Angel, J. L., Bandeen-Roche, K., Thorpe Jr, R. J., Han, H. R., Winch, P. J., & Szanton, S. L. (2022). Longer residence in the United States is associated with more physical function limitations in African immigrant older adults. *Journal of Applied Gerontology, 41*(2), 411–420. https://doi.org/10.1177/0733464820977608

Office of Disease Prevention and Health Promotion. (n.d.-a). *About disparities data.* Retrieved February 2, 2024, from https://health.gov/healthypeople/objectives-and-data/about-disparities-data

Office of Disease Prevention and Health Promotion. (n.d.-b). *Healthy People 2023: Home page.* Retrieved February 2, 2024, from https://health.gov/healthypeople

Office of Disease Prevention and Health Promotion. (n.d.-c). *Social determinants of health.* Retrieved February 2, 2024, from https://health.gov/healthypeople/objectives-and-data/social-determinants-health

Park, Y. J., & Martin, E. G. (2018). Geographic disparities in access to nursing home services: Assessing fiscal stress and quality of care. *Health Services Research, 53*, 2932–2951. https://doi.org/10.1111/1475-6773.12801

Putney, J. M., Keary, S., Hebert, N., Krinsky, L., & Halmo, R. (2018). "Fear runs deep:" The anticipated needs of LGBT older adults in long-term care. *Journal of Gerontological Social Work, 61*(8), 887–907. https://doi.org/10.1080/01634372.2018.1508109

Raj, M., Oleschuk, M., Chapman-Novakofski, K., & Levine, S. K. (2023). Perceived facilitators and barriers to implementing culturally inclusive diets into hospitals and long-term care facilities. *Journal of the American Medical Directors Association, 24*(10), 1503–1507. https://doi.org/10.1016/j.jamda.2023.04.018

Recognize, Assist, Include, Support and Engage Family Caregivers Act of 2017, H.R. 3759, Pub. L. No. 115–119, 132 Stat 23 (2018). https://acl.gov/sites/default/files/about-acl/2018-10/PLAW-115publ119%20-%20RAISE.pdf

Reinhard, S. C., Caldera, S., Houser, A., & Choula, R. B. (2023, March). *Valuing the invaluable: 2023 update strengthening supports for family caregivers.* AARP Public Policy Institute. https://archrespite.org/wp-content/uploads/2023/03/valuing-the-invaluable-2023-update.doi_.10.26419-2Fppi.00082.006.pdf

Rochon, P. A., Kalia, S., & Higgs, P. (2021). Gendered ageism: Addressing discrimination based on age and sex. *The Lancet, 398*(10301), 648–649. https://doi.org/10.1016/S0140-6736(21)01636-6

Rowen, N. P., Van Stekelenburg, B., Nohria, R., Saunders, R. S., & Whitaker, R. G. (2022, September 14). *How to improve race, ethnicity, and language data and disparities interventions.* Health Affairs Forefront. https://www.healthaffairs.org/content/forefront/improve-race-ethnicity-and-language-data-and-disparities-interventions

Rozenfeld, Y., Beam, J., Maier, H., Haggerson, W., Boudreau, K., Carlson, J., & Medows, R. (2020). A model of disparities: Risk factors associated with COVID-19 infection. *International Journal for Equity in Health, 19*(1), 1–10. https://doi.org/10.1186/s12939-020-01242-z

Sanghavi, P., & Chen, Z. (2023). Underreporting of quality measures and associated facility characteristics and racial disparities in US nursing home ratings. *JAMA Network Open, 6*(5), e2314822. https://doi.org/10.1001/jamanetworkopen.2023.14822

Scales, K. (2021). It is time to resolve the direct care workforce crisis in long-term care. *The Gerontologist, 61*(4), 497–504. https://doi.org/10.1093/geront/gnaa116

Scambler, G., & Higgs, P. (1999). Stratification, class and health: Class relations and health inequalities in high modernity. *Sociology, 33*(2), 275–296. https://doi.org/10.1177/S0038038599000176

Schwartz, L. B., Lieblich, C., Laxton, C. E., Kaes, L., Barnett, D. P., Port, C., & Pace, D. D. (2023). COVID-19 in assisted living: Protecting a critical long-term care resource. *Journal of the American Medical Directors Association, 24*(2), 134–139. https://doi.org/10.1016/j.jamda.2022.12.012

Sengupta, M., Lendon, J. P., Caffrey, C., Melekin, A., & Singh, P. (2022). *Post-acute and long-term care providers and services users in the United States, 2017–2018*. https://stacks.cdc.gov/view/cdc/115346

Shippee, T. P., Akosionu, O., Ng, W., Woodhouse, M., Duan, Y., Thao, M. S., & Bowblis, J. R. (2020). COVID-19 pandemic: Exacerbating racial/ethnic disparities in long-term services and supports. *Journal of Aging & Social Policy*, *32*(4–5), 323–333. https://doi.org/10.1080/08959420.2020.1772004

Shippee, T. P., Ng, W., & Bowblis, J. R. (2020). Does living in a higher proportion minority facility improve quality of life for racial/ethnic minority residents in nursing homes? *Innovation in Aging*, *4*(3), igaa014. https://doi.org/10.1093/geroni/igaa014

Siconolfi, D., Shih, R. A., Friedman, E. M., Kotzias, V. I., Ahluwalia, S. C., Phillips, J. L., & Saliba, D. (2019). Rural-urban disparities in access to home- and community-based services and supports: Stakeholder perspectives from 14 states. *Journal of the American Medical Directors Association*, *20*(4), 503–508. https://doi.org/10.1016/j.jamda.2019.01.120

Silverstein, N. M., Whitbourne, S. K., Bowen, L. M., Montepare, J. M., Jansen, T., Beaulieu, C., & Prasad, A. (2022). Assessing age inclusivity in higher education: Introducing the Age-Friendly Inventory and Campus Climate Survey. *The Gerontologist*, *62*(1), e48–e61. https://doi.org/10.1093/geront/gnab090

Smith, D. B., Feng, Z., Fennell, M. L., Zinn, J. S., & Mor, V. (2007). Separate and unequal: Racial segregation and disparities in quality across US nursing homes. *Health Affairs*, *26*(5), 1448–1458. https://doi.org/10.1377/hlthaff.26.5.1448

Travers, J. L., Dick, A. W., & Stone, P. W. (2018). Racial/ethnic differences in receipt of influenza and pneumococcal vaccination among long-stay nursing home residents. *Health Services Research*, *53*(4), 2203–2226. https://doi.org/10.1111/1475-6773.12759

University of Pittsburgh. (2020). *Effects of COVID-19 on family caregivers: A community survey from the University of Pittsburgh*. https://ucsur.pitt.edu/files/center/covid19_cg/COVID19_Full_Report_Final.pdf

Ver Ploeg, M., & Perrin, E. (Eds.). (2004). *Eliminating health disparities: Measurement and data needs* (pp. 83–98). National Academies Press. https://www.ncbi.nlm.nih.gov/books/NBK215742

Waymouth, M., Siconolfi, D., Friedman, E. M., Saliba, D., Ahluwalia, S. C., & Shih, R. A. (2023). Barriers and facilitators to home-and community-based services access for persons with dementia and their caregivers. *The Journals of Gerontology: Series B*, *78*(6), 1085–1097. https://doi.org/10.1093/geronb/gbad039

Weng, S. S., & Landes, S. D. (2017). Culture and language discordance in the workplace: Evidence from the National Home Health Aide Survey. *The Gerontologist*, *57*(5), 900–909. https://doi.org/10.1093/geront/gnw110

Whitfield, K. E., Allaire, J. C., Belue, R., & Edwards, C. L. (2008). Are comparisons the answer to understanding behavioral aspects of aging in racial and ethnic groups? *The Journals of Gerontology Series B: Psychological Sciences and Social Sciences*, *63*(5), P301–P308. https://doi.org/10.1093/geronb/63.5.P301

World Health Organization. (n.d.). *Social determinants of health*. Retrieved February 2, 2024, from https://www.who.int/health-topics/social-determinants-of-health

Zarit, S. H., Todd, P. A., & Zarit, J. M. (1986). Subjective burden of husbands and wives as caregivers: A longitudinal study. *The Gerontologist*, *26*(3), 260–266. https://doi.org/10.1093/geront/26.3.260

Zephyrin, L. (2021, November 18). *New Health Equity Scorecard: State-by-state scorecard of racial and ethnic disparities finds all states' health systems are failing people of color*. The Commonwealth Fund. https://www.commonwealthfund.org/press-release/2021/new-health-equity-scorecard-state-state-scorecard-racial-and-ethnic-disparities

Zhang, X., Pérez-Stable, E. J., Bourne, P. E., Peprah, E., Duru, O. K., Breen, N., Berrigan, D., Wood, F., Jackson, J. S., Wong, D. W. S., & Denny, J. (2017). Big data science: Opportunities and challenges to address minority health and health disparities in the 21st century. *Ethnicity & Disease*, *27*(2), 95. https://ethndis.org/archive/files/ethndis-27-95.pdf

CHAPTER 10

ADDRESSING HEALTHCARE DISPARITIES IN LONG-TERM CARE: CHALLENGES AND STRATEGIES

Darren Liu

Learning Objectives

After completing this chapter, each learner will be able to:

- Identify the key challenges faced by people with disabilities in long-term care (LTC) settings and the strategies for addressing these challenges.
- Understand the concepts of person-centered care planning and its benefits in LTC settings.
- Analyze the potential benefits and challenges of consumer-centric care models compared to traditional models.
- Evaluate the importance of data collection, root cause analysis, and quality improvement initiatives in reducing healthcare disparities in LTC.
- Assess the challenges that healthcare providers and LTC facilities may face when implementing culturally and linguistically appropriate services (CLAS) standards and strategies for addressing these challenges.

INTRODUCTION

The aging population and individuals with disabilities are increasingly intertwined groups within the context of long-term care (LTC), presenting unique challenges and considerations. Those aged 65 and older, along with individuals with disabilities, frequently require extensive support due to a higher prevalence of chronic conditions and functional limitations. This convergence of aging and disability necessitates a comprehensive approach to long-term services and supports (LTSS) that can accommodate their specific needs. However, addressing healthcare disparities among individuals with disabilities in LTC is a pressing concern, as emphasized by the National Council on Disability (2023b).

In the United States, about 27% of adults grapple with a disability, and face substantial barriers when seeking healthcare services. Notably, nearly 25% of those aged 18 to 44 lack a designated healthcare provider due to financial constraints. Additionally, one in six adults aged 45 to 64 with disabilities forego routine check-ups, heightening health risks (Centers for Disease Control and Prevention [CDC], 2024). This demographic contends with a range of functional limitations encompassing vision, mobility, cognition, hearing, self-care, and independent living, contributing to elevated rates of chronic conditions such as obesity, smoking, heart disease, and diabetes (Froehlich-Grobe et al., 2016). Therefore, ensuring equitable access to quality LTSS is paramount for individuals with disabilities, as it plays a crucial role in promoting their well-being and independence.

This chapter delves into the critical issue of healthcare disparities experienced by individuals with disabilities within LTC settings, emphasizing the urgent need for interventions and policies to address these inequities. Additionally, the chapter underscores the importance of recognizing and understanding these disparities as a collective effort among stakeholders. By comprehensively addressing the challenges outlined in this chapter and implementing the strategies discussed, stakeholders can collaboratively work toward fostering a healthcare system that is truly inclusive and equitable for all users, especially those reliant on LTC services.

HEALTHCARE DISPARITIES AMONG PEOPLE WITH DISABILITIES

The disparities in healthcare experienced by individuals with disabilities are deeply rooted in avoidable disadvantages and intersecting forms of marginalization. Those with disabilities often face poorer health conditions and higher utilization of healthcare services compared to their counterparts without disabilities. This systemic failure to deliver adequate care has led to lower-quality services, insufficient preventive care, and an increased prevalence of chronic conditions (Seervai et al., 2019).

Iezzoni and Agaronnik (2020) emphasize the significance of recognizing diverse definitions of disability, incorporating various perspectives and priorities. Civil rights law defines *disability* as "a physical or mental impairment that substantially limits one or more of the life activities of such individual" (U.S. Department of Health & Human Services [HHS], n.d., "Definitions of Who is Protected"). This widely accepted definition, aligned with the Americans with Disabilities Act (ADA) and the World Health Organization's International Classification of Functioning, Disability, and Health (ICF) model, prioritizes impairments that significantly impede major life activities. This definition guides healthcare settings in identifying individuals who require special accommodations to ensure equal access to healthcare.

Disparities disproportionately affect Black and Latinx adults with intellectual and developmental disabilities (IDD; Mitra et al., 2022), compounded by limited access to healthcare, socioeconomic hurdles, and social exclusion (Krahn et al., 2015). LGBTQI+ individuals with disabilities also report lower health-related quality of life than their non-LGBTQI+ counterparts (Mitra et al., 2022), often experiencing depression, chronic health issues, and diminished well-being. These disparities suggest systemic connections to various forms of marginalization, including limited healthcare access, treatment disparities, socioeconomic challenges, and social exclusion, highlighting the *intersectional* nature of marginalized identities and systemic factors influencing the health outcomes of individuals with disabilities.

The ADA serves as a federal statute mandating civil rights for people with disabilities, providing protections for accessing healthcare services, and stipulating that patients with disabilities must receive reasonable accommodations. However, a survey of 714 U.S. physicians revealed alarming gaps in knowledge, with 35.8% reporting little or no awareness of their legal responsibilities under the ADA, and 71.2% answering incorrectly regarding who determines reasonable accommodations (Iezzoni, Rao, et al., 2022). These findings underscore the existence of healthcare disparities for individuals with disabilities.

Ableism, as delineated in Chapter 9, constitutes systemic discrimination against individuals with disabilities, intensifying healthcare disparities. Prevalent negative attitudes and biases perpetuate substandard care, diagnosis delays, and restricted access to essential medical interventions (Iezzoni, 2023). Furthermore, the physical, cognitive, or sensory impediments associated with disabilities create additional hurdles, including inaccessible facilities and communication challenges, impeding the equitable and prompt delivery of healthcare services.

Persisting healthcare disparities for individuals with disabilities often stem from inaccessible care and a lack of accommodations, which significantly impact their ability to access quality healthcare services. Accommodations refer to modifications or adjustments made to healthcare facilities, services, or procedures to ensure equitable access for individuals with disabilities. These accommodations may include physical modifications to facilities, such as wheelchair ramps, accessible examination tables, or visual aids for individuals with vision impairments. Additionally, accommodations can involve communication supports, such as sign language interpreters, alternative formats for written materials, or assistive listening devices, to facilitate effective communication between healthcare providers and patients with disabilities.

Barriers to care, rooted in physicians' biases, inadequate training, and a general reluctance to care for individuals with disabilities, contribute to ongoing healthcare inequalities (Lagu et al., 2022). Research highlights that physicians are often insufficiently trained in legal requirements for equitable care, leading to potential misunderstandings of their responsibilities (Agaronnik et al., 2019). Overcoming these barriers requires a cultural shift within the medical community, emphasizing awareness, education, and inclusive practices. By implementing accommodations and addressing these barriers, healthcare providers can better meet the needs of individuals with disabilities and ensure they receive the same quality of care as their counterparts without disabilities.

Iezzoni, Rao, et al. (2022) underscores the imperative to eliminate disparities, advocating for policies, training, and technology to bridge gaps in care. A comprehensive approach involves cultural competency training for healthcare professionals and institutional changes. Improved data collection and accessible communication are vital components in enhancing healthcare for people with disabilities.

Data collection facilitates the identification of barriers and challenges faced by people with disabilities in accessing healthcare services (Akobirshoev et al., 2022). These data can be utilized at institutional or community levels to train staff, improving their awareness and responsiveness to the unique needs of people with disabilities. Such initiatives will help healthcare providers deliver more person-centered and culturally responsive LTC services, ultimately enhancing the quality and safety of care for people with disabilities in discussions and decisions about their healthcare arrangements (Donelan et al., 2020).

Policy and system-level interventions emerge as crucial strategies. Policymakers, healthcare providers, and LTC administrators need to take several steps to address the healthcare disparities and meet the needs of people with disabilities. This includes investing in disability research, promoting disability inclusion in healthcare training, and collecting disability data to develop and implement effective policies (Iezzoni, McKee, et al., 2022). These steps involve a multifaceted approach, including increased physical access, competency training for healthcare professionals, home- and community-based supports, nondiscriminatory insurance benefit design, and a revisit to the 2006 United Nations Convention on the Rights of Persons with Disabilities.

Addressing healthcare disparities necessitates a multifaceted strategy that directly confronts ableism, advocates for disability-inclusive healthcare practices, enhances sensitivity and training for healthcare professionals, refines communication modalities, and ensures a physically accessible environment (Iezzoni, 2011). To effectively tackle these disparities, substantial systemic and policy changes are imperative, as well as extending beyond the conventional scope of medical care provisions.

The Vital Role of Medicaid Waivers

Medicaid waivers play a vital role in supporting people with disabilities by offering essential services and support beyond what traditional Medicaid programs offer. A Medicaid waiver is a program that allows states to waive certain Medicaid requirements to provide services not typically covered by traditional Medicaid, particularly for individuals with disabilities or those in need of LTC. These waivers, such as home- and community-based services (HCBS) waivers, or Section 1915 (c) waivers, cater not only to individuals with disabilities but also to those coping with Alzheimer disease and related dementias. By delivering essential services within homes or communities, these waivers align with the preferences of many individuals to live independently, preventing unnecessary institutionalization and enhancing quality of life.

For example, the waivers enable eligible individuals to receive care in their homes or community settings, promoting independence and autonomy. Many states offer Medicaid waivers tailored to the needs of specific populations, providing additional services and supports to enhance access to LTC while allowing individuals to remain in their preferred living environments. These services encompass assistance with daily activities such as bathing, dressing, eating, and mobility, tailored to individual preferences and needs. Offered in various settings including home-based care, community programs, or institutional settings such as assisted living facilities or nursing homes, Medicaid waivers promote independence and community integration.

Furthermore, Medicaid waivers prioritize *autonomy* and *self-determination* by allowing states to customize support services, offering a cost-effective alternative to institutional care. With flexible services provided in home and community settings, individuals gain control over their lives and the services they receive, ensuring equitable distribution of resources and care.

Maintaining uninterrupted coverage during transitions from pandemic-related Medicaid enrollment is crucial to address disparities in coverage and care. Federal and state governments, guided by the Biden administration (Centers for Medicare & Medicaid Services, 2022), advocate for waivers that extend coverage, reduce healthcare disparities, and promote comprehensive "whole-person care" by addressing health-related social needs (HRSN) and key social determinants of health (SDOH; Guth, 2022).

Understanding the effectiveness of HCBS is essential to tailor service delivery to meet the diverse needs of individuals with disabilities, including those with IDD (Friedman, 2023). Ensuring their entitled coverage for equitable healthcare access is imperative, underscoring the importance of addressing their substantial healthcare needs (Rubenstein et al., 2024).

Health Equity Framework

The health equity framework for people with disabilities, as proposed by the National Council on Disability (2023a), presents a robust strategy to tackle healthcare disparities experienced by individuals with disabilities. Comprising five components—special medically underserved population (SMUP) designation, health disparities population designation, comprehensive disability clinical-care curricula, accessible medical diagnostic equipment, and improved data capturing—the framework offers 39 practical guides for implementing policy changes tailored to the unique needs of people with disabilities. Notably, the framework also recommends a *competency-based curriculum* to educate medical, nursing, and other healthcare professional students on clinical perspectives for serving individuals with disabilities and cultivate skills toward *patient-centered care.*

Effectively addressing healthcare disparities for individuals with disabilities requires collaborative efforts from policymakers, healthcare practitioners, patient advocacy groups, and researchers. Recommendations include increased accessibility, cultural competency training, promotion of disability inclusion in healthcare training, and comprehensive data collection. Eliminating healthcare disparities is an ongoing challenge, but with concerted efforts, it is possible to build a more inclusive and equitable healthcare landscape for all individuals, regardless of their backgrounds and abilities. In the following sections, we will outline strategies aimed at mitigating disparities in LTC.

THE TRANSFORMATIVE SHIFT TOWARD "PERSON-CENTERED CARE"

Despite the advent of various reform initiatives, progress in mitigating the outlined disparities highlighted in Chapter 9 and the initial section of this chapter has been sluggish. This prompts a critical examination of whether a comprehensive overhaul or incremental interventions are necessary to foster substantial improvements. Given the urgency of the situation, it is imperative to carefully deliberate the most effective approach to bridge the existing gaps in LTC provision.

Multiple reports from the Institute of Medicine (IOM) have consistently emphasized the paramount importance of placing consumers at the forefront of care delivery within nursing homes. This sentiment traces back to the 1986 report, which underscored the significance of honoring consumer preferences whenever possible (IOM, 1986, p. 172), a principle echoed in subsequent reports such as those from 2001 and 2022 (Wunderlich & Kohler, 2001, p. 28; National Academies of Sciences, Engineering, and Medicine [NASEM], 2022[1]). Moreover, seminal reports such as *Crossing the Quality Chasm* (IOM, 2001, p. 40) and *Unequal Treatment* (Smedley et al., 2003) underscore the critical nature of patient-centeredness in healthcare, challenging traditional models that often prioritize diseases and professional knowledge over patients' unique values and preferences.

Embracing a consumer-centric approach entails recognizing and addressing individuals' multifaceted needs, spanning physical, emotional, social, and spiritual dimensions, while also considering personal circumstances and diverse cultural influences, values, and socioeconomic backgrounds. Prioritizing patient-centered care within LTC frameworks signals a deliberate effort to promote fairness and equality, requiring a transformation of the overarching cultural landscape. This endeavor involves actively identifying and remedying disparities stemming from cultural diversity, economic inequalities, or unequal access to essential resources. For instance, offering financial incentives to empower consumers in healthcare decision-making becomes crucial as it aims to broaden choices, heighten satisfaction, and reduce costs (Konetzka & Werner, 2009).

DIMENSIONS OF CULTURAL TRANSFORMATION IN LONG-TERM CARE

Healthcare disparities within LTC settings often stem from cultural distinctions, underscoring the critical role of cultural competence training and education. These endeavors are pivotal in advancing patient-centered care, especially for diverse populations (Betancourt et al., 2005). LTC residents come from diverse cultural backgrounds, each with distinct values, beliefs, and preferences that significantly shape their care experiences. Cultural competence training empowers healthcare providers with the knowledge, skills, and sensitivity necessary to understand and respect these differences, ensuring that care delivery aligns with each resident's unique needs. By cultivating a culturally responsive environment, LTC facilities can foster inclusivity, facilitate effective communication, and enhance overall care quality.

Table 10.1 provides an in-depth exploration of various key dimensions related to cultural transformation within LTC, spanning from individual-focused care to organizational or systemic strategies. For instance, individual-focused care approaches prioritize tailoring healthcare to individual needs, while communication strategies in healthcare relationships foster active patient participation in decision-making (dyadic). Empowerment through consumer-directed services empowers individuals to choose and oversee their healthcare, enhancing independence. Organizational cultural competency targets healthcare systems to provide diverse care, while alignment in culture concordance aims to match cultural backgrounds between providers and patients to enhance communication and trust.

Promoting *cultural awareness* in practice involves acknowledging and integrating diverse cultural perspectives into healthcare. Implementing cultural sensitivity training for staff in healthcare facilities heightens awareness and fosters respectful practices in patient care. These strategies collectively provide a robust framework to cultivate more effective, empathetic, and equitable care within long-term healthcare settings.

[1] "RECOMMENDATION 1E: Nursing home owners, with the support of federal and state governmental agencies, should construct and reconfigure (renovate) nursing homes to provide smaller, more home-like environments and/or smaller units within larger nursing homes that promote infection control and person-centered care and activities" (NASEM, 2022, p. 507).

TABLE 10.1 Key Dimensions of Cultural Transformation in Long-Term Care

TERMS	SCALE	DEFINITIONS	APPROACH (TO ADDRESS DISPARITIES)
Cultural awareness	Individual and organizational	Recognition and understanding of diverse cultural perspectives, norms, and values	By fostering respectful integration of diverse cultural perspectives into healthcare practices at both individual and organizational levels
Cultural humility	Individual and organizational	A willingness to engage in self-evaluation, critique, and lifelong learning to address power imbalances and enhance cultural competency	By fostering continuous self-reflection, recognizing power differentials, and promoting cultural sensitivity at both individual and organizational levels
Consumer-directed services	Individual (empowering for service users)	Assessing one's own needs, choosing service providers, and monitoring service quality	By empowering individuals to determine their care needs, potentially reducing disparities
Patient–physician relationships, patient–provider relationships, patient–provider communication	Individual, dyadic (patient–physician)	Historical model emphasizing professional expertise over patient autonomy	By evolving to engage patients in decision-making, promoting patient involvement in care, training in communication skills
Culture concordance[a]	Individual (relational)	Alignment of healthcare providers' cultural background with that of the patients	By matching patients and providers' cultural backgrounds to improve communication and trust
Cultural competency	Organizational	Ability of organizations to provide care to patients with diverse values, beliefs, and behaviors	By enhancing understanding of cultural differences, improving care delivery to diverse groups
Consumer-centered care, patient-centered care, resident-centered care	Individual (patient-focused)	Healthcare closely congruent and responsive to patient wants, needs, and preferences; shift from professional-driven care to incorporating individual perspectives	By recognizing and accommodating individual needs and preferences

[a]Culture concordance: Expanding on the concept of *concordance*, various perspectives beyond culture can be considered. These include racialconcordance, genderconcordance, religiousconcordance, and language concordance. Each of these facets emphasizes alignment or similarity in racial background, gender identity, religion, or linguistic proficiency between individuals involved in healthcare interactions. These forms of concordance are crucial as they aim to bridge potential disparities, enhance understanding, and improve communication, ultimately fostering more effective and empathetic care.

Recent strides in addressing healthcare disparities signify a shift from conventional cultural competency training to a focus on *cultural humility* (Lekas et al., 2020). Cultural humility, characterized by continuous self-reflection, promotes *ongoing self-evaluation* and learning to rectify *power imbalances*, emphasizing self-reflexivity, valuing patients' lay expertise, and sharing power with them (Tervalon & Murray-Garcia, 1998). This transition acknowledges existing power imbalances and advocates for reevaluating institutional barriers.

Unlike *cultural competence* training, which may perpetuate stereotypes and implicit biases, cultural humility fosters continuous self-reflection and critique rooted in humility. This approach aims to replace detached cultural competence practices with a dynamic, empathetic connection between healthcare providers and patients. This transformative approach challenges traditional categorizations in medical anthropology, fostering a more inclusive and equitable healthcare environment.

COMPREHENSIVE APPROACHES TO ENHANCING PERSON-CENTERED CARE IN LONG-TERM SETTINGS

To enhance person-centered care in LTC settings, it is crucial to employ both organizational and systemic strategies. Organizational strategies focus on internal practices, empowering staff and fostering cultural competence. Systemic strategies address broader structural factors and policy interventions to promote equitable access to quality care. Integrating these approaches ensures a comprehensive effort to prioritize residents' needs while addressing systemic healthcare challenges.

Organizational Strategies

The organizational approach to cultural competence hinges on the organization's level of cultural literacy and its dedication to the process. While there is evidence to suggest that organizations with higher levels of cultural competence may provide more effective and equitable care (Saha et al., 2008), the direct impact on patient outcomes remains an area of ongoing research.

Studies have shown that culturally competent healthcare organizations are more likely to engage in patient-centered care practices (Carthon et al., 2020), which can lead to improved patient satisfaction, adherence to treatment plans, and better health outcomes overall (Engle et al., 2021). Additionally, organizations that prioritize cultural competence often experience higher levels of patient trust, communication, and engagement, which are all factors associated with better health outcomes. However, more research is needed to establish a direct causal relationship between organizational cultural competence and specific health outcomes.

While each concept has its unique focus and emphasis, they are not mutually exclusive. Instead, they can complement each other to create a more holistic and culturally responsive approach to healthcare delivery. For example, cultural humility informs cultural competency by encouraging healthcare providers to approach their interactions with patients with humility, openness, and a willingness to learn. Likewise, patient-centered care aligns with consumer-directed services by empowering individuals to actively participate in decisions about their care. By integrating these concepts, healthcare providers can strive to deliver more effective, equitable, and patient-centered care to diverse populations.

Figure 10.1 illustrates a spectrum representing an organization's cultural literacy or their perceived level of complexity (or difficulty) associated with implementing each concept or strategy, showing the breadth of its incorporation of these principles. "Low complexity" refers to concepts or strategies that are relatively simple to understand and put into practice, requiring minimal resources and organizational change. "Medium complexity" involves concepts or strategies that are moderately challenging to implement, requiring a deeper understanding and some degree of organizational adjustment. "High complexity" encompasses concepts or strategies that are particularly challenging, demanding significant effort, resources, and substantial organizational change to successfully implement. This classification aids in assessing the relative difficulty and resource requirements associated with different healthcare initiatives, guiding decision-making and prioritization in healthcare delivery.

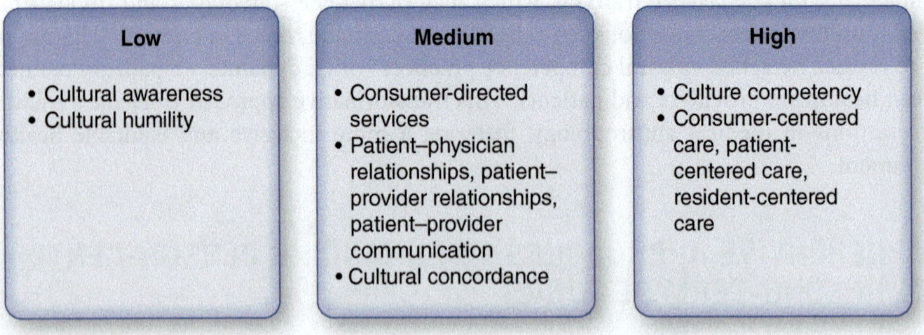

FIGURE 10.1. Level of complexity for cultural transformation strategies.

It is recommended that organizations begin with foundational concepts on the left side of Figure 10.1, which are typically adopted earlier in their cultural competency journey. As cultural literacy improves, organizations can advance toward embracing concepts on the right side, signifying a deeper commitment to addressing healthcare disparities through nuanced cultural considerations. Importantly, the positioning on the spectrum is flexible, enabling organizations to prioritize different aspects based on their unique circumstances, priorities, and readiness for cultural competency initiatives.

Systemic Strategies

Navigating the intricate landscape of LTC demands a *systems thinking* approach that recognizes the interconnectedness of various healthcare components. This approach, detailed in Chapter 12, underscores the importance of understanding the profound interdependence of SDOH, requiring holistic interventions to address disparities effectively across diverse healthcare settings.

Earlier in this chapter, we explored the literature advocating for individuals with disabilities, emphasizing the need for person-centered approaches and the importance of addressing barriers to access and quality of care. Insights from a 2023 report on dementia care (National Institute on Aging, 2023) underscore six strategic elements, aligning with recommendations on addressing systemic racism in a recent published article (Shippee et al., 2022), emphasizing a systemic thinking approach in LTSS for addressing healthcare disparities among persons living with dementia.

The recommendations presented in Table 10.2 highlight key strategies for addressing disparities in LTC, underlining the necessity of a comprehensive and inclusive approach to improve healthcare outcomes for marginalized communities. For instance, increasing Medicaid and Medicare reimbursement rates can alleviate financial challenges faced by providers serving vulnerable populations, facilitating investments in staff training, technology, and infrastructure, and ultimately enhance care quality.

Reconsidering pay-for-performance (P4P) programs involves incorporating SDOH to adopt a more holistic approach. This calls upon policymakers to consider social determinants, fostering a comprehensive understanding of the distinct needs of underserved populations and promoting a more equitable healthcare system. While P4P or *value-based* systems were not initially tailored for LTC, they hold the potential to alleviate disparities by incentivizing quality improvements (Norton, 2018). Research by Konetzka et al. (2018) underscore that higher weights on clinical outcomes in P4P bonuses generally result in more substantial improvements, whereas smaller weights may lead to no improvement or even deterioration of specific clinical outcomes. However, the goal is *not to eliminate* all health distinctions but *to mitigate* avoidable and unjust differentials, addressing issues such as unequal resource allocation,

TABLE 10.2 Strategic Recommendations for Addressing Disparities in Long-Term Care

STRATEGY	IMPORTANCE
Increase Medicaid and Medicare reimbursement rates	Provide *additional financial resources* to providers who serve the most vulnerable and underserved populations.
Reconsider P4P programs	Incorporate SDOH such as socioeconomic status, race, ethnicity, and rurality in P4P.
Integrate culturally sensitive measures in public reporting	Develop *culturally sensitive quality measures* and overall *health equity measures* in public reporting.
Expand access to Medicaid-waivered HCBS services	Provide *broader access to crucial HCBS*, and promote inclusivity, so older adults will be able to remain in their homes as long as possible.
Adopt culturally appropriate HCBS practices with special attention to family caregivers	*Culturally appropriate HCBS practices* meet the needs of diverse populations who need LTC and rely on family caregivers.
Increase promotion of integrated HCBS programs	*Valuing community health workers* enhances cultural competence and improves access to care for underserved older adults.
Implement culture change for person-centered care	Adopt both *culture change* and *job pay or career ladder* at the same time.

HCBS, home- and community-based services; LTC, long-term care; P4P, pay-for-performance; SDOH, social determinants of health.

Source: Data from Shippee, T. P., Fabius, C. D., Fashaw-Walters, S., Bowblis, J. R., Nkimbeng, M., Bucy, T. I., Duan, Y., Ng, W., Akosionu, O., & Travers, J. L. (2022). Evidence for action: Addressing systemic racism across long-term services and supports. *Journal of the American Medical Directors Association, 23*(2), 214–219. https://doi.org/10.1016/j.jamda.2021.12.018

cultural insensitivity, and insufficient support (Whitehead, 1992). Thoughtful metric selection is crucial to prevent unintended exacerbation of disparities.

Currently, the public reporting system, Care Compare, lacks consumer voices (see Chapter 6). Incorporating culturally sensitive measures into public reporting signals a commitment to understanding and addressing cultural intricacies in healthcare delivery, establishing a transparent system that assesses both quantitative outcomes and qualitative aspects of cultural competency and responsiveness among healthcare providers. One avenue to incorporate consumer voices on cultural competency is by integrating feedback mechanisms within the reporting system; for instance, distributing surveys or feedback forms to patients and their families, specifically probing their experiences with cultural sensitivity and responsiveness during interactions with healthcare providers. Furthermore, establishing focus groups or advisory councils comprised of diverse community members could provide ongoing input and recommendations for enhancing cultural competency in healthcare settings. By actively engaging consumers in assessing and enhancing the cultural competency practices, the public reporting system can better reflect the perspectives and needs of diverse populations receiving LTC.

Recommendations pertaining to HCBS focus on several key areas. First, expanding access to Medicaid-waivered HCBS can foster inclusivity and potentially reduce healthcare expenses. Second, tailoring support services to align with diverse cultural norms and practices acknowledges the vital role of family caregivers in the overall well-being of individuals receiving LTC. Furthermore, advocating for integrated HCBS programs that value community health workers aims to enhance cultural competence and strengthen community engagement. For a more detailed discussion on HCBS, please refer to Chapter 2.

Facilitating culture change for person-centered care requires implementing strategies that concurrently address both culture transformation and career progression. By embracing this approach, LTC facilities aim to cultivate a transformative environment that pivots toward person-centered care while concurrently acknowledging the significance of providing a supportive workplace for staff. This includes incentivizing the retention of direct care workers through opportunities for career advancement and professional growth. Moreover, the culture change strategy serves as the foundational framework for implementing all other recommended approaches to enhancing LTC practices.

AN IMPLEMENTATION FRAMEWORK FOR CULTURAL TRANSFORMATION

The conventional model of LTC has historically placed emphasis on institutional efficiency and task-based routines, often at the expense of personalized, resident-centric approaches essential for delivering high-quality care and ensuring resident satisfaction. Governed by regulatory and reimbursement structures, this model has frequently overlooked the diverse needs and preferences of consumers. To transition toward a person-centered care approach in LTC, a fundamental shift in organizational culture is necessary.

Recognizing the urgent need for this cultural transformation underscores a growing awareness of the importance of valuing autonomy, dignity, and holistic well-being in LTC settings. The journey toward "person-centered care" represents a significant cultural evolution within LTC, highlighting the need to redefine organizational values, attitudes, and practices to prioritize and personalize the care experience for each resident.

Drawing from prior literature, this chapter delineated 10 key components essential to this cultural transformation, metaphorically depicted in Figure 10.2 as the "beehive analogy." These components form an interconnected network, collectively contributing to the overarching objective of delivering individualized and holistic care.

Consumer Empowerment: Effective LTC hinges on consumer empowerment, where residents and their families actively participate in decision-making. This approach ensures that residents have a voice in determining their daily routines, preferred activities, and meal selections. By involving residents and their families in decision-making, a sense of autonomy and control is fostered, enhancing their experience within care settings. This empowerment not only improves the quality of care but also promotes dignity and fulfillment for those receiving care. Going forward, LTC facilities can prioritize consumer empowerment, fostering a culture of respect, autonomy, and person-centered care.

Holistic Relationship Building: Establishing meaningful connections between care receivers and staff is foundational to fostering continuity and emotional support. This process of building a holistic relationship can be achieved by assigning specific staff members to individual residents, cultivating relationships that extend beyond routine caregiving interactions. These connections, rooted in cultural concordance where possible, contribute to a compassionate and enduring support system, enhancing the overall well-being of care recipients.

Empowering Person-Centered Care: Empowering person-centered care involves the active participation of consumers and their families in crafting personalized care plans. Through this collaborative effort, care plans are precisely tailored to align with the unique needs and preferences of each consumer. Regular reviews and updates to these plans accommodate evolving requirements, maintaining continuous alignment with changing circumstances.

Investing in Staff Training: Investing in staff training and education is essential for successful cultural change. Ongoing training initiatives equip staff with the necessary skills and knowledge to navigate the complexities of person-centered care delivery. Through targeted educational

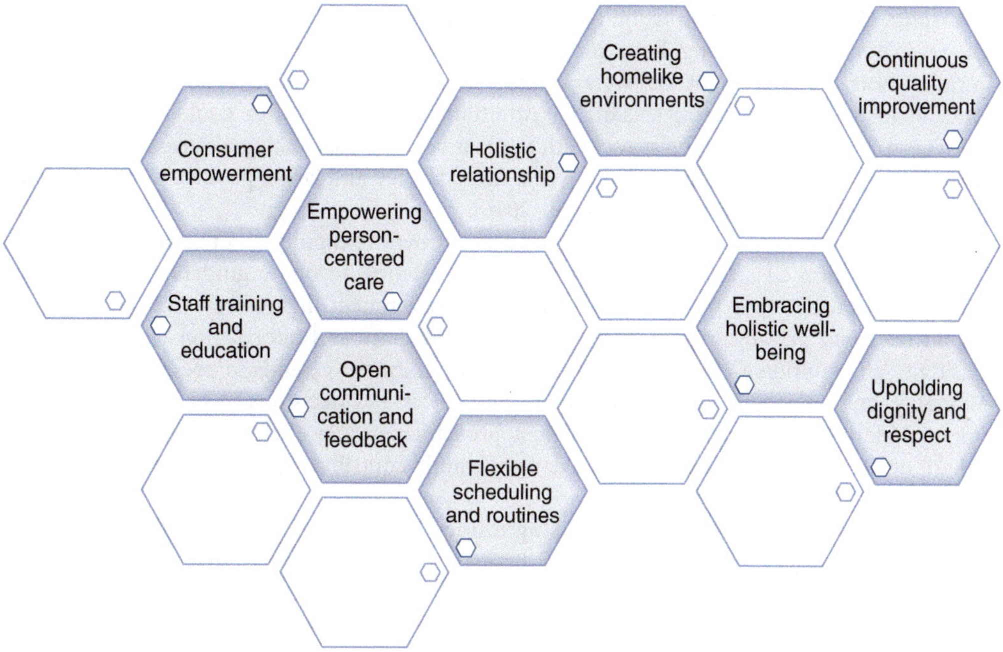

FIGURE 10.2 The beehive analogy: Components of cultural change in long-term care.

Note: Much like the complex formation of a beehive, where each hexagonal cell is vital to the overall structure, these components in person-centered care interact and depend on each other to achieve the overarching goal of individualized and holistic care. Just as bees collaboratively contribute to the construction of the hive, the person-centered care components collaborate to create a transformative environment in LTC facilities. This analogy emphasizes that the success of person-centered care is not achieved through isolated efforts but through the seamless integration and collaboration of these interconnected elements. It underscores the idea that the effectiveness of the strategy lies in the synergy of these components, working in harmony to shape a comprehensive and supportive framework.

Sources: Data from Hartmann, C. W., Snow, A. L., Allen, R. S., Parmelee, P. A., Palmer, J. A., & Berlowitz, D. (2013). A conceptual model for culture change evaluation in nursing homes. *Geriatric Nursing, 34*(5), 388–394. https://doi.org/10.1016/j.gerinurse.2013.05.008; Quality Partners of Rhode Island & Nursing Home Quality Improvement Support Center 8th Scope of Work, Task 1a: Individualized care training curriculum, the Holistic Approach to Transformational Change (HATCh) 2005. *Report of Contract HHSM-500-2006-RI002C*; Koren M. J. (2010). Person-centered care for nursing home residents: the culture-change movement. *Health Affairs, 29*(2), 312–317. https://doi.org/10.1377/hlthaff.2009.0966; Veterans Affairs. (n.d.). *HATCh model brochure.* Retrieved February 17, 2024, from https://www.va.gov/covidtraining/docs/HATCh_model_brochure_for_staff.pdf; White-Chu, E. F., Graves, W. J., Godfrey, S. M., Bonner, A., & Sloane, P. (2009). Beyond the medical model: The culture change revolution in long-term care. *Journal of the American Medical Directors Association, 10*(6), 370–378. https://doi.org/10.1016/j.jamda.2009.04.004

modules, employees are empowered to cultivate empathy, cultural sensitivity, and a deep understanding of each resident's unique needs and background. Specialized training sessions focusing on active listening techniques and responsive communication strategies further enhance staff proficiency in addressing diverse consumer needs with compassion and efficacy.

Flexible Scheduling and Routines: Embracing flexibility in scheduling and daily routines lies at the heart of promoting resident autonomy and individualized care experiences. Rather than adhering to rigid schedules, LTC facilities should prioritize adaptable frameworks. This approach allows residents to shape their daily routines according to their personal preferences and natural rhythms, fostering a sense of independence and agency. Whether it is selecting meal times, participating in recreational activities, or engaging in personal care routines, offering flexibility ensures that each resident's voice is heard and respected. Ultimately, this approach contributes to a more personalized and enriching care environment, where residents feel empowered and valued as active participants in their own care journey.

Creating Homelike Environments: Redesigning physical spaces to emulate homelike atmospheres is not only comforting, but it provides spaces for social interaction and personalization. In practical terms, this might involve arranging communal areas with comfortable seating for residents to gather, encouraging socializing. Additionally, personalization could involve allowing residents to decorate their living spaces with familiar belongings, creating a sense of comfort and belonging. Such modifications contribute to a more homey ambiance, positively impacting the overall well-being of residents (Bowers et al., 2016).

Upholding Dignity and Respect: A steadfast commitment to dignity and respect permeates all interactions within LTC settings. This commitment extends beyond a guideline, becoming an integral part of the ethos that permeates the care environment. It involves a vigilant effort to uphold residents' privacy and safeguard their personal space and information with the utmost sensitivity and confidentiality. Concurrently, this commitment extends to preserving residents' autonomy, granting them the authority to make choices and decisions in harmony with their unique preferences and values. This holistic approach creates an environment where residents feel not only cared for but also empowered, significantly contributing to their overall well-being and quality of life.

Embracing Holistic Well-Being: Addressing residents' social, emotional, and spiritual needs alongside physical care is essential for well-being. This commitment aligns with the HATCh model, developed in 2005 to enhance nursing home culture by promoting a holistic approach to transformational change. The model aims to facilitate personal, organizational, community, and systems changes, fostering a shift from institutional to individual care. It outlines six interrelated domains crucial for this transformation: workplace practice, care practice, environment, leadership, family and community, and regulatory/government. Practical applications of the HATCh model include integrating holistic therapies such as music or art therapy into the care regimen.

Open Communication and Feedback: Advancing care practices in LTSS hinges on fostering open communication and feedback mechanisms that actively involve consumers. This collaborative engagement empowers individuals, allowing them to articulate their preferences, concerns, and aspirations regarding their care journey. Through transparent and inclusive communication, residents and their families become integral partners in decision-making processes, ensuring that care plans are tailored to meet their unique needs and preferences.

Continuous Quality Improvement: Establishing a culture of continuous quality improvement ensures that care practices evolve in response to the changing needs and expectations of service users. By embracing a philosophy of ongoing learning and adaptation, organizations can systematically identify areas for enhancement and innovation within their care delivery systems. This entails creating mechanisms for collecting and analyzing feedback, both from residents and staff, and leveraging this information to drive meaningful improvements in care quality and outcomes. By prioritizing responsiveness and accountability, organizations can cultivate an environment where feedback is not only welcomed but actively sought after, fostering a culture of excellence and innovation in LTC settings.

In summary, the holistic approach outlined in this chapter emphasizes the need for a comprehensive, systems thinking strategy to tackle healthcare disparities in LTC. Success in implementing these approaches relies heavily on robust support from administrative leadership and integration of insights from diverse health professionals (White-Chu et al., 2009). Additionally, involving consumers, particularly residents themselves, as active participants in driving cultural transformation is crucial (Shura et al., 2011). By collectively addressing systemic barriers and fostering inclusive interventions, policymakers can work toward rectifying existing disparities and proactively preventing future inequalities. Policymakers must deepen their understanding of these factors to ensure successful implementation of policies aimed at advancing equitable LTC practices (Grabowski et al., 2014).

STRATEGIC IMPLEMENTATION FOR HEALTHCARE EQUITY IN LONG-TERM CARE: CASE STUDIES

LTC administrators can effectively translate strategic initiatives into actionable plans by adopting a systems approach and drawing inspiration from successful case studies. A valuable resource in this context is the *Building an Organizational Response to Health Disparities* report (Office of Minority Health, 2019), which presents insights from five diverse cases. These case studies, conducted with private-sector healthcare organizations, focus on their approaches for identifying and addressing healthcare disparities within their communities, detailing how each organization strategically planned and implemented initiatives to transform their service delivery models.

For instance:

- **Frederick Memorial Hospital** prioritized communication services for minority groups with *limited English proficiency* (LEP) and incorporated *American Sign Language* to enhance access to care.
- **Harvard Pilgrim Health Care** responded to customer requests by offering *transgender-inclusive care.*
- **Health Net of California** targeted healthcare disparities in the Latino population, addressing performance gaps in care for low-income subsidy-eligible individuals.
- **Highmark Health** utilized *self-reported data* to identify care gaps, initiating interventions in areas such as access to care, immunization, and preventive services.
- **Methodist Le Bonheur Healthcare** implemented *Familiar Faces* to reduce emergency department visits for high users of health services.

These case studies offer actionable business cases, providing detailed insights into specific steps, necessary resources, challenges faced, and lessons learned. While not tailored specifically for LTC, they remain relevant, highlighting the importance of understanding the needs of underserved populations, complying with regulations, fostering strong leadership, and utilizing data for continuous improvement.

Table 10.3 summarizes seven important actionable steps to effectively tackle healthcare disparities, providing a comprehensive roadmap for LTC administrators and policymakers to implement sustainable changes.

The integration of these approaches creates a powerful synergy, enhancing their impact when harmonized. At the core is data collection, guiding the identification of disparities and informing the development of precise strategies through root cause analysis. Implementing these strategies involves creating clear plans with timelines, resources, and responsibilities, while quality improvement initiatives track progress and ensure ongoing assessment of care quality. Collaboration and community engagement further fortify effectiveness by incorporating diverse perspectives, ensuring interventions are culturally appropriate and responsive to community needs. Continuous evaluation, incorporating feedback from patients and caregivers, allows for adjustments to be made based on real-world experiences. Finally, policy advocacy plays a crucial role in laying the groundwork for thriving strategies, advocating for policies that promote equitable access to care and address systemic barriers.

It should be noted that actionable plans at organizational level focus on establishing internal procedures, ensuring compliance with regulations, providing training, fostering a culture of continuous improvement, and effectively managing change within the organization. Change management is integral to this process, as it ensures smooth transitions and acceptance of new policies or procedures among employees.

TABLE 10.3 Actionable Steps for Addressing Healthcare Disparities

ACTIONABLE STEPS	APPROACHES
Data collection and analysis	• Collect and analyze data on population demographics and health outcomes. • Use data to identify disparities (objectives) and create targeted interventions. • Continuously monitor data for progress and areas needing improvement.
Root cause analysis	• Conduct root cause analysis to identify underlying determinants of the targeted disparities. • Identify other systemic barriers such as healthcare access or organizations' cultural competency.
Implement strategies	• Develop actionable strategies for addressing health disparities. • Create a clear implementation plan with timelines, resources, and responsibilities.
Quality improvement initiatives	• Implement quality improvement initiatives for diverse population needs. • Track quality metrics using data and regularly assess care quality.
Collaboration and community engagement	• Collaborate with stakeholders to create culturally appropriate interventions. • Engage the community to incorporate their perspectives in interventions.
Continuous evaluation	• Continuously evaluate intervention effectiveness using data. • Incorporate patient and caregiver feedback into evaluations.
Policy advocacy	• Advocate for policies promoting equitable care access. • Collaborate with policymakers using data to address systemic barriers to care.

Conversely, actionable plans in public policy advocacy entail conducting research and analysis, building coalitions, engaging with policymakers, and mobilizing public support to influence government policies. The steps in Table 10.3 are drawn from principles commonly found in public health policy advocacy (Hearne et al., 2023; Israel et al., 2010), aiming to address broader societal issues by advocating for specific policy solutions and leveraging collective action to shape policy decisions. Both types of plans involve taking tangible steps to achieve desired outcomes, tailored to the distinct contexts and objectives of organizational policy and public policy advocacy.

Case Study 10.1 illustrates the effectiveness of this synergy. The inclusion of real-world business case studies strengthens the practical application of theoretical frameworks. This holistic approach empowers LTC administrators and policymakers to proactively address healthcare disparities, fostering positive changes in services delivery and contributing to the continual enhancement of care delivery.

Case Study 10.1 Addressing Healthcare Disparities Through a Data-Driven Approach: Clubview Senior Care

Background

Clubview Senior Care serves a diverse population of older adult consumers. Administrators noticed disparities in health outcomes and access to care among demographic groups. They aimed to identify and address these disparities to ensure equitable healthcare provision.

Data Collection and Analysis Approach

Administrators initiated a comprehensive data collection and analysis to understand and rectify healthcare disparities among consumers.

Activities Undertaken

1. *Data Gathering:* Collected data on various health metrics, including prevalence rates of chronic conditions such as diabetes, heart disease, and mental health disorders across different demographic groups (e.g., by race/ethnicity, gender, and socioeconomic status).
2. *Access to Care Assessment:* Collected data on access to care elements such as transportation availability for medical appointments and the affordability of medication. This involved conducting surveys and analyzing records to pinpoint barriers faced by specific subgroups.
3. *Comparative Analysis:* Analyzed collected data to compare health outcomes and access to care among different demographic categories. Disparities were identified, revealing differences in chronic condition prevalence and access to essential medical services among various resident groups.
4. *Tailored Intervention Development:* Formulated targeted interventions based on data insights. For instance, they arranged transportation services for consumers facing mobility challenges and implemented cost-assistance programs for medications to ensure affordability.

Outcomes

The data-driven approach led to:

- recognition and addressing of disparities in chronic condition prevalence through tailored interventions,
- mitigation of access to care barriers for specific subgroups, such as transportation and medication costs, and
- improved health outcomes and equitable access to care among consumers.

Case Study Discussion Question

1. How do Clubview Senior Care's strategies align with the key steps in Table 10.3 for addressing healthcare disparities in LTC?

ENHANCING CULTURAL AND LINGUISTIC COMPETENCE IN LONG-TERM CARE: A COMPREHENSIVE GUIDE TO CLAS STANDARDS IMPLEMENTATION

The culturally and linguistically appropriate services (CLAS) standards, established by the Office of Minority Health within the HHS, offer a crucial framework for ensuring equitable care within LTC facilities (Barksdale et al., 2017). These standards address barriers such as varying levels of health literacy and language differences (NASEM, 2018), which can impede comprehension, decision-making, and access to appropriate care options for individuals and families (Mukherjea et al., 2020). Prioritizing health literacy and employing patient-friendly approaches are essential strategies to enhance communication, understanding, and patient engagement in care (Koh et al., 2013). Adhering to CLAS standards empowers LTC facilities to potentially improve care quality and address healthcare disparities (Periyakoil, 2019).

Table 10.4 outlines the specific focus and commitment of CLAS standards across key domains within LTC facilities, emphasizing areas for improvements in care quality and patient safety. While not binding regulations, CLAS standards serve as guiding beacons, promoting culturally sensitive care practices throughout healthcare settings.

Encouraging healthcare providers to offer services that are respectful and responsive to diverse cultural beliefs, practices, and languages, CLAS standards play a crucial role in recognizing and respecting varied health perspectives. Aligning with these standards empowers LTC facilities to address healthcare disparities through culturally competent care, language access, and trust-building between caregivers and recipients. This approach elevates care quality, improves health outcomes, and contributes to reducing disparities faced by marginalized groups within LTC settings.

Drawing insights from a successful adoption at a community health center (CHC), Case Study 10.2 illustrates potential activities for LTC facilities to implement CLAS standards. While specific evidence in the LTC context is still emerging, broader implementation of CLAS standards has demonstrated positive outcomes for healthcare providers, including reduced length-of-stay for Medicare patients (Schiaffino et al., 2020). Prioritizing language access and cultural competency enables LTC facilities to effectively tackle disparities in healthcare access and outcomes across diverse demographic groups. These achievements underscore the significance of integrating CLAS standards, emphasizing the pivotal role of cultural competence and language services in fortifying healthcare equity and quality across diverse communities.

TABLE 10.4 Integration of CLAS Standards in Long-Term Care: Key Domains and Applications

KEY DOMAIN	QUALITY OF CARE	PATIENT SAFETY
Cultural competence	Understanding diverse beliefs and practices	Ensuring accurate medication information
	Respecting cultural and linguistic needs	Addressing cultural beliefs impacting medication
Language access	Providing language services for proficiency	Utilizing interpreters for informed consent
	Offering translation services for materials	Using translated forms for procedure understanding
Organizational support	Incorporating cultural competence policies	Promoting medication safety through clarity
	Staff training for culturally sensitive care	Enhancing communication for consent
Community Engagement	Collaborating with community organizations	Engaging diverse communities in healthcare planning

CLAS, culturally and linguistically appropriate services.

Source: Data from U.S. Department of Health and Human Services. (n.d.). *National culturally and linguistically appropriate services standards*. Retrieved October 27, 2024, from https://thinkculturalhealth.hhs.gov/clas/standards

Case Study 10.2 Implementing CLAS Standards in a Community Health Center

Background

The CHC serves a diverse population with varying cultural and linguistic backgrounds. The administration noticed disparities in healthcare access and outcomes among different demographic groups and aimed to improve care through CLAS standards.

CLAS Standards Actionable Step: Language Access

Activities Undertaken

1. *Assessment of Language Needs:* The CHC conducted an assessment to identify the language needs of its patient population. They analyzed patient demographics to determine the languages spoken and the proficiency levels of non-English speakers.
2. *Implementing Language Services:* Based on the assessment, the CHC established a system to provide language services. They ensured the availability of trained interpreters and translated materials in commonly spoken languages within the community.
3. *Staff Training:* To comply with CLAS standards, the CHC provided cultural competency training for its staff. This training focused on understanding diverse cultural backgrounds, improving communication, and delivering respectful care.
4. *Community Engagement:* The CHC collaborated with local community organizations to engage diverse communities. They sought feedback from community leaders and patients to better understand their needs and preferences.

Outcomes

Through the implementation of CLAS standards, the CHC observed several positive outcomes:

- increased access to healthcare services for non-English speakers,
- improved patient–provider communication, leading to better health outcomes,
- enhanced patient satisfaction and trust within the diverse communities served, and
- reduced disparities in healthcare access and outcomes among different demographic groups.

Case Study Discussion Question

1. How did the implementation of CLAS standards, particularly focusing on language access, contribute to the observed positive outcomes in the CHC case study? Additionally, how might similar strategies be adapted in different healthcare settings to address disparities in access and outcomes for diverse populations?

SUMMARY

Chapter 10 discusses the pervasive disparities encountered by individuals with disabilities in LTC settings and presents viable strategies for addressing these pressing challenges. It underscores the critical need for swift interventions and policy reforms to address healthcare inequities faced by this vulnerable population, highlighting the collective efforts necessary among stakeholders to realize a truly inclusive and equitable healthcare system.

The chapter meticulously examines the key challenges confronting people with disabilities in LTC settings and underscores the paramount importance of person-centered care planning.

It critically evaluates the potential advantages and challenges of consumer-centric care models compared to traditional models.

Moreover, the chapter underscores the significance of robust data collection, root cause analysis, and quality improvement initiatives in ameliorating healthcare disparities in LTC. It also delves into the challenges healthcare providers and LTC facilities may encounter when implementing CLAS standards, offering actionable strategies for overcoming these obstacles.

In conclusion, the chapter asserts that healthcare administrators and policymakers play pivotal roles in fostering equity and inclusivity within LTC. It advocates for transformative change through active engagement with staff, consumers, and families, emphasizing the collective responsibility in championing the rights and dignity of individuals reliant on LTC services within the healthcare landscape.

END-OF-CHAPTER RESOURCES

DISCUSSION QUESTIONS

1. How can LTC settings be adapted to suit the unique needs of people with disabilities?
2. What does person-centered care planning involve, and how can consumers and their families actively participate in creating personalized care plans?
3. What are the potential benefits of the consumer-centric paradigm in LTC, and how does it differ from traditional models?
4. What specific strategies or interventions for reducing healthcare disparities in LTC are discussed in this chapter? Can you provide examples of organizations that have successfully implemented these interventions?
5. What are the potential challenges that healthcare providers and LTC facilities may face when implementing CLAS standards, and how can these challenges be addressed?
6. What is systems thinking, and how can it be applied in analyzing healthcare problems and proposing solutions that consider the interconnectedness of systems, feedback loops, and emergent properties?

SPRINGER PUBLISHING CONNECT™

A robust set of instructor resources designed to supplement this text is located at http://connect.springerpub.com/content/book/978-0-8261-4935-0. Qualifying instructors may request access by emailing textbook@springerpub.com.

REFERENCES

Agaronnik, N. D., Pendo, E., Campbell, E. G., Ressalam, J., & Iezzoni, L. I. (2019). Knowledge of practicing physicians about their legal obligations when caring for patients with disability. *Health Affairs*, *38*(4), 545–553. https://doi.org/10.1377/hlthaff.2018.05060

Akobirshoev, I., Vetter, M., Iezzoni, L. I., Rao, S. R., & Mitra, M. (2022). Delayed medical care and unmet care needs due to the COVID-19 pandemic among adults with disabilities in the US: Study examines delayed medical care and unmet care needs attributable to the COVID-19 pandemic among US adults with disabilities. *Health Affairs*, *41*(10), 1505–1512. https://doi.org/10.1377/hlthaff.2022.00509

Barksdale, C. L., Rodick, W. H., Hopson, R., Kenyon, J., Green, K., & Jacobs, C. G. (2017). Literature review of the national CLAS standards: Policy and practical implications in reducing health disparities. *Journal of Racial and Ethnic Health Disparities*, *4*, 632–647. https://doi.org/10.1007/s40615-016-0267-3

Betancourt, J. R., Green, A. R., Carrillo, J. E., & Park, E. R. (2005). Cultural competence and health care disparities: Key perspectives and trends. *Health Affairs*, *24*(2), 499–505. https://doi.org/10.1377/hlthaff.24.2.499

Bowers, B., Nolet, K., Jacobson, N., THRIVE Research Collaborative, Bowers, B., Brown, P., Cohen, L., Grabowski, D., Horn, S., Hudak, S., Nolet, K., Reed, D., & Zimmerman, S. (2016). Sustaining culture change: Experiences in the Green House model. *Health Services Research, 51*, 398–417. https://doi.org/10.1111/1475-6773.12428

Carthon, J. M. B., Brom, H., Poghosyan, L., Daus, M., Todd, B., & Aiken, L. (2020). Supportive clinical practice environments associated with patient-centered care. *The Journal for Nurse Practitioners, 16*(4), 294–298. https://doi.org/10.1016/j.nurpra.2020.01.019

Centers for Disease Control and Prevention. (2024, July). *Disability impacts all of us* [Infographic]. Retrieved September 26, 2024, from https://www.cdc.gov/ncbddd/disabilityandhealth/infographic-disability-impacts-all.html

Centers for Medicare & Medicaid Services. (2022, December 6). *Addressing health-related social needs in Section 1115 demonstrations*. https://www.medicaid.gov/sites/default/files/2023-01/addrss-hlth-soc-needs-1115-demo-all-st-call-12062022.pdf

Colello, K. J. (2023, October 2). *Overview of long-term services and supports*. Congressional Research Service. https://crsreports.congress.gov/product/pdf/IF/IF10427

Donelan, K., Chang, Y., Matulewicz, H., Warsett, K., Heaphy, D., & Iezzoni, L. I. (2020). Care plans, care teams, and quality of life for people with disabilities. *Journal of General Internal Medicine, 35*, 2274–2280. https://doi.org/10.1007/s11606-020-05908-w

Engle, R. L., Mohr, D. C., Holmes, S. K., Seibert, M. N., Afable, M., Leyson, J., & Meterko, M. (2021). Evidence-based practice and patient-centered care: Doing both well. *Health Care Management Review, 46*(3), 174–184. https://doi.org/10.1097/HMR.0000000000000254

Friedman, C. (2023). Medicaid home-and community-based services waivers for people with intellectual and developmental disabilities. *Intellectual and Developmental Disabilities, 61*(4), 269–279. https://doi.org/10.1352/1934-9556-61.4.269

Froehlich-Grobe, K., Jones, D., Businelle, M. S., Kendzor, D. E., & Balasubramanian, B. A. (2016). Impact of disability and chronic conditions on health. *Disability and Health Journal, 9*(4), 600–608. https://doi.org/10.1016/j.dhjo.2016.04.007

Grabowski, D. C., Elliot, A., Leitzell, B., Cohen, L. W., & Zimmerman, S. (2014). Who are the innovators? Nursing homes implementing culture change. *The Gerontologist, 54*(Suppl. 1), S650–S75. https://doi.org/10.1093/geront/gnt144

Guth, M. (2022, November 15). *Section 1115 waiver watch: Approvals to address health-related social needs*. KFF. Retrieved February 2, 2024, from https://www.kff.org/medicaid/issue-brief/section-1115-waiver-watch-approvals-to-address-health-related-social-needs

Hearne, S., Pollack Porter, K. M., & Forrest, K. S. (2023). *Policy engagement*. American Public Health Association.

Iezzoni, L. I. (2011). Eliminating health and health care disparities among the growing population of people with disabilities. *Health Affairs, 30*(10), 1947–1954. https://doi.org/10.1377/hlthaff.2011.0613

Iezzoni, L. I. (2023). Disability disparities and ableism in medicine. In I. U. Shehla & F. John (Eds.), *ABC of equality, diversity and inclusion in healthcare* (pp. 61–68). Wiley-Blackwell.

Iezzoni, L. I., & Agaronnik, N. D. (2020). Healthcare disparities for individuals with disability: Informing the practice. In L. M. Meeks & L. Neal-Boylan (Eds.). *Disability as diversity: A guidebook for inclusion in medicine, nursing, and the health professions* (pp. 15–31). Springer Nature.

Iezzoni, L. I., McKee, M. M., Meade, M. A., Morris, M. A., & Pendo, E. (2022). Have almost fifty years of disability civil rights laws achieved equitable care? Overview examines 50 years of US disability civil rights laws. *Health Affairs, 41*(10), 1371–1378. https://doi.org/10.1377/hlthaff.2022.00413

Iezzoni, L. I., Rao, S. R., Ressalam, J., Bolcic-Jankovic, D., Agaronnik, N. D., Lagu, T., Pendo, E., & Campbell, E. G. (2022). US physicians' knowledge about the Americans with Disabilities Act and accommodation of patients with disability: Study examines what physicians know about the Americans with Disabilities Act and what is done to accommodate patients with a disability. *Health Affairs, 41*(1), 96–104. https://doi.org/10.1377/hlthaff.2021.01136

Institute of Medicine. (1986). *Improving the quality of care in nursing homes*. National Academies Press. https://www.ncbi.nlm.nih.gov/books/NBK217556

Institute of Medicine. (2001). *Crossing the quality chasm: A new health system for the 21st century*. National Academies Press. https://www.ncbi.nlm.nih.gov/books/NBK222274

Israel, B. A., Coombe, C. M., Cheezum, R. R., Schulz, A. J., McGranaghan, R. J., Lichtenstein, R., Reyes, A. G., Clement, J., & Burris, A. (2010). Community-based participatory research: A capacity-building approach for policy advocacy aimed at eliminating health disparities. *American Journal of Public Health, 100*(11), 2094–2102. https://doi.org/10.2105/AJPH.2009.170506

Koh, H. K., Brach, C., Harris, L. M., & Parchman, M. L. (2013). A proposed 'health literate care model' would constitute a systems approach to improving patients' engagement in care. *Health Affairs, 32*(2), 357–367. https://doi.org/10.1377/hlthaff.2012.1205

Konetzka, R. T., Grabowski, D. C., Perraillon, M. C., & Werner, R. M. (2015). Nursing home 5-star rating system exacerbates disparities in quality, by payer source. *Health Affairs, 34*(5), 819–827. https://doi.org/10.1377/hlthaff.2014.1084

Konetzka, R. T., Skira, M. M., & Werner, R. M. (2018). Incentive design and quality improvements: Evidence from state Medicaid nursing home pay-for-performance programs. *American Journal of Health Economics, 4*(1), 105–130. https://doi.org/10.1162/ajhe_a_00095

Konetzka, R. T., & Werner, R. M. (2009). Disparities in long-term care: Building equity into market-based reforms. *Medical Care Research and Review, 66*(5), 491–521. https://doi.org/10.1177/1077558709331813

Krahn, G. L., Walker, D. K., & Correa-De-Araujo, R. (2015). Persons with disabilities as an unrecognized health disparity population. *American Journal of Public Health, 105*(S2), S198–S206. https://doi.org/10.2105/AJPH.2014.302182

Lagu, T., Haywood, C., Reimold, K., DeJong, C., Walker Sterling, R., & Iezzoni, L. I. (2022). 'I am not the doctor for you': Physicians' attitudes about caring for people with disabilities: Study examines physician attitudes about caring for people with disabilities. *Health Affairs, 41*(10), 1387–1395. https://doi.org/10.1377/hlthaff.2022.00475

Lekas, H. M., Pahl, K., & Fuller Lewis, C. (2020). Rethinking cultural competence: Shifting to cultural humility. *Health Services Insights, 13*. https://doi.org/10.1177/1178632920970580

Mitra, M., Long-Bellil, L., Moura, I., Miles, A., & Kaye, H. S. (2022). Advancing health equity and reducing health disparities for people with disabilities in the United States: Study examines health equity and health disparities for people with disabilities in the United States. *Health Affairs, 41*(10), 1379–1386. https://doi.org/10.1377/hlthaff.2022.00499

Mukherjea, A., Ali, S., & Smith, J. A. (2020). A human rights perspective on palliative care: Unraveling disparities and determinants among Asian American populations. *Topics in Language Disorders, 40*(3), 278–296. https://doi.org/10.1097/TLD.0000000000000222

National Academies of Sciences, Engineering, and Medicine. (2018). *Health literacy and older adults: Reshaping the landscape: Proceedings of a workshop*. National Academies Press. https://www.ncbi.nlm.nih.gov/books/NBK532464

National Academies of Sciences, Engineering, and Medicine. (2022). *The national imperative to improve nursing home quality: Honoring our commitment to residents, families, and staff*. National Academies Press. https://doi.org/10.17226/26526

National Council on Disability. (2023a, May 4). *Framework to end health disparities of people with disabilities*. https://www.ncd.gov/report/framework-to-end-health-disparities-of-people-with-disabilities

National Council on Disability. (2023b, October 31). *2023 progress report: Toward economic security: The impact of income and asset limits on people with disabilities*. https://www.ncd.gov/report/2023-progress-report-toward-economic-security-the-impact-of-income-and-asset-limits-on-people-with-disabilities

National Institute on Aging. (2023). *National research summit on care, services, and supports for persons living with dementia and their care partners/caregivers*. https://www.nia.nih.gov/sites/default/files/2023-07/caregiving-dementia-summit.pdf

Norton, E. C. (2018). Long-term care and pay-for-performance programs. *Review of Development Economics, 22*(3), 1005–1021. https://doi.org/10.1111/rode.12359

Office of Minority Health. (2019, July 1). *Building an organizational response to health disparities: Five pioneers from the field*. U.S. Department of Health & Human Services, Centers for Medicare & Medicaid Services. https://www.cms.gov/About-CMS/Agency-Information/OMH/Downloads/Building-an-Organizational-Response-to-Address-Health-Disparaties-Executive-Summary.pdf

Periyakoil, V. S. (2019). Building a culturally competent workforce to care for diverse older adults: Scope of the problem and potential solutions. *Journal of the American Geriatrics Society*, *67*(S2), S423–S432. https://doi.org/10.1111/jgs.15939

Rubenstein, E., Tewolde, S., Levine, A. A., Droscha, L., Meyer, R. M., Michals, A., & Skotko, B. (2024). Medicare, Medicaid, and dual enrollment for adults with intellectual and developmental disabilities. *Health Services Research*, *59*(3), e14287. https://doi.org/10.1111/1475-6773.14287

Saha, S., Beach, M. C., & Cooper, L. A. (2008). Patient centeredness, cultural competence and healthcare quality. *Journal of the National Medical Association*, *100*(11), 1275–1285. https://doi.org/10.1016/s0027-9684(15)31505-4

Schiaffino, M. K., Ruiz, M., Yakuta, M., Contreras, A., Akhavan, S., Prince, B., & Weech-Maldonado, R. (2020). Culturally and linguistically appropriate hospital services reduce Medicare length of stay. *Ethnicity & Disease*, *30*(4), 603–610. https://doi.org/10.18865/ed.30.4.603

Seervai, S., Shah, A., & Shah, T. (2019, April 16). *The challenges of living with a disability in America, and how serious illness can add to them*. The Commonwealth Fund. https://www.commonwealthfund.org/publications/fund-reports/2019/apr/challenges-living-disability-america-and-how-serious-illness-can

Shippee, T. P., Fabius, C. D., Fashaw-Walters, S., Bowblis, J. R., Nkimbeng, M., Bucy, T. I., Duan, Y., Ng, W., Akosionu, O., & Travers, J. L. (2022). Evidence for action: Addressing systemic racism across long-term services and supports. *Journal of the American Medical Directors Association*, *23*(2), 214–219. https://doi.org/10.1016/j.jamda.2021.12.018

Shura, R., Siders, R. A., & Dannefer, D. (2011). Culture change in long-term care: Participatory action research and the role of the resident. *The Gerontologist*, *51*(2), 212–225. https://doi.org/10.1093/geront/gnq099

Smedley, B. D., Stith, A. Y., & Nelson, A. R. (Eds.). (2003). *Unequal treatment: Confronting racial and ethnic disparities in health care*. National Academies Press.

Tervalon, M., & Murray-Garcia, J. (1998). Cultural humility versus cultural competence: A critical distinction in defining physician training outcomes in multicultural education. *Journal of Health Care for the Poor and Underserved*, *9*(2), 117–125. https://doi.org/10.1353/hpu.2010.0233

U.S. Department of Health & Human Services. (n.d.). *Section 504 of the Rehabilitation Act of 1973 final rule: Section by section fact sheet for recipients of financial assistance from HHS*. Retrieved September 26, 2024, from https://www.hhs.gov/civil-rights/for-individuals/disability/section-504-rehabilitation-act-of-1973/ocr-detailed-504-fact-sheet/index.html

White-Chu, E. F., Graves, W. J., Godfrey, S. M., Bonner, A., & Sloane, P. (2009). Beyond the medical model: The culture change revolution in long-term care. *Journal of the American Medical Directors Association*, *10*(6), 370–378. https://doi.org/10.1016/j.jamda.2009.04.004

Whitehead, M. (1992). The concepts and principles of equity and health. *International Journal of Health Services*, *22*(3), 429–445. https://doi.org/10.2190/986L-LHQ6-2VTE-YRRN

Wunderlich, G. S., & Kohler, P. O. (Eds.). (2001). *Improving the quality of long-term care*. National Academies Press. https://www.ncbi.nlm.nih.gov/books/NBK224500

CHAPTER 11

IMPLEMENTING EVIDENCE-BASED PRACTICES IN LONG-TERM SERVICES AND SUPPORTS

Miranda C. Kunkel, Katherine M. Abbott, Natalie F. Douglas, and Kimberly S. Van Haitsma

Learning Objectives

After completing this chapter, each learner will be able to:

- Understand the significance of implementation science in long-term care (LTC), recognize the barriers and facilitators to the implementation of evidence-based practices (EBP), and demonstrate knowledge of the consolidated framework for implementation research and its application in the nursing home setting.
- Comprehend the pivotal role of individuals in the implementation process and recognize the challenges posed by staff shortages and turnover in LTC settings.
- Recognize the critical importance of the preimplementation stage in the process of implementing EBP in LTC, including creating an appropriate implementation team, assessing needs and context, planning, and tailoring strategies before engaging in innovation.
- Understand the critical influence of macro-level factors—including policy dynamics, organizational factors, and community influences—on the successful implementation of EBP in LTC settings.
- Use the practical tools and recommendations provided for EBP implementation in care delivery.

INTRODUCTION

If our collective goal is to improve the quality of care individuals receive, then it is vital that we utilize evidence-based healthcare practices. Evidence-based practices (EBP) are "the conscientious and judicious use of current best evidence in conjunction with clinical expertise and patient values to guide healthcare decisions" (Titler, 2008, p. 113). Evidence can come from a continuum of sources ranging from rigorous research studies to expert opinion (see Figure 11.1). The field of implementation science grew out of the realization that it was taking, on average, 17 years for 14% of EBPs to be incorporated into every-day care (Morris et al., 2011). This has been termed the *know-do gap*. Essentially, we know outcomes could be better if we did a specific practice. However, many implementation efforts fail for a whole host of reasons. Implementation science provides us with theories, methods, and frameworks to systematically identify and remediate barriers to implementation. Implementation science is an exciting and emerging field whose approach offers broad and novel insights into the gap between research and practice. Implementation science is commonly defined as the study of methods and strategies to promote the uptake of interventions that have proven effective in routine practice, with the aim of improving population health.

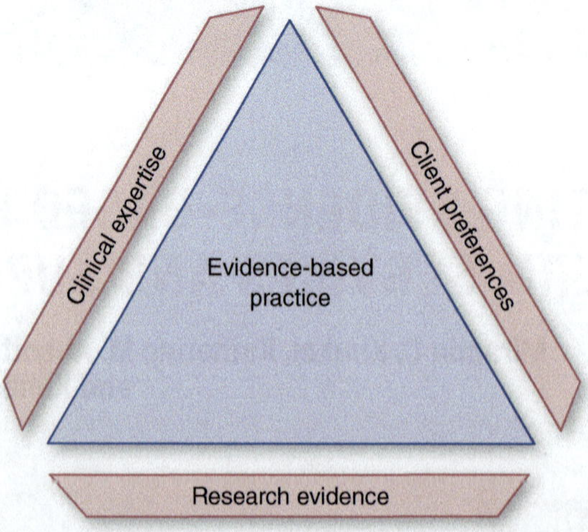

FIGURE 11.1. Integration of elements for evidence-based practice.

Therefore, *implementation research* is used to understand the approaches that work best to translate research to the real world, and *implementation practice* applies and adapts these approaches in different settings to achieve outcomes. The purpose of this chapter is to introduce you to the field of implementation science, explain why it is important to quality and safety, and suggest context-specific considerations when implementing new initiatives in the nursing home setting via the consolidated framework for implementation research (CFIR). The CFIR was selected because it is the most cited framework (Damschroder et al., 2009, 2022; Skolarus et al., 2017) and widely applicable to the nursing home setting (Abbott et al., 2022).

CFIR provides a comprehensive approach to identifying the barriers and facilitators to implementation efforts (Damschroder et al., 2022). This framework is a determinant framework because the included domains and constructs determine the outcomes of the implementation effort. Ideally, CFIR can be used to help you identify barriers and facilitators throughout implementation, or to explain differences in implementation outcomes. The original CFIR framework was developed in 2009 and revised with input from users in 2022 (Damschroder et al., 2009, 2022). Of particular note is how the authors centered the individual's/client's/patient's health equity as a foundation for the changes in CFIR 2.0. What follows is a description of the CFIR 2.0 domains, facilitators and barriers that have been found in the nursing home setting by domain, and examples of work to illustrate the central role that implementation science should play in the nursing home setting.

BARRIERS AND FACILITATORS TO THE IMPLEMENTATION OF EVIDENCE-BASED PRACTICES IN LONG-TERM CARE

Studying EBPs in nursing home settings is crucial for several reasons, especially when considering their impact on quality and safety. Implementing EBPs can lead to higher-quality care for residents, contribute to more efficient and cost-effective care delivery, and help long-term care (LTC) providers meet regulatory requirements and avoid penalties (Connor et al., 2023). When considering EBPs, it is important to understand the barriers and facilitators to their implementation. The CFIR 2.0 offers practitioners and researchers a method for systematically and accurately tracking barriers and facilitators to innovations. The following section will detail each of the five CFIR 2.0 domains (i.e., characteristics of the innovation, characteristics of the individual, the process of implementing, the inner setting, and the outer setting). For each domain, we address common barriers and facilitators that nursing home providers may encounter when implementing innovations in their community, as well as an illustrative example related to that domain.

Characteristics of the Innovation to Be Implemented

According to the CFIR 2.0, the innovation is the "thing" being implemented and has traits such as adaptability, complexity, cost, trialability, and design that may either help or hinder implementation (Damschroder et al., 2022). Innovations that are too complex, time-consuming, expensive, or confusing may be quickly abandoned (Abbott et al., 2022). Nursing home staff typically have heavy workloads and limited time to provide care to residents (Hoedl et al., 2022). If EBPs are overly time-consuming or burdensome, they may detract from the time available for direct resident care, leading to dissatisfaction with the innovation and/or inadequate resident care. In contrast, interventions that are flexible, understandable, and fit into existing workflows are more likely to be successful (de Veer et al., 2021). Simplified and clear practices are more likely to be consistently applied by all staff, regardless of their level of expertise (Abu-Baker et al., 2021). Similarly, the added work associated with an implementation (e.g., additional time, staffing, and paperwork) should be carefully considered. Some increases to staff workload are reasonable; however, whenever possible, innovations should be designed in a way to leverage information that is already available and/or being collected (e.g., the Minimum Data Set interview information). To limit added burden on staff, it is important that innovations provide sufficient training and continued support for the nursing home staff (Tappen et al., 2017). A one-time training is rarely sufficient; innovation models that offer accessible program managers and regular check-ins are preferred (Rolland et al., 2021). Follow-up communication between the innovation researchers/developers and the nursing home staff actually implementing the innovation allows for rapport building, sharing success stories, and troubleshooting issues.

While it may also be a barrier if the innovation requires significant adaptation to achieve the best fit with the community's local context, this is a reality that most EBPs in nursing homes face (Koerner et al., 2021). In nursing home settings, innovations should be tailored around the resources, workflow, and priorities of an organization (Barrera et al., 2017). It is also important to take into consideration the unique physical, emotional, cognitive, and social needs and preferences of the nursing home residents (Vikström et al., 2015). Another element of achieving fit with the local context involves goal-alignment, as disconnects often exist between the priorities and outcomes of the innovation and the priorities of the daily care demands in the nursing home (Abbott et al., 2022). This disconnect often leads to innovations being adapted; however, it is necessary to ensure innovations are being adapted appropriately (Wiltsey Stirman et al., 2019). Poorly executed adaptations, such as those that disregard the core components of the innovation or fail to align with the needs of the target population, may be less effective (Pérez et al., 2015). Models such as the Framework for Reporting Adaptations and Modifications to Evidence-based Implementation Strategies (FRAME-IS) can be used to systematically monitor and document adaptations to EBPs (C. Miller et al., 2021). The FRAME-IS includes the following four core modules: (1) the description of the adaptation, (2) what is being adapted, (3) the nature of the adaptation, and (4) the main goal and rationale for the adaptation. Please see Table 11.1 for a full list of barriers and facilitators related to the first CFIR domain, characteristics of the innovation.

As an example of the right (and wrong) way to adapt an innovation, consider a recent study on the Individualized Positive Psychosocial Interaction (IPPI) program (Kunkel et al., 2024). The IPPI is a nonpharmacologic, behavioral intervention that trains care partners to engage people living with dementia (PLWD) in brief, one-on-one, preference-based tailored activities. There are three core elements, or components, necessary to maintain fidelity of the IPPI program: (1) staff complete emotion-focused communication training and IPPI delivery training, (2) 1:1 interaction format between staff and resident, and (3) the IPPI activity is based on a preferred activity of the PLWD. Please see Figure 11.2 for a sample IPPI protocol. While the IPPI is an intervention that allows and even encourages adaptation, if the adaptation deviates from one of the three core components it would be considered fidelity-inconsistent.

In the study by Kunkel et al. (2024), the FRAME-IS is used to understand how and why nursing homes choose to adapt the IPPI program in their community. Findings showed that

TABLE 11.1 Characteristics of the Innovation: Barriers and Facilitators

DOMAIN AND CONSTRUCTS	BARRIER	FACILITATOR
Characteristics of the Innovation • Innovation source • Evidence base • Relative advantage • Adaptability • Trialability • Design • Cost	• Cannot be applied without adaptation to the local context • Unfamiliar implementation methods • Complexity of intervention, time-consuming, expensive, confusing, impractical/not pragmatic • Increased paperwork • Disconnect between intervention goals and nursing home organization goals	• Flexible, transparent, understandable, perceived ease • Clear activities/goals aligned with mission/values of organization • Seeing positive results • Advantages are clear to staff • Sufficient training • Fits into existing workflow • Clearly defined champion(s) • Ability to tailor the intervention to the needs of the physical, emotional, cognitive, and social needs of residents • Well-designed strategies and protocols where literacy and experience levels of end users are taken into consideration • Data are collected on the impact and reported regularly

adaptations helped the IPPI program achieve a greater fit with nursing home residents, as many providers adapted existing IPPIs or created new activities depending on residents' culture, religion, physical ability, and personal preferences. Additionally, adaptations helped lower the costs associated with implementation as nursing homes were able to reuse materials from other activities or EBPs. Other nursing homes were able to find ways to seamlessly integrate the IPPI into their daily care demands (as opposed to adding the IPPI as an additional activity throughout the day), which made implementation more efficient, took up less time, and posed less of an additional burden on staff. The only fidelity-inconsistent adaptation found was deviating from the one-to-one format of the IPPI.

By using the core modules of the FRAME-IS, Kunkel et al. (2024) were able to gain highly detailed and contextual information on adaptations providers were making to the IPPI program. While findings showed various ways in which adaptations helped the IPPI program achieve a greater fit with the community and residents, an arguably more valuable finding was the ways in which nursing homes adapted the innovation in fidelity-inconsistent ways. Information such as this can be considered in future iterations of the IPPI and training for future nursing home implementers. Other EBPs can similarly use tools like the FRAME-IS to systematically track adaptations and capitalize on their benefits, and simultaneously understand if innovations are being adapted in ways that disregard the core components.

Characteristics of the Individual Delivering the Innovation

The individuals responsible for implementation greatly impact the overall success of an innovation. In the nursing home setting, the majority of implementation responsibility falls to staff. Currently, nursing homes across the United States are facing severe staff shortages and rates of turnover, and overwhelmed workloads for those tasked with daily care pose a significant barrier to implementation (Mudallal et al., 2017). Some research advocates for a single champion to lead implementation efforts; however, due to the aforementioned staff shortages and turnover, utilizing motivated cochampions with clear responsibilities is recommended (Abbott et al., 2022).

Picking Out an Outfit Activity

RESIDENT IDENTIFIED CHOOSING WHAT CLOTHES TO WEAR AS A PREFERENCE

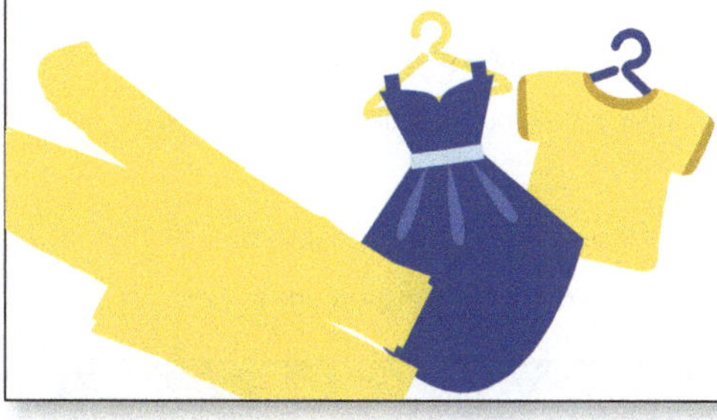

Supply Checklist

- ☑ Assistive devices, as needed:
  - Resident's glasses or magnifying glass, hearing aids, walker, or other assistive devices
- ☑ Wipes
- ☑ The resident's clothes and accessories
- ☑ Feeling Faces Emotion Assessment form

Preference Based Living

Activity Introduction

[APPROACH] Approach the resident from the front, on eye level, and smile.

[GREET] Greet the resident using their name.

[INTRODUCE] Introduce yourself using your name, and point to yourself.

[ASK] Ask how the resident is doing today.
» Say: "How are you doing today?"

[ASSESS] Complete the **'before'** portion of the Emotion Assessment form.
» Say: "Which face shows how you feel right now?"
» Do: Present the resident with the Emotion Assessment **'before'** Feeling Faces.

[RESPOND] Respond to and validate their response.
» Say: "So glad to hear you're well today." or "I'm sorry you're not feeling well."
» Do: Address the person's needs, if applicable.

Activity Questions

Question Suggestions:

- What are your favorite colors to wear?
  - Why are those your favorite colors? Do they have a special meaning to you?
- Do you have a favorite outfit or item of clothing?
  - Why is that your favorite? Does it remind you of something?
- What do you like about this outfit?
- What do you usually like to wear for the day?

FIGURE 11.2. Sample Individualized Positive Psychosocial Interaction (IPPI) program protocol.

Source: Courtesy of Preference Based Living.

Activity Instructions

[INTRODUCE] Introduce the personal care activity.
- » Say: "I know it's important for you to choose your clothes. Would you like me to help you pick out an outfit?"
- » Do: Gesture 'you' (point to person) and 'I' (point to self). Show the materials or a picture of the activity.

[EXPLAIN] Use the activity as a conversation starter.
- » Say: "Let's look through your clothes together and you can pick out an outfit you'd like to wear."
- » Do: Gesture to the resident's closet or dresser.
- » Do: Do your best to honor the preferences of the resident when picking out an outfit with the resident.

[CHOICE] Ask the resident what they would like to wear.
- » Say: "Is there a certain color you want to wear today?"
- » Do: Explain what season it is, what the weather is like, and if there are any upcoming holidays/events. Point to different options as you list them.
- » Variation: If more help is needed, pick out 2 options at once, as to not overwhelm the resident. If they are unable to choose, then pick one that aligns with their preferences.

Activity Instructions continued

[CHOICE] Ask the resident if they want to wear any accessories.
- » Say: "Are there any accessories you want to wear today?"
- » Do: List different options such as jewelry, bag, watch, wallet, hat, ring, etc. Point to the options as you list them.
- » Variation: If more help is needed, pick out two options at once, as to not overwhelm the resident. If they are unable to choose, then pick one that aligns with their preferences.

[BEGIN] Begin picking out an outfit with the resident.

[ENCOURAGE] Encourage the resident (remember: engagement over correctness).
- » Say: "That's a great outfit." or "I love your [shirt/pants/shoes/accessory/etc]!"
- » Do: Smile and nod, point to the clothing item.
- » Do: Respond to the resident based on their emotional cues.

Activity Instructions continued

[ASK QUESTIONS] See question card for ideas.

[OFFER] Offer to assist the resident with the activity, if needed.
- » Say: "I will be right here if you need any help."
- » Do: Observe the resident and, if they are struggling, offer to help.

  For example, if a resident does not respond to which item of clothing they prefer, see if they respond to the color or texture of one more than the other.
- » Variation: If more help is needed, continue to encourage choice, but offer suggestions of outfits.

Activity Closing

[THANK] Thank the resident for doing the activity with you.

[ASK] Ask for feedback:
- » Say: "How did you feel about picking out an outfit today?"

[ASSESS] Complete the **'after'** portion of the Emotion Assessment form
- » Say: "Which face shows how you feel right now?"
- » Do: Present the resident with the Emotion Assessment **'after'** Feeling Faces.

[ASK] Ask if the resident needs anything before you leave and wipe down materials before storing the supplies.

great job!

FIGURE 11.2. *(continued)*

While most innovations relating to direct care will be delivered by direct care staff such as LPNs and certified nursing assistants (CNAs), there can be other "implementation deliverers" in the community based on the targeted innovation.

Also, informal opinion leaders, implementation facilitators, implementation team members, those who support implementation, and innovation recipients can all help or hinder the implementation process (Damschroder et al., 2022). When the weight of implementation falls entirely on the shoulders of direct care staff, there is a missed opportunity for collaboration across the organization. Even in instances where the champion is self-efficacious and determined, the support of an entire team and organization should not be overlooked (Kunkel, Kasler, et al., 2023). Other team members can help spread the word about the innovation to residents and family, participate in training, and aid in other aspects of implementation such as gathering resources and redistribution of workload (Demes et al., 2020). Across all levels of staff in an organization, a concerted effort to prioritize an innovation and roll it out across a community is an incredible facilitator to implementation (Gilster et al., 2021).

Even if other levels of staff are involved in implementation, barriers may still exist. Misalignment on the goals and objectives of an innovation as well as lack of clarity on logistics like the innovation rollout and aspects of timing could be detrimental (Karrer et al., 2020). For example, if several levels of staff in a nursing home are on board with implementation, but the administrator and other influential leaders in the organization do not see the value or support the innovation, it will be difficult to gain traction for long-term implementation. Leadership involvement helps to create the appropriate climate for implementation, which several scholars have deemed as a necessity for success (Helfrich et al., 2007; Weintraub & McKee, 2018). On the other hand, if leadership does support the innovation but cannot find staff willing and able to deliver the innovation, implementation will likely not succeed either. In an ideal scenario, all levels of staff will be involved and supportive. This goes for roles outside of the organization as well, such as the implementation facilitators, or individuals who developed an innovation and are helping coach a nursing home throughout the process of implementation. These facilitators should prioritize helping the community succeed and collect data secondarily and/or in ways that are not an added burden on top of the innovation. Please see Table 11.2 for a full list of barriers and facilitators related to the second CFIR domain. characteristics of the individual.

TABLE 11.2 Characteristics of the Individual: Barriers and Facilitators

DOMAIN AND CONSTRUCTS	BARRIER	FACILITATOR

Characteristics of the Individual
• Roles
  • High-level leaders
  • Mid-level leaders
  • Opinion leaders
  • Implementation facilitators
  • Implementation team members
  • Other implementation support
  • Innovation deliverers
  • Innovation recipients
• Project characteristics
  • Need
  • Capability
  • Opportunity
  • Motivation
	• Inadequate training, expertise, or awareness
	• Being task-focused
	• Reluctance to change daily routine
	• Lack of confidence in skills/lack of interest, negative attitude
	• Staff lack information about intervention
	• Time constraints
	• Inadequate access to resident clinical information
	• Perceived threats to autonomy and expertise
	• Moral distress
	• Resistant to working with external collaborators (e.g., academic researchers)
		• Staff knowledge (confidence) and skills (competence)
		• Staff motivation and openness (positive attitudes) to innovation, curiosity
		• Past experience with QI initiatives
		• External expertise to coach champion
		• Champion given protected time and resources to implement
		• Multiple cochampions support effort who are accessible to staff

QI, quality improvement.

In a recent study by Kunkel, Kasler, et al. (2023), the authors used only the characteristics of the individual domain from the CFIR to help understand the barriers and facilitators to a person-centered, evidence-based program in the nursing home setting called preference for activities and leisure (PAL) cards. PAL cards are laminated 5 × 7 cards that display a nursing home resident's important preferences for activity and leisure (Abbott et al., 2018; Van Haitsma et al., 2013). PAL cards are created after doing a preference interview, such as the Preferences for Everyday Living Inventory (PELI). The PELI is a questionnaire designed to elicit older adults' important preferences for various domains of day-to-day life, in order to integrate those preferences into care delivery (Van Haitsma et al., 2013). The PELI was developed and rigorously tested through cognitive interviewing techniques and partnership with nursing homes in order to ensure the words used in the PELI elicited the intended meaning (Van Haitsma et al., 2013). Please see Figures 11.3 and 11.4 for an example front and back of a PAL card.

PAL cards can be secured to a resident's wheelchair, walker, or door so staff, visitors, and other residents can see the information quickly and engage in conversation or activities related to the

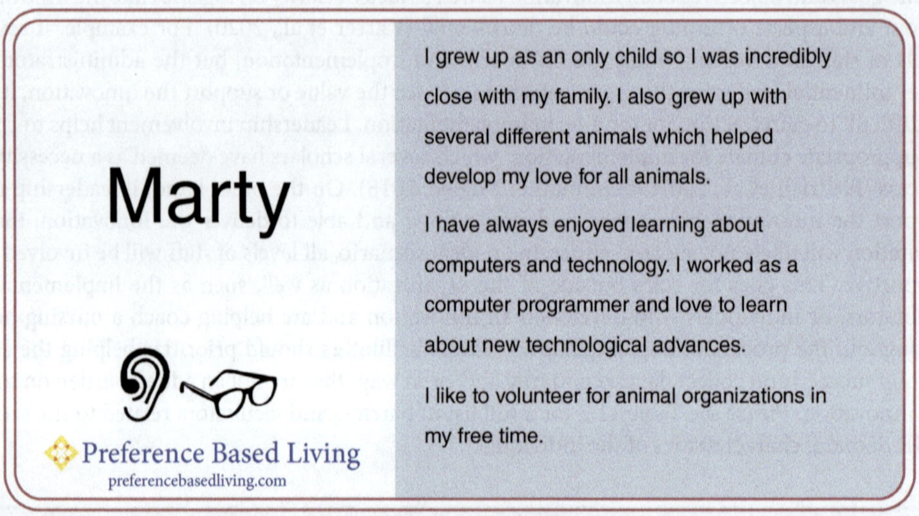

FIGURE 11.3. Sample front of preferences for activity and leisure (PAL) card.
Source: Courtesy of Preference Based Living.

Animals	Reading
I love any and all animals. I like to walk, pet, play, and watch all different kinds of animals. I grew up with big dogs so am not afraid of big animals.	I love to read on the kindle. My favorite genres of books are historical and nonfiction books.
Technology	**Reminiscing**
I enjoy learning about new technology so would enjoy having access to a computer and the internet.	I love group activities, especially board games or bingo. I have a competitive spirit and like to share it with others.
Volunteering	**Communication preferences**
I love to spend my time giving back to the community by volunteering. I would love to participate in any and all volunteering opportunities.	When communicating with me, I prefer to wear my hearing aids and my glasses.

FIGURE 11.4. Sample back of preferences for activity and leisure (PAL) card.
Source: Courtesy of Preference Based Living.

individual's preferences. For the PAL card project, champions are tasked with delegating responsibility of direct care staff to complete the preference interviews and create the cards, organize all the cards either in a central location or individually for each resident, and engage in monthly check-in calls with the PAL card project manager. Several important findings related to the champion and other individuals arose. When champions believed PAL cards would instigate a lasting change in their community, they were more inclined to "make it work" in their organization, even if that meant making changes to current workflow processes. Even for the most motivated and self-efficacious champions, the presence and support of their team was invaluable to implementation. Champions whose values aligned ideologically with the preference-based focus of the PAL card quality improvement project (QIP) were especially conscientious in their implementation efforts.

The Process of Implementing the Innovation

Attention to the actual process of implementation is required for optimal uptake of EBP in nursing homes. Perhaps contrary to popular belief, this process begins far before actively engaging in an innovation. In order for an innovation to be as effective as possible, it is necessary for the implementing organization to take the time to create an appropriate implementation team, assess needs and context, plan, and tailor strategies all before engaging in the innovation. Therefore, a barrier to implementation is jumping right into the innovation process without properly planning beforehand. In the preimplementation stage, it is crucial to get enough team members on board and trained so that they have ownership over the innovation and will see it through (Abbott, Heppner, et al., 2021). As implementation is underway, it's important to have check-in meetings at regularly scheduled intervals in order to make sure implementation is on track and account for any potential barriers (Oosterveld-Vlug et al., 2019). After engaging and implementing the innovation, it is equally important to reflect, evaluate, and adapt.

Quality improvement (QI) initiatives and implementation science have many overlaps, with the main being QI initiatives are designed to improve the targeted outcome within the community where the initiative is being studied. Implementation science, on the other hand, would traditionally result in more generalizable knowledge that could be applied in multiple settings. We recognize the tension here as the conversation about adaptation and tailoring to local needs in implementation science clearly could mirror that of a QI initiative. In fact, the CFIR 2.0 process domain is similar to a popular framework in QI called the Plan-Do-Study-Act (PDSA) cycle. When possible, it is helpful when staff who have experience with QI or planning cycles can be involved in implementation. The added time it takes to plan and do all the steps before implementation will actually help get more mileage out of the innovation, hopefully improving care and creating a long-lasting change in the community. Implementation facilitators falling under the CFIR process domain include the involvement of multiple disciplines with a structured and guided implementation process (Hirt et al., 2021). In addition, staff engagement across the entire community facilitates implementation, including staff not traditionally included in implementation efforts such as housekeeping and maintenance (Mills et al., 2019). Considering CNAs as champions and facilitators can assist with both retention of CNAs and successful implementation. Please see Table 11.3 for a full list of barriers and facilitators related to the third CFIR domain, the process of implementing.

The Inner Setting Where the Innovation Is Being Delivered

The inner setting, or the setting in which the innovation is implemented, encompasses various factors such as the organization's size, age, composition, the quality of internal communication, and the prevailing organizational culture and climate. In a nursing home, the staff play a key role in the inner setting, especially in implementation efforts as they are the primary executors of innovations. Furthermore, nursing homes often feature multiple internal layers of management, including in-house administration, nursing management, and potentially external rehabilitation management entities, all vying for the attention and commitment of direct care workers (DCWs; Abbott et al., 2022). This multiplicity of roles can lead to role confusion, hindering effective

TABLE 11.3 Process: Barriers and Facilitators

DOMAIN AND CONSTRUCTS	BARRIER	FACILITATOR
Process • Teaming • Assessing needs • Assessing context • Planning • Tailoring strategies • Engaging • Doing • Reflecting and evaluating • Adapting	• Lack of consistency in the identification and training of implementation champions in the nursing home setting • Lack of QI expertise • Lack of time for staff to take on additional responsibilities/competing priorities • Lack of planning/jumping right into implementation	• Involvement of multiple disciplines • Structured and guided implementation process • Opportunity for role modeling and mentoring • Staff engagement (including staff that are not traditionally included; e.g., housekeeping) • CNAs as champions • Actively providing encouragement • Reinforcing use of protocols through reminders, chart audits, and meetings

CNAs, certified nursing assistants, QI, quality improvement.

cooperation and teamwork. Similarly, poor communication is an additional barrier to implementing EBPs in nursing homes (Kong et al., 2022). Communication breakdowns can occur among different levels or roles of staff, or between staff, residents, and family (Kolanowski et al., 2015). Effective communication is a cornerstone of person-centered care (PCC) in nursing homes, and when residents and families feel they are kept informed and involved, they are more likely to trust the community, its staff, and the care provided (Kwame & Petrucka, 2021). Challenges such as staff shortages, elevated turnover rates, and suboptimal staff satisfaction levels can exert a detrimental impact on the implementation process. Inadequate staffing resources can result in an overwhelming workload, conflicting priorities, and a heightened risk of staff burnout (Mudallal et al., 2017). It is worth noting that the issues of staff shortages and turnover have become especially salient barriers, further exacerbated by the challenges brought about by the COVID-19 pandemic.

Further, staff shortages, high turnover, and poor staff satisfaction can negatively affect implementation. Inadequate staffing can contribute to an overloaded workload, competing priorities, and burnout (McArthur et al., 2021). Additionally, the COVID-19 pandemic exacerbated staff shortages and turnover in nursing homes due to increased staffing needs, staff burnout, health and safety concerns, infection control measures, staff illness, competitive job markets, and ongoing challenges. These factors led to increased turnover and recruitment difficulties in the industry, impacting the continuity and quality of care (Brazier et al., 2023). Consider Donabedian's (1966/2005) model for quality care, which includes structure, process, and outcomes. In this model, the structure is where the innovation is embedded or implemented into, the process is the innovation itself, and the outcomes are hopefully positive changes at the individual and organizational level. Despite adaptations to the process or innovation, if the structure does not support the implementation of EBP, it simply will not be implemented. We argue that nursing homes are facing unprecedented challenges since the COVID-19 pandemic. While we advocate for structural changes (e.g., staffing, interprofessional practice, improved wages, benefits, and working conditions), we also must acknowledge that these structural problems practically preclude the implementation of most innovations in the current climate.

Staff considerations can also play a crucial role in facilitating implementation. When all levels of staff (e.g., DCWs, administrators, and nursing management) are in sync/harmony on goals, communication, and workload, implementation runs smoothly. Rather than hierarchical structures of leadership/organization, flexible structures that are more collaborative support shared decision-making and staff engagement that can support implementation (Karrer et al., 2020). Additionally, residents and family can be highly involved/active participants in implementation. In order to effectively communicate with and engage with residents and families, DCWs often require culturally responsive and emotionally intelligent skills (Abbott, Elliot, et al., 2021). Leadership support and commitment are paramount to prioritizing resources necessary for implementation (e.g., staff time; Tappen et al., 2017). Open, frequent, scheduled times to discuss the delivery of services help to facilitate clear communication about the intervention across the community (Kaasalainen et al., 2010). Another consideration is if the nursing home is *ready* to take on implementation of a novel EBP. For example, readiness can be assessed through a tool such as the readiness assessment for pragmatic trials (RAPT; Baier et al., 2019). The success, validity, or impact of an intervention may fail if the nursing is simply not ready to take on implementation of a novel EBP (Baier et al., 2019). Therefore, conducting a readiness assessment before launching into implementation is a critical step in order to reduce cost by identifying potential barriers that may arise during implementation and help refine the innovation protocol (Talmage et al., 2024). Please see Table 11.4 for a full list of barriers and facilitators related to the fourth CFIR domain, inner setting.

Our example of the inner setting thus focuses on staff. In a forthcoming paper by Douglas et al. (2024), efforts were made to assess the inner setting prior to the implementation of a communication partner coaching intervention designed to support communication between nursing assistants and PLWD. Dementia collaborative coaching (DCC) is a communication partner coaching intervention administered by speech-language pathologists to nursing assistant and PLWD dyads (Douglas et al., 2023). It involves six-sessions designed to support communication of PLWD in nursing homes by maximizing sensory (e.g., vision, hearing) input, utilizing external memory aids, modifying the communication environment, and incorporating person-centered activities and routines. Although this intervention was designed with real-world

TABLE 11.4 Inner Setting: Barriers and Facilitators

DOMAIN AND CONSTRUCTS	BARRIER	FACILITATOR
Inner Setting • Structural characteristics • Relational connections • Communications • Culture • Tension for change • Compatibility • Relative priority • Incentive systems • Mission alignment • Available resources • Access to knowledge and information	• No family/negative attitudes from family • Lack of data/modes to collect data to inform • Plan, do, study, act cycle • Lack of a structured approach and the involvement of others • Higher staff ratios/ inadequate staffing • Multiple levels of management • Multiple competing demands/multiple projects going on simultaneously/ hectic pace of daily practice • Conflicts and misunderstandings, lack of formal meetings • Lack of communication and information flow between resident, family, and staff • Toxic team cultures/ lack of teamwork (lack of cooperation and role coordination) • Staff from different cultural backgrounds • Staff shortages • Leadership and direct care staff turnover	• Flexible organizational structures (less hierarchy, more collaborative to facilitate shared decision-making) • Planning and documentation of care • Readiness to implement • Person-centered culture and vision • Management and leadership support and commitment • Open communication • Collaborative teams • Staff education/learning culture • Well-functioning and stable care teams/positive team culture • Involving/engaging the networks of residents (e.g., families) • Staff time to attend education and practice new knowledge • Diverse educational strategies • Positive attitudes of relatives

conditions in mind, principles of implementation science indicate that inner contexts can differ dramatically, requiring the tailoring of any evidence-based intervention to that inner setting or local context. So in this case focus groups were conducted with nursing home managers, nursing assistants, administrators, and speech-language pathologists as a way to address barriers to the implementation of DCC proactively, as well as to capitalize on any facilitators to implementation that may be present.

These focus groups revealed that although nursing home employees felt positive about the potential of DCC to improve outcomes for PLWD in their communities, there were barriers in the inner setting that tempered their optimism. Participants noted that severe staffing shortages including the use of unregulated agency staff would preclude the implementation of a person-centered communication intervention such as DCC. This was illustrated by the following nursing assistant quote:

> *The biggest issue is staffing. When facilities do not have enough in-house staff, staffing is supplemented by registry or travelers. These staff members rotate shifts and buildings, and typically have minimal investment in the building and residents. Lack of consistent staff results in sporadic instruction/education of programming with poor carryover between shifts. (Interviewee #1, personal communication, March 18, 2023)*

Further, employee participants noted that the implementation of any evidence-based intervention would require planning, buy-in across leadership and direct care providers, and explicit implementation plans that allow for both accountability and team building. As a speech-language pathologist said, "For this project, we're going to have to identify support and structure" (Douglas et al., 2024, Table A). Participants also noted that ideally documentation of DCC would be part of the medical record or attached to a responsibility that the employee had to do as a task in their usual workday. For instance, when documenting how much a person ate that day, one could also document if they were wearing their glasses and/or hearing aids.

One way to structure a plan to account for the inner setting is to use the *Learn. Engage. Act. Process. QI learning program (LEAP)*. Born out of the Ann Arbor Veterans Administration (VA) and designed by Damschroder et al. (2021), the LEAP program is a tool to engage direct care providers in QI initiatives such as the implementation of an intervention like DCC. The program is designed to last 21 weeks and provide hands-on opportunities for engagement. Key features of LEAP include a LEAP improvement coach who facilitates learning (done virtually), written and video guidance, and data to help teams assess progress and make adjustments as needed. Resources such as handouts, a sample calendar, and overview videos are available on the VA marketplace innovations website. While there may be less control over the staffing concerns, a program such as LEAP would allow nursing home employees to engage with DCC in a way that is meaningful and tailored to employee needs.

The Outer Setting Where the Innovation Is Being Delivered

The outer setting includes all macro-level factors related to the inner setting. For example, if the inner setting is the nursing home itself, the outer setting may include the local healthcare/hospital network that the nursing home is situated within and the local community, as well as state-level and national-level policies and programs that impact the nursing home's care. All of these factors can contribute to pressuring nursing homes to implement and to adapt care (Damschroder et al., 2009). A barrier to the implementation of EBP in nursing homes is the increasingly medically complex nature of the residents residing in them; for example, individuals living with dementia. The medical and care needs of individuals with dementia are frequently changing and require care that is responsive and adaptive of those changing needs (Karrer et al., 2020). This barrier was further complicated by the COVID-19 pandemic, which drastically disrupted, and at times halted, EBP implementation in nursing homes (Yingling, 2020). In many nursing homes, the adoption of PCC and novel interventions was forced to take a backseat to the basic needs of simply keeping residents alive, safe, and healthy (Morgan et al., 2023).

External policies that incentivize completion of tasks over relationship-building (e.g., meals done by noon, medications passed by 8:45; Abbott et al., 2022) take a problematic transactional approach to PCC. This is further challenged by the constantly shifting pay-for-performance (P4P) and reimbursement guidelines, and an overwhelming lack of funding to support the LTC workforce (Abbott et al., 2016). On the other hand, external policies and incentives that advocate for implementing EBPs are needed for successful implementation (Abbott, Elliot, et al., 2021; S. C. Miller et al., 2018). The outer setting can further facilitate implementation of EBPs in several ways related to the needs, preferences, and resources of Nnursing homeresidents and family (McArthur et al., 2021). The pressure to adopt person-centered EBPs can come from other local nursing homes or the culture change movement at large (Jacobs et al., 2018). Finally, including nursing home residents and their families in implementation efforts wherever possible can greatly help shift the focus of an EBP away from rote completion to the person-centered processes and outcomes behind the intervention. Please see Table 11.5 for a full list of barriers and facilitators related to the fifth CFIR domain, outer setting.

A recent case study of an Ohio P4P program highlights the importance of proper support versus rote incentivization of PCC (Abbott, Elliot, et al., 2021). In 2015, the Ohio Department of Medicaid (ODM) adopted a new five-point system of quality indicators featuring pressure ulcers, antipsychotics, hospital admissions, employee retention, and the use of the PELI (ODM). The revised P4P asked nursing homes to simply report through a Yes/No checkbox if they "[u]tilize the nursing home version of the PELI for all of its residents, and indicate in section eight of the nursing facility's annual cost report that it was used" (Ohio Department of Medicaid, 2018, p. 3). By checking this box, nursing homes were eligible for the financial incentive in the form of an increased reimbursement rate per resident per day.

Unfortunately, this checkbox was the only way for ODM to measure nursing homes' adoption of PELI, and as such led to a lack of differentiation in who received the payment incentive. Because of this, in 2019 a new administration deimplemented the PELI as a P4P indicator. While well-intentioned, this is an example of an ineffective incentive for PCC. Rather than incentivizing a checkbox with no real action, an effective P4P structure should incentivize positive change in provider circumstances and reduce disparities (Werner et al., 2016). The thresholds of performance for payment should be isometric and realistically attainable, so low-performing nursing homes are motivated to participate and able to achieve (Werner et al., 2016). It is also important that financial incentives meet or exceed the expected investment costs of starting a new initiative or QI program in order to motivate participation and change (Abbott et al., 2016).

TABLE 11.5 Outer Setting: Barriers and Facilitators

DOMAIN AND CONSTRUCTS	BARRIER	FACILITATOR
Outer Setting • Critical incidents • Local attitudes • Local conditions • Partnerships & connections • Policies and laws • Financing • External pressure	• Resident complexity (multiple comorbidities, serious mental illness, high care needs (e.g., dementia), and frequently changing needs • Limited information about resident social and medical history • Ageism • Financing issues (e.g., no clear reimbursement, lack of funding for workforce) • Governmental regulations (task orientation) • Lack of rigorously defined EBP • Frequently changing COVID-19 restrictions	• P4P initiatives • Advocate for implementation of EBP • Information about the preferences of the individual receiving care • Resident engagement • Education, knowledge, and experience of the resident and family members • Pressure from culture change movement

EBP, evidence-based practice; P4P, pay-for-performance.

Subsequent research by Kunkel et al. (2022), using five sources of publicly available data on Ohio NHs, found that nursing homes with complete PELI implementation were more likely to have a four- or five-star deficiency star rating, lower deficiency scores, and were more likely to be deficiency-free. Additionally, nursing homes with complete PELI implementation were less likely to have any complaints and any substantiated complaints as compared to partial PELI implementers (Kunkel, Bowblis, et al., 2023). These findings point to the fact that person-centered initiatives take time to see fruits of the labor. Research on implementation outcomes takes longer than policy makers would like, which is why initiatives often lose funding before those benefits are fully realized.

RECOMMENDATIONS FOR PROVIDERS IMPLEMENTING NEW INITIATIVES

In this section we outline recommendations and resources to consider when implementing a new safety initiative in a nursing home. As stated earlier, we certainly acknowledge the structural issues that may make some of these resources less practical; however, we aim to present a menu of options that could be tailored to your local community. We structure this section according to three main areas—leadership, existing resources, and the iterative nature of implementing any such initiative.

Leadership

Time and again the literature has shown the critical nature of leadership to any implementation effort (Brodtkorb et al., 2019). While many nursing home administrators may excel in the technical aspects of leadership, adaptive aspects of leadership may present an opportunity for growth. Kuluski et al. (2020) argue that, "the defining feature of adaptive leadership is the separation of technical solutions (ie applying existing knowledge and techniques to problems) from adaptive solutions (ie requiring shifts in how people work together, not just what they do)" (p. 176). Adaptive leadership has been described as the four As—(1) *anticipation* of future needs, (2) *articulation* of those needs to build understanding and support for action, (3) *adaptation* or continuous learning and adjustment, and (4) *accountability* including transparency in decision-making and openness to challenges and feedback (Ramalingam et al., 2020).

Nursing homes are certainly volatile, uncertain, complex, and ambiguous (VUCA) environments (Cousins, 2018), and the ability to respond nimbly was clearly evident in the throes of the COVID-19 pandemic. Nursing home staff looked to their leaders for direction, help, and support, but it could be argued that the pandemic uncovered an overreliance on technical solutions and technical leadership. Consider the second "A" (articulation) and the fourth "A" (accountability or transparency in decision-making). With the long history of lack of trust and open communication between nursing home leaders and direct care providers, it is not surprising that there was serious resistance to uptake of the COVID-19 vaccine (Sadarangani et al., 2021). Luthans and Broad (2022) outline the role of positive psychologic capital or PsyCap in supporting people working and living in a VUCA environment (arguably all of us). PsyCap consists of the "HERO within" or **H**ope, **E**fficacy, **R**esilience, and **O**ptimism (Luthans & Broad, 2022). An updated definition includes, "[a]n individual's positive psychological state of development characterized by (1) having confidence (efficacy) to take on and put in the necessary effort to succeed at challenging tasks; (2) making a positive attribution (optimism) about succeeding now and in the future; (3) persevering toward goals and, when necessary, redirecting paths to goals (hope) in order to succeed; and (4) when beset by problems and adversity, sustaining and bouncing back and even beyond (resiliency) to attain success" (Luthans et al., 2015, p. 2). A potential resource to apply PsyCap is located in the Appendix of Luthans and Broad (2022), and there are several other psychologic capital and adaptive leadership trainings that may benefit not only nursing home administrators but also DCWs in the service of implementing safety innovations.

Existing Resources

There are several resources available to support the implementation of safety initiatives, and while not exhaustive, we offer a few key examples here that may be useful in your community.

Project charters: A project charter states the purpose of any safety initiative and can serve as an informal contract (Johnson, 2021). Usually key components of a project charter include the problem statement, the case for change, performance measures, milestones, and noted barriers to success. Other important aspects include assembling the team, which should include anyone who is impacted by the project (e.g., DCWs). The Agency for Healthcare Research and Quality (2009) have freely available templates including a toolkit on their website.

Benjamin Rose Institute on Aging: The Benjamin Rose Institute on Aging (https://benrose.org) supports care partners of individuals living with dementia. They boast a rich library of freely available training resources including webinars on how to develop a quality workforce and how to make the transition to LTC successful. Further, their Center for Research and Education outlines best practices in caregiving, which can be sorted and compared by program name. All programs listed in this database have at least some level of evidence for their use and may support the implementation of safety initiatives.

Enabling research in care homes (ENRICH): The National Institute for Health and Care Research (n.d.) in the UK supports ENRICH, which provides resources for PLWD, their families, and nursing home staff. Freely available modules review basics of nursing homes along with case studies where resources are applied. A value of ENRICH is to collaborate with researchers to integrate the realities of nursing home care provision with research in practical ways. For instance, there is a case study about "how to improve the experience for everyone involved," that may offer helpful ideas for the implementation of safety initiatives in your particular nursing home community.

Implementation support practitioners: The focus of implementation support practitioners, a newer construct, is the tailoring of implementation to the local setting. Nursing home administrators or relevant staff may benefit from a number of implementation support practitioner trainings. Many are available from the University of North Carolina at Chapel Hill or the Center for Implementation. Metz et al. (2020) developed a practice guide to supporting implementation and key competencies that includes cocreation and engagement, ongoing improvement, and sustaining change, all factors key to any safety innovation implementation. They further describe six principles that should drive implementation practice: empathy, curiosity, commitment, equity, critical thinking, and cross-disciplinary approaches. Many resource documents are open-access and may indeed support adaptive leadership skills as well as discussed earlier.

The Iterative Nature of the Work

Finally, we encourage the "long-view" regarding the implementation of these initiatives. Much of what we focused on in this chapter involves defining a key aspect to change, implementing something, studying the result of that implementation, and then adjusting and trying again. The nature of nursing home practice requires such an iterative approach, and while the job may never be "done," it is critical to celebrate the wins, however small. Nursing homes are complex organizations where some of our most vulnerable citizens live; as such, it is critical that we draw from the literature to support both the people who live there and the people who work there in the best ways we know how. The implementation of innovations, particularly safety ones, is a way that we can participate in achieving high-quality outcomes for individuals but with ripple effects that could ultimately positively impact nursing home organizations as a whole.

SUMMARY

The topic of safety innovation and adaptive leadership is highly relevant in the field of LTC, and this chapter provides crucial insights into how to navigate this complex process. The chapter examines the issue of the know-do gap and highlights the importance of understanding the barriers and facilitators to successful implementation. By discussing the field of implementation science, the chapter facilitates an understanding of the theoretical underpinning of successful implementation and provides tools that can be used to foster change within the LTC setting.

Furthermore, the chapter offers details on practical initiatives that can be employed to improve the quality of care and safety in LTC communities. Project charters and training programs are discussed as effective tools to guide change initiatives and facilitate staff engagement. In addition, the chapter highlights the Benjamin Rose Institute on Aging and ENRICH as well as preference-based living's valuable resources for both care partners and nursing home staff, noting the accessibility and quality of their training programs.

Ultimately, the aim of this chapter is to support the efforts of LTC administrators and DCWs toward improving quality of care and safety by honoring residents' important preferences. Through the provision of valuable training resources and detailed explanations of implementation science, the chapter offers a comprehensive guide for those seeking to navigate the complexities of implementing change within the nursing home setting.

Take-Home Points

- *Barriers and facilitators awareness:* Understand the barriers and facilitators that may influence the implementation of EBP in LTC settings, and consider the need for proactive strategies to overcome challenges and leverage supportive factors.
- *Preimplementation stage importance:* Recognize the critical importance of the preimplementation stage, including the creation of a suitable implementation team, thorough assessment of needs and context, strategic planning, and customization of approaches. Success in this stage significantly influences the overall implementation process.
- *Macro-level factors' influence:* Appreciate the broad impact of macro-level factors, such as policy dynamics, organizational influences, and community factors, on the successful implementation of EBP in LTC. Understanding and navigating these factors are crucial for achieving successful implementation outcomes.
- *Practical tools:* Equip yourself with practical tools and recommendations for implementing EBP in care delivery. Develop a commitment to continuous improvement in care delivery by applying these tools effectively.

END-OF-CHAPTER RESOURCES

DISCUSSION QUESTIONS

1. What are our organization's values regarding PCC?
2. What is our current care planning process? Does our current process incorporate some form of preference assessment?
3. Do we currently integrate preference information into the care plan? If so, how?
4. Who is involved in the care planning process? Are all relevant departments represented?
   a. Do we include CNAs in care plan meetings? If not, how can we gain their input?
   b. How do we create a welcoming environment for all knowledge holders during care plan meetings?
5. If you had to receive LTC services and supports, which important preferences would you want to inform and guide your care?

6. Do we invite family members, close friends, or other trusted care partners when we cannot learn about preferences directly from the resident?
7. Do we review a completed PELI or another preference assessment during the care plan meeting?
8. How does our team collaborate to come up with solutions to learn about and honor preferences?

TOOLS FOR FURTHER LEARNING

- Quality Assurance Performance Improvement (QAPI) training
  https://www.preferencebasedliving.com/training-videos/quality-assurance-and-performance-improvement-training-videos
- Integrating preferences into care planning
  https://www.preferencebasedliving.com/training-videos/integrating-preferences-into-care-planning
- Engaging family and friends in assessing preferences
  https://www.preferencebasedliving.com/training-videos/engaging-family-and-friends-to-assess-preferences
- Interviewing older adults
  https://www.preferencebasedliving.com/training-videos/interviewing-older-adults-using-the-peli
- The process for care planning for resident choice
  https://www.preferencebasedliving.com/training-videos/the-process-for-care-planning-for-resident-choice
- Preference for activities and leisure (PAL) cards
  https://www.preferencebasedliving.com/pal-cards
- Emotion-focused communication training
  https://www.preferencebasedliving.com/emotion-focused-communication-training
- PELI questionnaires
  https://www.preferencebasedliving.com/for-practitioners/practitioner/assessment/peli-questionnaires
- IPPI
  https://www.preferencebasedliving.com/ippi/individualized-positive-psychosocial-intervention-protocol-ippi

SPRINGER PUBLISHING CONNECT™ A robust set of instructor resources designed to supplement this text is located at http://connect.springerpub.com/content/book/978-0-8261-4935-0. Qualifying instructors may request access by emailing textbook@springerpub.com.

REFERENCES

Abbott, K. M., Douglas, N., & Van Haitsma, K. (2022). A rising tide lifts all boats: Equitable nursing home policy through implementation science. *Public Policy & Aging Report*, *32*(1), 6–12. https://doi.org/10.1093/ppar/prab030

Abbott, K. M., Elliot, A., & Van Haitsma, K. (2021). Lessons learned from Ohio's statewide implementation of the preferences for everyday living inventory as a pay for performance initiative to enhance person-centered care. *Journal of the American Medical Directors Association*, *22*(10), 2074–2078. https://doi.org/10.1016/j.jamda.2021.06.011

Abbott, K. M., Elliot, A., & Van Haitd care. *Clinical Gerontologist, 39*(3), 190–209. https://doi.org/10.1080/07317115.2016.1151968

Abbott, K. M., Heppner, A., Hicks, N., Hermesch, A., & Van Haitsma, K. (2021). Evaluating the implementation of a pragmatic person-centered communication tool for the nursing home setting: PAL cards. *Clinical Gerontologist, 45*(3), 634–646. https://doi.org/10.1080/07317115.2021.1929632

Abbott, K. M., Klumpp, R., Leser, K. A., Straker, J. K., Gannod, G. C., & Van Haitsma, K. (2018). Delivering person-centered care: Important preferences for recipients of long-term services and supports. *Journal of the American Medical Directors Association, 19*(2), 169–173. https://doi.org/10.1016/j.jamda.2017.10.005

Abu-Baker, N. N., Abu Alrub, S., Obeidat, R. F., & Assmairan, K. (2021). Evidence-based practice beliefs and implementations: A cross-sectional study among undergraduate nursing students. *BMC Nursing, 20*(1), 13. https://doi.org/10.1186/s12912-020-00522-x

Agency for Healthcare Research and Quality. (2009, December 23). *Project charter template: Version 1.5.* Texas Project Delivery Framework. https://www.ahrq.gov/sites/default/files/wysiwyg/professionals/systems/hospital/qitoolkit/d2-projectcharter.pdf

Baier, R. R., Jutkowitz, E., Mitchell, S. L., McCreedy, E., & Mor, V. (2019). Readiness assessment for pragmatic trials (RAPT): A model to assess the readiness of an intervention for testing in a pragmatic trial. *BMC Medical Research Methodology, 19*(1), 156. https://doi.org/10.1186/s12874-019-0794-9

Barrera, M., Jr., Berkel, C., & Castro, F. G. (2017). Directions for the advancement of culturally adapted preventive interventions: Local adaptations, engagement, and sustainability. *Prevention Science, 18*(6), 640–648. https://doi.org/10.1007/s11121-016-0705-9

Brazier, J. F., Geng, F., Meehan, A., White, E. M., McGarry, B. E., Shield, R. R., Grabowski, D. C., Rahman, M., Santostefano, C., & Gadbois, E. A. (2023). Examination of staffing shortages at US nursing homes during the COVID-19 pandemic. *JAMA Network Open, 6*(7), e2325993. https://doi.org/10.1001/jamanetworkopen.2023.25993

Brodtkorb, K., Skaar, R., & Slettebø, A. (2019). The importance of leadership in innovation processes in nursing homes: An integrative review. *Nordic Journal of Nursing Research, 39*(3), 127–136. https://doi.org/10.1177/2057158519828140

Connor, L., Dean, J., McNett, M., Tydings, D. M., Shrout, A., Gorsuch, P. F., Hole, A., Moore, L., Brown, R., Melynyk, B. M., & Gallagher-Ford, L. (2023). Evidence-based practice improves patient outcomes and healthcare system return on investment: Findings from a scoping review. *Worldviews on Evidence-Based Nursing, 20*(1), 6–15. https://doi.org/10.1111/wvn.12621

Cousins, B. (2018). Design thinking: Organizational learning in VUCA environments. *Academy of Strategic Management Journal, 17*(2), 1–18. https://www.abacademies.org/articles/design-thinking-organizational-learning-in-vuca-environments-7117.html

Damschroder, L. J., Aron, D. C., Keith, R. E., Kirsh, S. R., Alexander, J. A., & Lowery, J. C. (2009). Fostering implementation of health services research findings into practice: A consolidated framework for advancing implementation science. *Implementation Science, 4*(1), 50. https://doi.org/10.1186/1748-5908-4-50

Damschroder, L. J., Reardon, C. M., Opra Widerquist, M. A., & Lowery, J. (2022). Conceptualizing outcomes for use with the consolidated framework for implementation research (CFIR): The CFIR outcomes addendum. *Implementation Science, 17*(1), 7. https://doi.org/10.1186/s13012-021-01181-5

Damschroder, L. J., Yankey, N. R., Robinson, C. H., Freitag, M. B., Burns, J. A., Raffa, S. D., & Lowery, J. C. (2021). The LEAP program: Quality improvement training to address team readiness gaps identified by implementation science findings. *Journal of General Internal Medicine, 36*, 288–295. https://doi.org/10.1007/s11606-020-06133-1

Demes, J. A. E., Nickerson, N., Farand, L., Montekoi, V. B., Torres, P., Dube, J. G., Coq, J. G., Pomey, M.-P., Champagne, F., & Jasmin, E. R. (2020). What are the characteristics of the champion that influence the implementation of quality improvement programs? *Evaluation and Program Planning, 80*, 101795. https://doi.org/10.1016/j.evalprogplan.2020.101795

de Veer, A. J. E., Fleuren, M. A. H., Voss, H., & Francke, A. L. (2021). Sustainment of innovations in palliative care: A survey on lessons learned from a nationwide quality improvement program. *Journal of Pain and Symptom Management, 61*(2), 295–304. https://doi.org/10.1016/j.jpainsymman.2020.07.035

Donabedian, A. (2005). Evaluating the quality of medical care. *Milbank Quarterly, 83*(4), 691–729. https://doi.org/10.1111/j.1468-0009.2005.00397.x (Original work published 1966)

Douglas, N. F., Browning, S., & Claypool, K. (2023). Preliminary evidence for dementia collaborative coaching. *American Journal of Speech-Language Pathology, 32*(5), 2146–2157. https://doi.org/10.1044/2023_AJSLP-22-00367

Douglas, N. F., Snell, A., & Carpenter, J. (2024). Staff perspectives on dementia care in nursing homes: A pre-implementation, content analysis study guided by the Practical, Robust Implementation and Sustainability Model. *Journal of Gerontological Nursing, 50*(2), 5–9. https://doi.org/10.3928/00989134-20231215-01

Gilster, S. D., Langhout, K. J., & Dalessandro, J. L. (2021). Staff stability through service: Promoting a "person-centered" culture for work and care in long-term services and supports environments. *Journal of Gerontological Nursing, 47*(11), 6–10. https://doi.org/10.3928/00989134-20211012-01

Helfrich, C. D., Weiner, B. J., McKinney, M. M., & Minasian, L. (2007). Determinants of implementation effectiveness adapting a framework for complex innovations. *Medical Care Research and Review, 64*(3), 279–303. https://doi.org/10.1177/1077558707299887

Hirt, J., Karrer, M., Adlbrecht, L., Saxer, S., & Zeller, A. (2021). Facilitators and barriers to implement nurse-led interventions in long-term dementia care: A qualitative interview study with Swiss nursing experts and managers. *BMC Geriatrics, 21*(1), 159. https://doi.org/10.1186/s12877-021-02120-1

Hoedl, M., Thonhofer, N., & Schoberer, D. (2022). COVID-19 pandemic: Burdens on and consequences for nursing home staff. *Journal of Advanced Nursing, 78*(8), 2495–2506. https://doi.org/10.1111/jan.15193

Jacobs, M. L., Snow, A. L., Parmelee, P. A., & Davis, J. A. (2018). Person-centered care practices in long-term care in the deep south: Consideration of structural, market, and administrator characteristics. *Journal of Applied Gerontology, 37*(3), 349–370. https://doi.org/10.1177/0733464816642583

Johnson, H. (2021). Novel application of Six Sigma in a skilled nursing facility. *Journal of Nursing Care Quality, 36*(1), 67–73. https://doi.org/10.1097/NCQ.0000000000000492

Kaasalainen, S., Williams, J., Hadjistavropoulos, T., Thorpe, L., Whiting, S., Neville, S., & Tremeer, J. (2010). Creating bridges between researchers and long-term care homes to promote quality of life for residents. *Qualitative Health Research, 20*(12), 1689–1704. https://doi.org/10.1177/1049732310377456

Karrer, M., Hirt, J., Zeller, A., & Saxer, S. (2020). What hinders and facilitates the implementation of nurse-led interventions in dementia care? A scoping review. *BMC Geriatrics, 20*(1), 127. https://doi.org/10.1186/s12877-020-01520-z

Koerner, J., Johnston, N., Samara, J., Liu, W. M., Chapman, M., & Forbat, L. (2021). Context and mechanisms that enable implementation of specialist palliative care Needs Rounds in care homes: Results from a qualitative interview study. *BMC Palliative Care, 20*(1), 118. https://doi.org/10.1186/s12904-021-00812-4

Kolanowski, A., Van Haitsma, K., Penrod, J., Hill, N., & Yevchak, A. (2015). "Wish we would have known that!" Communication breakdown impedes person-centered care. *The Gerontologist, 55*(Suppl. 1), S50–S60. https://doi.org/10.1093/geront/gnv014

Kong, E. H., Kim, H., & Kim, H. (2022). Nursing home staff's perceptions of barriers and needs in implementing person-centred care for people living with dementia: A qualitative study. *Journal of Clinical Nursing, 31*(13–14), 1896–1906. https://doi.org/10.1111/jocn.15729

Kuluski, K., Reid, R. J., & Baker, G. R. (2020). Applying the principles of adaptive leadership to person-centred care for people with complex care needs: Considerations for care providers, patients, caregivers and organizations. *Health Expectations, 24*(2), 175–181. https://doi.org/10.1111/hex.13174

Kunkel, M. C., Bowblis, J. R., Straker, J., Van Haitsma, K., & Abbott, K. M. (2022). Impact of implementing the preferences for everyday living inventory on nursing home survey deficiencies. *Journal of the American Medical Directors Association, 24*(1), 113–118. https://doi.org/10.1016/j.jamda.2022.10.021

Kunkel, M. C., Bowblis, J. R., Straker, J., Van Haitsma, K., & Abbott, K. M. (2023). Can implementing person-centered care tools reduce complaints? Evidence from the implementation of PELI in Ohio nursing homes. *Journal of Aging and Social Policy*. Advance online publication. https://doi.org/10.1080/08959420.2023.2265775

Kunkel, M. C., Kasler, K., Heppner, A., Van Haitsma, K., & Abbott, K. M. (2023). Implementing preference-based communication tools in nursing homes: Influence of champions. *Activities, Adaptation, & Aging, 48*(3), 393–408. https://doi.org/10.1080/01924788.2023.2213022

Kunkel, M. C., Talmage, L., Noble, M., Van Haitsma, K., & Abbott, K. M. (2024). "It's what would work for her": An analysis of adaptations to the Individualized Positive Psychosocial Interaction program in US nursing homes. *The Gerontologist*, gnae122. Advance online publication. https://doi.org/10.1093/geront/gnae122

Kwame, A., & Petrucka, P. M. (2021). A literature-based study of patient-centered care and communication in nurse-patient interactions: Barriers, facilitators, and the way forward. *BMC Nursing, 20*, 158. https://doi.org/10.1186/s12912-021-00684-2

Luthans, F., & Broad, J. D. (2022). Positive psychological capital to help combat the mental health fallout from the pandemic and VUCA environment. *Organizational Dynamics, 51*(2), 100817. https://doi.org/10.1016/j.orgdyn.2020.100817

Luthans, F., Youssef, C. M., & Avolio, B. J. (2015). *Psychological capital and beyond.* Oxford University Press.

McArthur, C., Bai, Y., Hewston, P., Giangregorio, L., Straus, S., & Papaioannou, A. (2021). Barriers and facilitators to implementing evidence-based guidelines in long-term care: A qualitative evidence synthesis. *Implementation Science, 16*(1), 70. https://doi.org/10.1186/s13012-021-01140-0

Metz, A., Burke, K., Albers, B., Louison, L., & Bartley, L. (2020, December). *A practice guide to supporting implementation: What competencies do we need?* National Implementation Research Network. https://nirn.fpg.unc.edu/sites/nirn.fpg.unc.edu/files/resources/ISP%20Practice%20Guide-v1-10.27.22.pdf

Miller, C., Barnett, M. L., Baumann, A. A., Gutner, G. A., & Wiltsey-Stirman, S. (2021). The FRAME-IS: A framework for documenting modifications to implementation strategies in healthcare. *Implementation Science, 16*, 36. https://doi.org/10.1186/s13012-021-01105-3

Miller, S. C., Schwartz, M. L., Lima, J. C., Shield, R. R., Tyler, D. A., Berridge, C. W., Gozalo, P. L., Lepore, M. J., & Clark, M. A. (2018). The prevalence of culture change practice in US nursing homes: Findings from a 2016/17 nationwide survey. *Medicare Care, 56*(12), 985–993. https://doi.org/10.1097/MLR.0000000000000993

Mills, W. L., Pimentel, C. B., Snow, A. L., Allen, R. S., Wewiorski, N. J., Palmer, J. A., Clark, V., Roland, T. M., McDannold, S. E., & Hartmann, C. W. (2019). Nursing home staff perceptions of barriers and facilitators to implementing a quality improvement intervention. *Journal of the American Medical Directors Association, 20*(7), 810–815. https://doi.org/10.1016/j.jamda.2019.01.139

Morgan, J. C., Ahmad, W., Chen, Y.-Z., & Burgess, E. O. (2023). The Impact of COVID-19 on the person-centered care practices in nursing homes. *Journal of Applied Gerontology, 42*(7), 1582–1587. https://doi.org/10.1177/07334648231154544

Morris, Z. S., Wooding, S., & Grant, J. (2011). The answer is 17 years, what is the question: Understanding time lags in translational research. *Journal of the Royal Society of Medicine, 104*(12), 510–520. https://doi.org/10.1258/jrsm.2011.110180

Mudallal, R. H., Othman, W. M., & Al Hassan, N. F. (2017). Nurses' burnout: The influence of leader empowering behaviors, work conditions, and demographic traits. *Inquiry, 54*, 46958017724944. https://doi.org/10.1177/0046958017724944

National Institute for Health and Care Research. (n.d.). *Enabling research in care homes (ENRICH).* Retrieved September 21, 2023, from https://enrich.nihr.ac.uk

Ohio Department of Medicaid. (2018). *Nursing facilities (NFs): Quality indicators and per medicaid day quality payment rate.* https://www.registerofohio.state.oh.us/pdfs/5160/0/3/5160-3-58_PH_OF_A_RU_20180626_1031.pdf

Oosterveld-Vlug, M., Onwuteaka-Philipsen, B., ten Koppel, M., van Hout, H., Smets, T., Pivodic, L., Tanghe, M., Van den Noortgate, N., Hockley, J., Payne, S., Moore, D. C., Kijowska, V., Szczerbinska, K., Kylanen, M., Leppaaho, S., Mercuri, C., Rossi, P., Mercuri, M., Gambassi, G., … Van den Block, L. (2019). Evaluating the implementation of the PACE Steps to Success Programme in long-term care facilities in seven countries according to the RE-AIM framework. *Implementation Science, 14*(1), 107. https://doi.org/10.1186/s13012-019-0953-8

Pérez, D., Van der Stuyft, P., Zabala, M., Castro, M., & Lefèvre, P. (2015). A modified theoretical framework to assess implementation fidelity of adaptive public health interventions. *Implementation Science, 11*, 91. https://doi.org/10.1186/s13012-016-0457-8

Ramalingam, B., Nabarro, D., Oqubuy, A., Carnall, D. R., & Wild, L. (2020, September 11). *5 Principles to guide adaptive leadership*. Harvard Business Review. https://hbr.org/2020/09/5-principles-to-guide-adaptive-leadership

Rolland, B., Resnik, F., Hohl, S. D., Johnson, L. J., Saha-Muldowney, M., & Mahoney, J. (2021). Applying the lessons of implementation science to maximize feasibility and usability in team science intervention development. *Journal of Clinical and Translational Science, 5*(1), e197. https://doi.org/10.1017/cts.2021.826

Sadarangani, T. R., David, D., & Travers, J. (2021). Engaging nursing assistants to enhance receptivity to the coronavirus disease 2019 vaccine. *Journal of the American Medical Directors Association, 22*(6), 1125–1127. https://doi.org/10.1016/j.jamda.2021.03.016

Skolarus, T. A., Lehmann, T., Tabak, R. G., Harris, J., Lecy, J., & Sales, A. E. (2017). Assessing citation networks for dissemination and implementation research frameworks. *Implementation Science, 12*, 97. https://doi.org/10.1186/s13012-017-0628-2

Talmage, A., Kunkel, M. C., Kasler, K., Keiser, C., Akter, N., Van Haitsma, K., & Abbott, K. M. (2024). *"I think we just saw happier residents"*: Nursing home provider reported readiness assessment of the Individualized Positive Psychosocial Interaction (IPPI) program. *Aging & Mental Health*. Advance online publication. https://doi.org/10.1080/13607863.2024.2401960

Tappen, R. M., Wolf, D. G., Rahemi, Z., Engstrom, G., Rojido, C., Shutes, J. M., & Ouslander, J. G. (2017). Barriers and facilitators to implementing a change initiative in long-term care using the INTERACT® quality improvement program. *The Health Care Manager, 36*(3), 219–230. https://doi.org/10.1097/HCM.0000000000000168

Titler, M. G. (2008). The evidence for evidence-based practice implementation. In R. G. Hughes (Ed.), *Patient safety and quality: An evidence-based handbook for nurses* (pp. 113–161). Agency for Healthcare Research and Quality. https://www.ncbi.nlm.nih.gov/books/NBK2659

Van Haitsma, K., Curyto, K., Spector, A., Towsley, G., Kleban, M., Carpenter, B., Ruckdeschel, K., Feldman, P. H., & Koren, M. J. (2013). The preferences for everyday living inventory: Scale development and description of psychosocial preferences responses in community-dwelling elders. *The Gerontologist, 53*(4), 582–595. https://doi.org/10.1093/geront/gns102

Vikström, S., Sandman, P. O., Stenwall, E., Boström, A. M., Saarnio, L., Kindblom, K., Edvardsson, D., & Borell, L. (2015). A model for implementing guidelines for person-centered care in a nursing home setting. *International Psychogeriatrics, 27*(1), 49–59. https://doi.org/10.1017/S1041610214001598

Weintraub, P., & McKee, M. (2018). Leadership for innovation in healthcare: An exploration. *International Journal of Health Policy and Management, 8*(3), 138–144. https://doi.org/10.15171/ijhpm.2018.122

Werner, R. M., Skira, M., & Konetzka, R. T. (2016). An evaluation of performance thresholds in nursing home pay-for-performance. *Health Services Research, 51*(6), 2282–2304. https://doi.org/10.1111/1475-6773.12467

Wiltsey Stirman, S., Baumann, A. A., & Miller, C. J. (2019). The FRAME: An expanded framework for reporting adaptations and modifications to evidence-based interventions. *Implementation Science, 14*, 58. https://doi.org/10.1186/s13012-019-0898-y

Yingling, J. K. (2020). Rationing evidence-based nursing practice: Considering a resource-based approach. *The Online Journal of Issues in Nursing, 26*(1). https://doi.org/10.3912/OJIN.Vol26No01PPT62

CHAPTER 12

EFFECTIVE MANAGEMENT AND LEADERSHIP IN LONG-TERM CARE QUALITY AND SAFETY

Michael Lin

Learning Objectives

After completing this chapter, each learner will be able to:

- Identify the roles of nursing home managers that are associated with leadership.
- Contrast different systems-related concepts as they pertain to nursing home dynamics and performance.
- Analyze how nursing home managers affect quality and safety of care.
- Synthesize the importance of a nursing home manager's skills, style, and traits to improving nursing home quality.

INTRODUCTION

In this chapter, the central perspective is that a nursing home's environment is integrally intertwined with how effectively resident needs are met, and that a nursing home manager's role is largely one of managing both the internal and external environment while addressing performance issues such as quality and resident safety. Although the nursing home is an organization with an internal environment that requires a great deal of attention to ensure that operational challenges are met, a key observation is that a manager must also be deliberate in interacting with the external environment that provides key resources such as supplies, financing, staff, and certification to keep the nursing home open for business. Although quality and resident safety are very meaningful to all stakeholders, these are not the only concerns that demand attention from organizational leaders who must deftly navigate a complex environment in which there are multiple priorities and goals to consider. We explore how managers must balance competing needs of different stakeholders and how they must embrace both learning and change in the dynamic environments that affect their organization's performance (Figure 12.1).

To be effective leaders, managers should employ systems thinking when identifying and prioritizing activities and investments. Systems thinking conceptualizes the action of individual components as being interconnected to some extent, rather than being isolated, independent components. When thinking of quality improvement (QI), especially those strategies that pertain to developing the staff and organizational routines which ultimately influence the quality and safety of services, systems thinking takes into account the nature of relationships among and across different individuals and subsystems, recognizing the complexities of indirect relationships and feedback loops. A systems orientation includes concepts such as context, situational behaviors, multiple environments, just culture, learning and evaluation, and collaborations to maintain and improve the organization. From a practical perspective, there is evidence that leadership style

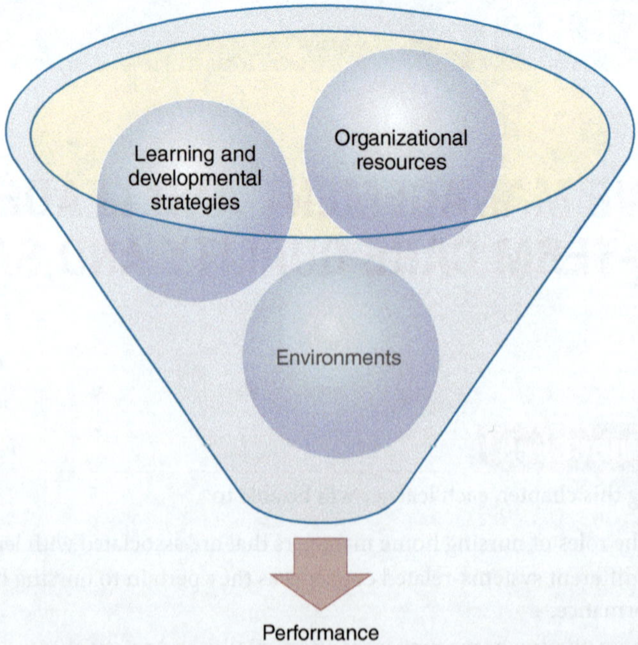

FIGURE 12.1. Key elements that affect nursing home performance.

matters, but personal characteristics (e.g., emotional intelligence, integrity, authenticity, honesty, and humility) and context (e.g., culture, team structure, regulatory and economic factors) matter because they create a climate for development, accountability, and collaboration.

MANAGING ESSENTIAL RESOURCES IN NURSING HOME OPERATIONS

When considering the complexity of resident needs and importance of nursing homes in a disjointed healthcare ecosystem, managers must address many competing demands. For managers and leaders, the routine daily activities include challenges related to checking in on essential resources such as staff, residents, supplies, medications, food, and information. These resources are integral to both operational and strategic success, and it is rare that a nursing home manager would have an abundance of these essential resources readily available.

Figure 12.2 depicts the connection between resources, routines, and performance in nursing homes. This figure provides examples of how resources such as staffing, supplies, and information systems influence operational routines and ultimately impact organizational performance. The supply or inventory of these resources, whether physical plant, personnel, supplies, money, brand/reputation, and/or information, affects the organization's ability to meet the needs of key stakeholders such as residents, families, ownership, and neighboring communities. Caring for a vulnerable population that requires 24-hour supervision, personal care, medical care, and social services requires a broad range of supplies to engage and improve the health of the nursing home's residents. Besides overseeing accounts payable and managing inventory, the nursing home needs staff to develop and maintain relationships with various suppliers. With many nursing home physical plants being old, repairing and replacing equipment and furniture, while updating the buildings and grounds, may place a heavy demand on the budget. Between scheduling bids and meeting with various contractors, there are often several meetings to work through the various purchasing and financing decisions prior to the implementation and monitoring processes.

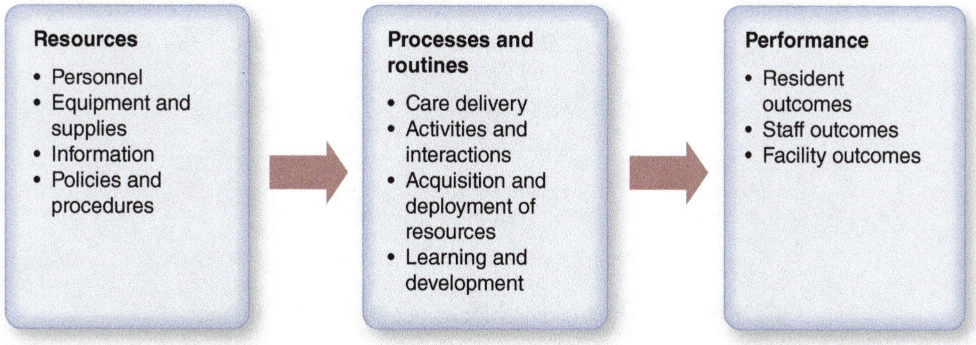

FIGURE 12.2. Connection between resources, routines, and performance.

As for staffing, with the current shortage of staff expected to increase in the coming years, developing relationships with training programs, hosting internal training programs, and contracting with agency staff are but a few of the activities that a manager must engage in to establish and maintain high quality and safety.

As it is for all organizations, money is an essential resource for a nursing home, especially because it is expensive to operate a healthcare facility that is open 365 days a year, 24 hours a day. Money is needed to pay for licensed and certified staff, maintain the physical plant, and ensure an adequate inventory of all the essential supplies. In order to generate revenue, the nursing home needs to complete resident assessments for the payment-driven payment model (PDPM), and then collect on accounts payable, whether from Medicaid, Medicare, or private payers. Similarly, a nursing home needs to establish relationships with referring providers, discharge planners, payors, and survey agencies not only to maintain status to be certified to provide care, but to attract residents and staff. Managing the quality and reputation of the nursing home is no trivial task, and often requires investments in training, membership and attendance at conferences, and meeting with external community members and groups to exchange information and establish a shared understanding.

One resource that is often underappreciated but is increasingly recognized as critical to nursing home operations and quality is pertinent information in the form of data. Obtaining, storing, analyzing, and making decisions with relevant data requires expensive information systems and specialized staff to stay in compliance with the myriad regulations for payment and security. Data such as the Minimum Data Set (MDS), payroll-based journal, Medicare and Medicaid claims, and complaints may all provide insights into nursing home performance. Perhaps more importantly, knowledge and wisdom are resources that require investments in the personnel, equipment, time, and processes that acquire, deploy, and evaluate information regarding the nursing home's quality. Rather than a comprehensive and exhaustive list of resources, let's turn the focus to the manager to better understand how these individuals affect quality and safety.

ROLE OF THE MANAGER

Given the complex needs of residents and the array of resources that must be acquired and deployed, the nursing home may be considered a machine that delivers care to vulnerable individuals, but it needs an operator and key inputs in order to provide high-quality care in a safe manner. Obtaining these resources requires exchange with the environment because it is an open rather than closed system (W. R. Scott & Davis, 2006).

Further complicating matters, nursing homes operate in an environment characterized by numerous regulatory requirements from state and federal laws, and complex governance situations stemming from ownership arrangements and frequent leadership changes (Werner et al., 2021).

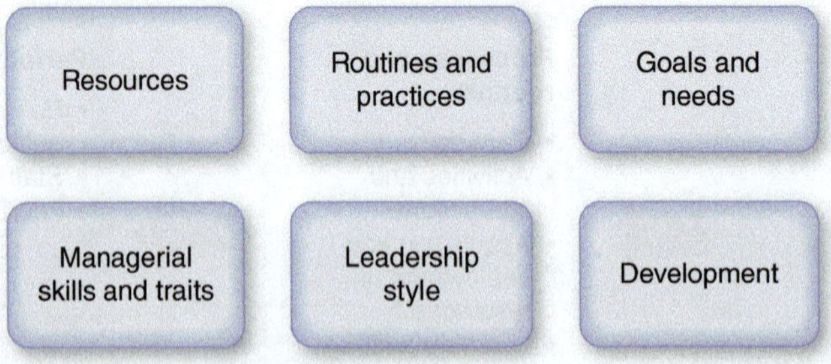

FIGURE 12.3. The building blocks of effective governance.

Figure 12.3 describes how effective governance can be achieved considering such complications, outlining the six key building blocks that contribute to strong leadership and oversight. While ensuring that processes are in compliance with regulations, nursing home managers must also contend with recruitment, selection, and training of staff amid historically high turnover and minimum nurse staffing ratio laws (Shen et al., 2023). Consequently, managers must recruit both front-line and administrative staff with the appropriate credentials and, given resource constraints, must often select from a pool with limited setting-specific experience. This is a daunting challenge due to low numbers of applicants despite rather minimal education requirements, potentially due to such factors as low wages, limited benefits, and heavy workloads (Scales, 2022).

Adding to the burden of limited budgets, nursing home managers must maintain if not update their aging physical plant to attract new clients. Thus, nursing home managers must manage relationships with not only internal stakeholders such as residents and staff, but a slew of external ones such as residents' family members, referring providers, lawyers, hospital discharge planners, and home health agency staff. The environment provides resources, but the environment is also a market for which there is competition for scarce resources such as money, residents, providers, and physical space. In fact, it would be fair to say that nursing homes exist in a resource-scarce environment when one considers Medicaid financing, staffing shortages, and heavy competition for a limited number of residents.

It would be desirable to consider the supply of staff and resources as being sufficient to have high quality and create a high safety environment, but the resource limitations require nursing home managers to take on boundary-spanning roles, scanning and perceiving the environment and subsequently taking the perceived steps to secure needed resources so that critical resources are available to address core operational concerns. For instance, relationships with hospital staff and insurers facilitate a flow of short-stay residents who require short-term rehabilitation services offered by the skilled nursing facility (SNF). Having a good reputation for high-quality care can facilitate referrals from hospital discharge planners and managed care network leaders who want their vulnerable clients to receive safe and effective care. Managing the reputation through good processes and consistent attainment of desirable outcomes that are listed on public reporting sites requires a commitment to hiring the right staff, training them in organizational routines, and ensuring that they have the necessary technologies and equipment to achieve good outcomes. This may require nurturing relationships with training programs to pique the interest of nurses, aides, and therapists in training.

Similarly, managers may need to scan the environment by reading trade journals, attending conferences, and meeting with vendors to evaluate and test out new technologies such as new electronic record systems. Furthermore, the constant flux in technologies and medications will require associated workflow changes to integrate these innovations into standard operating procedures, which may also affect performance reviews, training programs, and communication among staff members. These intraorganizational and interorganizational system dynamics are sufficiently complex as to warrant both specialized roles and specific skills to address the flow of these resources and clients. In fact, the array of quality metrics used to gauge nursing home quality are subject to change, with revisions to the regulatory process that focus on quality assurance and performance improvement, infection control, emergency preparedness, and minimum nurse staffing ratios (Centers for Medicare & Medicaid Services, 2023). Managers play a critical role because they often have to fill in gaps and do a little bit of everything to make sure that there are sufficient resources and functional processes to address all of the various activities that keep the nursing home running smoothly on a daily basis. Deploying the resources often requires motivating, educating, disciplining, and coordinating people, and while managers do not have to do everything, they have to ensure that such matters are completed in a satisfactory and timely manner. Hence, quality and safety may be compromised, especially in situations with limited resources and challenging environmental conditions.

Because the environment is multifaceted and changing, how a nursing home and its members interact with environment to achieve its goals is a constantly evolving challenge. To prepare the system for achieving performance goals such as high-quality care, the manager must facilitate change processes to not only acquire resources, but also deploy them in a sustainable manner that is consistent with the nursing home's mission and financial situation. Some nursing homes can stockpile resources because they have sufficient money to invest in an excess supply of key resources such as inventory and personnel. Furthermore, for the sake of ensuring a supply of resources, the organization can establish linkages, whether formal or informal, to suppliers and buyers in the ecosystem (Pfeffer & Salancik, 1978). The environment, both internal and external to a nursing home, have technical and cultural elements, and are in constant flux, with important considerations including high staff turnover, changing social norms about aging and dying, and continued development of evidence-based practices. Amid shifting expectations about how to deliver care and provide a safe environment, market relationships are ever changing due to the economics of modern healthcare and political battles over funding entitlement programs like Medicare and Medicaid.

SYSTEMS THINKING

In this section, we consider the system—the nursing home—as a multidimensional social construct which has task characteristics like roles, standards, protocols, and goals, as well as social characteristics such as culture, values, norms, and ceremonies with both symbolic and practical benefits for learning and strategizing. Systems thinking is a holistic method involving understanding, analyzing, and solving problems by considering the interconnectedness of complex systems (Atun, 2012). One of the major orientations for a systems thinker is to consider a network of relationships, necessarily embracing that people, groups, and organizations are interdependent with their environment near and far, and that behavior is based on both person and situational factors.

Thinking about nursing homes as systems includes conceiving of networks of relationships, with patterns of behavior like routines and protocols, and the arrangements between and among groups, departments, and programs that form an organizational chart and menu of services. These patterns become social norms and operational protocols that are learned and sustained so that the nursing home has some durability of identity and reliability in processes. Rather than blaming errors or mistakes solely on a person, systems thinking means that performance—whether desirable like profits or undesirable like infectious outbreaks—are a function of system characteristics, with accountability being partially if not largely on the underlying infrastructure including the assumptions and beliefs that guide work, rather than just a person or piece of equipment that is successful or fails to do its job. Hence, when trying to understand how an error, mistake, or undesirable outcome occurred in a nursing home, it is impossible to detach the person or equipment from the organizational context in which the failure, oversight, or ignorance occurred. Such an orientation is a departure from a blame-and-shame approach which focuses on individual responsibility for errors and undesirable outcomes, and management approaches that solve problems by firing the employee(s) involved.

Perhaps equally important to recognize is that changing a person or piece of equipment may not be sufficient to prevent errors; rather, sometimes the fix requires altering not only the organization's infrastructure (staff, policy, and goals) and the processes (standard operating procedures), but also the underlying mental model or set of assumptions about the appropriate goals and objectives. These root causes are subject to much scrutiny and experimentation in systems thinking. Such an approach to QI and safety embraces the importance of the network structure and dynamics; thus, efforts to improve quality and performance are associated with system design or systems engineering rather than simply improving (or replacing) a person or piece of equipment.

Awareness that a staff member's behavior is intertwined—more specifically, interdependent—with their situation does not mean that individual employees don't have accountability for their capabilities and actions. In fact, such recognition means that paying attention to one's competencies, behaviors, and the environment—both physical and social—needs to be nurtured and developed as a mindset. For the former two, self-awareness and soliciting feedback from others is critical. As for the latter, while certain environmental conditions are easily managed and respond to efforts to change them, others may be difficult to change and may actually resist efforts to alter existing dynamics. One of the most frequent applications for systems thinking is the focus of our next section on quality management. The emphasis should not be restricted to what can be done better, but what can be done differently and what different things can be done (Argyris, 1991).

QUALITY MANAGEMENT

QI methods such as lean, for which there is a great deal of attention to processes, focus on the activities that are necessary to complete tasks, whether resident/resident-focused or on the supply chain. These activities ensure that essential medications, supplies, and equipment are available when needed, but neither too early nor too late; this lowers the chances of excess inventory or tardiness. For instance, the tools, activities, and mind-set associated with lean thinking is a systematic approach to value and improvement. A major source of innovation and QI develops when different stakeholders are involved in mapping out a process to assess value and waste in processes.

Another QI approach, known as root cause analysis, has roots in systems engineering. By examining interrelationships, in particular the causal mechanisms that affect how undesirable outcomes come about, this assessment traces the root causes, which are the target of improvement activities. In a system, rather than just the immediate proximal cause, sometimes distal, indirect influences are the root of the problem. Similarly, a system is not just the formalized elements, but also the informal groups and interactions among different elements. In addition, a change in one part of the system may potentially lead to unintentional repercussions, leading to unintended consequences. More generalized system mapping approaches which study precursors or the aftermath of events, both positive and negative, include fishbone diagrams, customer experience mapping, logic models, and change models to dissect the pathways that lead to particular outcomes.

In contrast to systems characterized by managers who are effective in creating a high-performing, high-quality, and safety-minded climate, Vaughan et al. (2019) studied struggling healthcare organizations and identified some issues that may lead to low performance, low quality, and low resident safety. These include the dysfunctions of a noncollaborative culture, recurrent problems caused by an inadequate technological and human resource infrastructure, a disjointed mission that leads to conflicting directions, external shocks to the system that create operational and strategic challenges, and dysfunctional relationships with the local healthcare ecosystem that affect the flow of resources. These characteristics are especially important because meaning, fulfillment, success, and reputation all hinge on sensing the environment, responding to changing norms, and addressing the internal issues that are also dynamic (e.g., person-centered care, trauma-informed care, and cultural sensitivity). These demonstrate the need for nursing homes to balance different needs and secure different resources.

ORGANIZATIONAL CULTURE AND CLIMATE

Organizational culture and its relative, climate, have been the subject of organizational sociologists and anthropologists, and are often used to characterize an organization. Among the many tools for assessing organizational culture, one particularly useful framework is the Competing Values Framework (CVF), which provides a taxonomy of organizational cultures (Cameron & Quinn, 1999; T. Scott et al., 2003). Emphasizing dualities such as collaboration and competition, differentiation and integration, discretion and control, the framework adheres to the "one size *does not* fit all" mentality that open systems experts described as a contingency approach (Lawrence & Lorsch, 1967). In the CVF, the primary axes of a two-dimensional chart reflect how an organization is a system for which there are both internal and external dimensions to consider, and both stability/rigidity and innovation/flexibility issues when considering organizational cultures. As a system, every organization must address elements in all four quadrants, though some organizations will elect to emphasize certain values more than others (e.g., the internal, rigid quadrant is known as the bureaucratic or hierarchical culture). While used in many healthcare studies, nursing homes typically fall in the hierarchical/bureaucratic or team/group culture, reflecting an internal emphasis (Scott-Cawiezell et al., 2005).

Another important characteristic of systems that is related and similar to culture is climate, which is an employee's perception of the meaning and significance of their work (Glisson, 2015). Climate is similar to culture in that individuals from the same organization may have different opinions, though a strong culture or climate is one for which the perceptions are shared. Similarly, both can be used to describe an organization and the contextual expectations about behavior, though culture is typically focused on norms, while climate focuses on engagement, functionality, and stress in the organization.

To foster a development-focused climate associated with a learning health system (Agency for Healthcare Research and Quality [AHRQ], 2019) and implementation science, both external linkages and internal reactions influence what employees believe matter (Aase et al., 2021; Vindrola-Padros et al., 2017). A learning health system, as defined by the AHRQ, is a system where "internal data and experience are systematically integrated with external evidence, and that knowledge is then applied to practice" (2019, para. 1). This approach enables higher quality, safer, and more efficient care for patients, while also improving the work environment for healthcare staff. A learning health system is characterized by leadership committed to continuous learning and improvement, real-time evidence integration, the use of IT to inform clinical decision-making, active patient inclusion, and continuous data analysis to refine processes and outcomes. The result is a feedback loop that drives ongoing learning and care improvement (AHRQ, 2019).

Internally, creating a nonpunitive work environment and open communication about adverse events are important components of creating a climate associated with a high resident safety culture (Bonner et al., 2009). In a study of the association between work climate and resident safety-related behaviors, efficient and smooth-functioning work processes, social support, and cohesion were positively associated with behavior, while work stress and insufficient time to complete tasks were negatively associated with behavior (Arnetz et al., 2011).

Given the significance of the situation or context, nursing home managers must invest in the structures and processes that influence quality and safety. However, it is not always the formal, stated structure and standard operating practices that are sufficient to ensure high quality. For instance, DiMartino et al. (2018) evaluate the influence of policies and practices on the implementation of palliative care, finding that formal policies and procedures, such as training, guidelines, and protocols, may not necessarily create a strong implementation climate, while informal policies and practices such as spontaneous feedback and frequent reinforcement through communication can create a strong implementation climate.

TRANSFORMATIONAL LEADERSHIP

The previous sections presented an image of an organization that functions like a machine, needing resources to operate. However, it is also a living organism with a lifecycle—encompassing birth and a death—along with key biological issues such as longevity, growth, composition, experience, and successful performance, all of which can be quite uncertain (Morgan, 1986/2006). Comprehending the nursing home as a multidimensional social construct which has characteristics like culture, values, roles, rituals, and ceremonies has both symbolic and practical benefits for learning and strategizing. How does a manager balance all of the competing dynamic demands? Rather than approach the nursing home manager's job as too complex, too unstable, or too challenging, this section explores the leadership styles, individual traits, and daily routines that enable a nursing home manager to not only survive, but thrive, in such an environment.

A keen and enduring interest in leadership and leadership styles has led to a variety of management studies. The previous sections have highlighted a *contingency* or situational leadership model. These are in contrast to the studies of leadership that were focused on heroes and their traits (Borkowski, 2016). Contemporary leadership models provide a balance of the preceding ones, incorporating the individual leader, the follower, the environment/situation, and goals/objectives. These perspectives are more focused on integrating "ideological, moral, and value applications" (Borkowski, 2016, p. 246). They attempt to draw some practical conclusions about what works and what does not work, with one of the most relevant frameworks focusing on the distinction between *transformational* and *transactional* leadership (Burns, 1978). Transformational leadership (Bass, 1985) is based on the idea that some leaders are able to appeal to the greater good when motivating employees to go beyond a transactional mind-set of "what's in it for me?" to a focus on "this is for the greater good" approach to group rewards and systemic change. Poels et al. suggest that transformational leadership is characterized by leaders motivating employees "to do more than what is expected of them" (2020, p. 2). In contrast to transformational leadership, the transactional leadership model is characterized by a task focus that offers contingent reward (whether material and/or psychologic) when obligations are fulfilled, as well as monitoring the work of followers so that corrective action can be taken when errors are observed.

> "Transformational leadership occurs 'when leaders broaden and elevate the interests of their employees, when they generate awareness and acceptance of the purposes and mission of the group and when they stir their employees to look beyond their own self-interest for the good of the group' (Bass, 1991, p. 21)." (Ree & Wiig, 2019, p. 257).

In terms of research, there is a growing body of evidence that finds that transformational leadership style—or at least some of the characteristics associated with this style—is associated with high-quality nursing homes. For instance, Castle and Decker (2011) found that transformational and consultative authoritarian leadership styles were most associated with higher quality in nursing homes. In a review of transformational leadership, Dewar et al. (2019) found that this leadership style creates enduring relationships and a strong commitment to development that creates conditions for success. McKinney et al. (2016) focused on leadership styles, and found that the consultative and consensus styles were associated with lower odds of deficiencies for resident behavior and facility practices, quality of life, quality of care, and nursing services. This is hypothesized to have occurred through expanded information gathering, a verity of interactions, and the subsequent deeper understanding of systems and more creative generation of resident-centered solutions. Likewise, in a study of Veterans Affairs (VA) nursing homes, communication and responsiveness to safety issues raised by direct care staff were important differentiators that distinguished organizations with high safety climate ratings from those with low to medium safety climate ratings (Engle et al., 2023). Song et al. (2020) found that staff on units with more favorable work environments were less likely to miss or rush care tasks in a sample of 93 urban nursing homes in Western Canada.

TRAITS STILL MATTER

This chapter has characterized long-term care (LTC)/nursing home managers as leaders and strategists that affect quality and safety in LTC through their focus on certain issues, their perception and detection of opportunities for improvement, the criteria they use in decision-making, their approach to implementing innovations and corrective actions, and their evaluation of what worked and what didn't work in their performance improvement activities. However, we have not devoted much attention to who the managers and leaders are, why they work in a nursing home, how they develop into effective managers, or what differentiates them from other nursing home staff in charge of certain resources.

Early studies of effective leaders focused on personality traits, such as the Big Five factors (openness, conscientiousness, extraversion, agreeableness, and neuroticism), and delved into the question of whether leaders are made or born, effectively distinguishing between innate traits and acquired traits (Digman, 1990). More recently, some traits/characteristics may be hard to develop, so it may be better to select leaders from the group that possess key attributes, such as high emotional intelligence, to work with other people—not just staff but clients and partners (Chopra & Kanji, 2010). Similarly, working in the nursing home setting requires empathy and compassion to help residents, staff, and family members during difficult times, such as managing end-of-life care and grieving after departures by residents and staff. Perhaps two of the most important lessons learned from a public health emergency are that resilience and perseverance are essential for navigating through difficult times. These traits are crucial, not only for continuing to show up at work but also for maintaining effective operations amid turnover and disrupted relationships. However, similar to other research presented in this textbook, none of these studies have demonstrated that these leadership traits and characteristics are *sufficient* to guarantee high quality. Rather, they may be necessary ingredients that, when coupled with supportive environments, can lead to high-quality outcomes.

PRACTICES TO DEVELOP AND ENHANCE THE SYSTEM

Aiming to create a safe environment for residents and staff—one that fosters desired outcomes and is perceived as a high functioning reputable organization—is a common pursuit across nursing homes. However, not everyone is equally effective at attaining such goals in the competitive and ever-evolving U.S. healthcare system. As previously discussed, nursing homes are systems in which the numerous transactions rely on various individuals to interact with one another, their equipment, information systems, and other resources in markets characterized by dynamic, if not chaotic conditions. Yet, on a daily basis, the short-term activities and needs are not only varied but also recurring and essential to maintaining a highly functional and effective system. This is where managers must lead, motivate, and train others to create a high probability of quality and safety.

Managers should ensure that short-term needs are addressed by providing support, guidance, and oversight of the system's functioning. For instance, to deliver timely care, it is important that staff understand who they are caring for, what each resident requires in terms of physical support, and have a schedule that aligns with resident wishes as documented in their care plan. Each interaction and step should not be restricted to just addressing immediate issues; rather, it is important—if not essential—to manage long-term concerns such as staff training and mentoring. This involves helping staff not only perform their assigned tasks but also consider their own long-term goals to prevent dissatisfaction and burnout. To be equitable, managers must be consistent with both staff and residents, adopting and/or developing a systematic approach that is scalable and sustainable, thereby addressing concerns about commitment, fairness, and competence.

Huddles are an effective way to engage team members on a routine and frequent basis, offering a valuable opportunity for bidirectional communication between administration and frontline staff. Options include standing, regularly scheduled huddles that may address myriad issues or ad hoc, temporary huddles to address some particular issue that affects operations, quality, and safety. Zubkoff et al. (2017) evaluated a Veterans Affairs Healthcare Administration (VHA) collaborative aimed at improving fall prevention, finding that the most commonly implemented interventions were postfall huddles designed to understand the root causes of falls. Other approaches to reduce falls, such as program evaluation to analyze the fall cases, staff education, improved documentation and communication, and intentional rounding, were also adopted with varying degrees of success.

Managers should regularly set aside time to be regularly available to meet with staff, sharing developments and news about the organization, its residents, and its staff. This practice demonstrates honesty and a genuine commitment to information sharing and analysis. For instance, despite having implemented high reliability organizational (HRO) practices and a just culture mind-set, McCain et al. (2023) found that there was a need to implement interdisciplinary team huddles to ensure the organization's goals regarding an increase in near miss reporting, resident satisfaction, and employee satisfaction were met. These huddles promoted situational awareness through routine communication about individual, system, and environmental concerns, and facilitated shared understanding and decision-making.

Equally important to fostering relationships among staff, these huddles build trust regarding high expectations and team excellence through transparent discussions about resident safety events without fear of retribution. Huddles provide an opportunity to practice a no-fault approach, developing and planning safe reporting systems that foster a fair and just culture of shared accountability (Vogelsmeier et al., 2010).

LEADERSHIP STRATEGIES FOR PROFESSIONAL GROWTH AND ORGANIZATIONAL DEVELOPMENT

In addition to task-specific training, leaders should ensure that the organization invests in people through mentoring and professional development, offering dedicated time and financial support for these growth-directed activities. While this is crucial for succession planning and professional development, nurturing relationships and networks with other organizations can also enhance the pursuit of person-centered, high-quality care. External partnerships with research, practice, policy-regulation, education, and consumer groups provide insights into system dynamics beyond the nursing home's physical boundaries (Siegel & Young, 2021). One study found that managers that experiment with new ideas, coach their staff, provide direct feedback, and constructively manage conflict were more likely to be rated highly as leaders (Backman et al., 2017).

Rounding is one way for leaders to assess the nursing home's internal environment and understand the challenges encountered by their colleagues. Defined as a structured approach, rounding involves nurses conducting checks on staff and residents to assess and manage their needs (Roberts et al., 2020). This practice helps leaders build relationships with staff and residents, enabling them to gain deeper knowledge about the internal environment while providing opportunities to motivate and train others. It demonstrates a commitment to understanding operational challenges, and helps identify developmental needs among staff, teams, units, and the organization as a whole.

The frequent, high touch interactions that daily rounding offers are not merely for show; they allow managers to model behaviors related to safety, systematically investigate the sources of problems, clarify what is acceptable, determine what requires attention, and collaborate on identifying and customizing solutions. Even if rounding is not performed daily, it can still convey a commitment to quality and safety, while engaging staff members across various departments and units.

Berta et al. (2018) conducted a path analysis using data collected from staff in LTC and community settings across Ontario, Canada. They discovered a complex interplay between job satisfaction, work engagement, and organizational commitment, which in turn influenced employees' intent to stay, organizational citizenship behaviors, and overall performance. These work attitudes were significantly impacted by perceived supervisor support and workplace safety.

DEVELOPMENT, LEARNING, AND COLLABORATION

One of the key ways in which leadership affects learning and collaboration pertains to the analytics that accompany QI planning and associated implementation processes. QI relies on objective identification of problems, investigation of the root causes of problems, and assessment of levers—whether barriers or facilitators—that will improve the system so that recurrence of the problem may be eliminated or greatly reduced with the implementation of an appropriate mitigation strategy. Continually improving as the environment changes, comprehensive analytic routines also create a culture that accumulates knowledge so that the QI leaders have the wisdom to know when to abandon certain initiatives, slow down the pace of implementation, or revisit basic assumptions.

Leaders should ensure their foundation is strong—in this case, the data should be valid and reliable as represented by the base of the quality assurance and performance improvement pyramid (Figure 12.4)—and if there is insufficient quantity or quality of data, it may be necessary to collect or wrangle data to fill in information gaps. Subsequently, developing the QI plans should reflect an understanding of system dynamics that will lead to implementation success or failure, and plans should consider what to do in the event that certain steps are unsuccessful or results are far from the intended objectives. In this case, it may be necessary to develop small tests of change via Plan-Do-Check-Act (PDCA) or Plan-Do-Study-Act (PDSA) cycles, also known as Shewhart cycles (Best & Neuhauser, 2006).

Mindful of the validity and reliability of data, leaders play a crucial role in making data-driven decisions across a wide array of departments and functions, including reimbursement, regulatory compliance, operational research, and performance evaluation of individuals, groups, other organizations, and the environment. Leadership and governance practices are essential in creating a safe climate for obtaining, storing, retrieving, analyzing, and interpreting data. As staff design and implement performance improvement efforts—whether through adding steps or removing barriers—these initiatives will not be effective unless leaders provide support by securing necessary resources and ensuring that different systems are aligned with the improvement goals.

Quality teams often collaborate closely, huddling together to review results, devise improvement projects, support implementation, and conduct ongoing evaluations in continuous circles, such as the PDSA or Shewhart cycles. Leadership should encourage collaborative thinking, bringing together individuals from across the nursing home and ensuring that the group avoids pitfalls

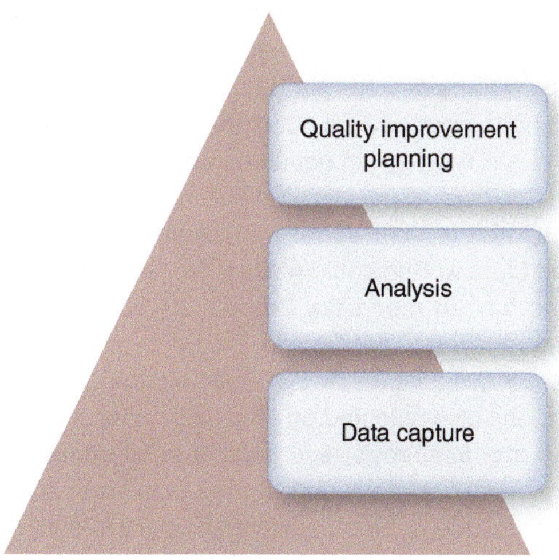

FIGURE 12.4. Quality assurance and performance improvement pyramid.

Note: Each of the elements are governed by a nursing home's leaders.

like groupthink or blind spots. This approach is essential when developing QI plans that are both evidence-based and feasible to implement.

Furthermore, it may be necessary for leadership to engage external stakeholders—such as family members, researchers, advocates, and community groups—in the planning process. To do so, leaders may need to allocate funds to ensure the right participants are involved. These funds resources can be used to facilitate communication and collaboration, whether for travel or hosting an event like focus groups, and supporting data collection, analysis, and interpretation of the results. Ultimately, the governance of the system and the resultant quality of the nursing home will depend on whether leadership has a strong foundation of data to make informed decisions related to QI (Case Study 12.1).

Case Study 12.1 Adapting Leadership and Technology in Long-Term Care: The New Nursing Home Administrator's Dilemma

Melanie Stramel, the new nursing home administrator of Shadybrook Nursing Center in Springfield, Colorado, sighs as her cellphone rings. She is sitting at her desk, reviewing a bill flagged by the finance director—a notice of a significant increase in the monthly cost for Harpo, the facility's electronic health record system. What is more concerning is that training will no longer be free. The new options include three tiers: in-person training, live webinars with standard content, and live webinars with custom content, along with on-demand sessions.

It is 7:45 p.m., and Melanie has been working since 6:30 a.m. on this Tuesday. She is hungry, frustrated, and exhausted. Before checking the caller ID, she realizes it is time to pack up and head home to relieve the babysitter before 8 p.m.—after all, it is a school night.

She answers the phone and hears the familiar voice of her longtime friend, Jennifer Kurtz, Shadybrook's director of nursing. Melanie and Jennifer have known each other since grade school, attended the same nursing program, and worked together in the ED of a hospital after becoming RNs. Their paths diverged after fulfilling their loan forgiveness commitment, with Jennifer opting to work part-time in outpatient care while raising her three children. Jennifer started at Shadybrook two years before Melanie, first as a charge nurse, then taking on infection control and quality assurance roles before her promotion to director of nursing.

"Mel, are you still at work? Aren't you supposed to be reading Colton his bedtime story? Anyway, I just got a call from Dr. Hudson—Ms. Daniels is being admitted for surgery to repair her fractured pelvis. I'm not entirely sure what happened. Sandy and Ben said they followed protocol for her two-person transfer from the bath to her wheelchair. They got her dressed and were putting on her shoes when she fell out of the chair while Sandy was prepping for her oral hygiene routine. Ben's still new, so I'm not sure how comfortable he is with Ms. Daniels—you know how confused she gets, especially at night."

Melanie was disappointed to hear about Ms. Daniels' injury but relieved that Jennifer could handle the situation for now. She could make it home in time to tuck in her son. Figuring out what went wrong and how to report the incident to the state could wait until after she finished reading *The Little Red Train That Could*.

As she drove home, just five minutes away, Melanie thought about how lucky she was to have a reliable babysitter. She also reflected on the rising costs of Harpo. She had anticipated the price hike ever since the company's recent initial public offering (IPO). While the extra cost of the subscription was manageable, she worried that Harpo's shareholder-driven focus might lead to higher fees for modernization, pushing the burden onto clients. She learned that

(*continued*)

Case Study 12.1 Adapting Leadership and Technology in Long-Term Care: The New Nursing Home Administrator's Dilemma (*continued*)

Jennifer had always loved Harpo's training and support services before the IPO, appreciating their free, on-demand webinars and flexible scheduling for live virtual training.

Melanie, on the other hand, had reservations. She found Harpo's user interface clunky, and the analytics and reports were less intuitive than what she was used to from Maple, the electronic medical record (EMR) system she had used at her previous hospital. Maple's user-friendly design, easy navigation of reports, and built-in clinical decision support had set a high bar. Although Harpo excelled in analyzing SNF quality reporting program (QRP) measures and was efficient for MDS and point-of-care documentation, Melanie missed Maple's seamless functionality.

Maple had been publicly traded for nearly a decade and had never charged for virtual trainings. Additionally, it had a strong community of practice, with users willing to share tips and troubleshoot implementation issues. Recently, Melanie heard that Maple was expanding into long-term care with a product called MapleLTC. She thought it might be worth calling her corporate information technology (IT) director to learn more about its features, costs, and interoperability.

She was particularly curious about MapleLTC's potential use of artificial intelligence (AI) and machine learning (ML). She had heard that Maple was partnering with large tech companies to develop advanced models, like artificial neural networks, capable of predicting risks and recommending preventive actions. Although she wasn not trained in AI/ML, Melanie had heard that Maple's system was especially effective at predicting sepsis risk. Given that Shadybrook's quality scores were only average—particularly in hospital readmissions and falls—Melanie wondered if Maple could help Shadybrook improve from a three-star to a four-star facility. But first, she would have to convince Jennifer to part ways with Harpo!

Case Study Discussion Questions

1. How does the case study illustrate the chapter's orientation that nursing homes are "open" systems?
2. What do you think of Melanie's reaction to Jennifer's report about Ms. Daniels' fall? How does this end-of-day situation illustrate the practical realities of being a nursing home administrator?
3. In what ways does the environment play a role in Shadybrook's current challenges?
4. How does Melanie's interest in MapleLTC illustrate the complexity of making health technology-related decisions in the nursing home industry?

SUMMARY

Whether running a unit, managing all of the facility staff, or strategizing for a chain of nursing homes, the enduring challenge for nursing home leaders depends on the ability to secure and organize resources, train and motivate employees to cooperate with one another, and treat residents and external partners with integrity and fairness. In order to deliver high-quality and safe care, leadership must train, deploy, monitor, and reward staff for being attentive to residents' needs, among other things. These recurring challenges require fundamental technical and interpersonal skills, and a leadership style suitable for the context. Even experienced and well-respected managers must continue to evolve as their organization's flow of resources and strategic positioning shifts amid dynamic social, competitive, economic, regulatory, and technical environments. The integration of quality and safety into payment programs continues to evolve, with increasing attention to value and evaluation. Successfully managing personnel and valuable resources like physical plant, supplies, food, and reputation requires an ability to refine skills, knowledge, processes, and collaborations (both internal and external), especially with the role of technology and interoperable information to transform quality-related decision-making.

END-OF-CHAPTER RESOURCES

DISCUSSION QUESTIONS

1. How can effective management improve the quality and safety of LTC?
2. How does a systems orientation affect quality management in nursing homes?
3. What are some of the challenges associated with acquiring and deploying personnel in LTC facilities? How can technology be used to improve the quality of care in nursing homes?
4. What are some of the risks and benefits of integrating technology into care practices?
5. What role do regulatory bodies play in ensuring the quality and safety of LTC facilities? How can administrators navigate complex regulations and policies to provide the best possible care?

SPRINGER PUBLISHING CONNECT™ A robust set of instructor resources designed to supplement this text is located at http://connect.springerpub.com/content/book/978-0-8261-4935-0. Qualifying instructors may request access by emailing textbook@springerpub.com.

REFERENCES

Aase, I., Ree, E., Johannessen, T., Holen-Rabbersvik, E., Thomsen, L. H., Strømme, T., Ullebust, B., Schibevaag, L., Lyng, H. B., O'Hara, J., & Wiig, S. (2021). Strategies and lessons learnt from user involvement in researching quality and safety in nursing homes and homecare. *International Journal of Health Governance*, *26*(4), 384–396. https://doi.org/10.1108/IJHG-05-2021-0044

Agency for Healthcare Research and Quality (2019). *About learning health systems*. https://www.ahrq.gov/learning-health-systems/about.html

Argyris, C. (1991). Teaching smart people how to learn. *Harvard Business Review*, *69*(3), 99–110. https://hbr.org/1991/05/teaching-smart-people-how-to-learn

Arnetz, J. E., Zhdanova, L. S., Elsouhag, D., Lichtenberg, P., Luborsky, M. R., & Arnetz, B. B. (2011). Organizational climate determinants of resident safety culture in nursing homes. *Gerontologist*, *51*(6), 739–749. https://doi.org/10.1093/geront/gnr053

Atun, R. (2012). Health systems, systems thinking and innovation. *Health Policy and Planning*, *27*(Suppl. 4), iv4–iv8. https://doi.org/10.1093/heapol/czs088

Backman, A., Sjogren, K., Lindkvist, M., Lövheim, H., & Edvardsson, D. (2017). Characteristics of highly rated leadership in nursing homes using item response theory. *Journal of Advanced Nursing*, *73*(12), 2903–2913. https://doi.org/10.1111/jan.13353

Bass, B. M. (1985). *Leadership beyond expectations*. Free Press.

Bass, B. M. (1991). From transactional to transformational leadership: Learning to share the vision. *Organizational Dynamics*, *18*(3), 19–31. https://doi.org/10.1016/0090-2616(90)90061-S

Berta, W., Laporte, A., Perreira, T., Ginsburg, L., Dass, A. R., Deber, R., Baumann, A., Cranley, L., Bourgeault, I., Lum, J., Gamble, B., Pilkington, K., Haroun, V., & Neves, P. (2018). Relationships between work outcomes, work attitudes and work environments of health support workers in Ontario long-term care and home and community care settings. *Human Resources for Health, 16*(1), 15–25. https://doi.org/10.1186/s12960-018-0277-9

Best, M., & Neuhauser, D. (2006). Walter A Shewhart, 1924, and the Hawthorne factory. *Quality & Safety in Health Care, 15*(2), 142–143. https://doi.org/10.1136/qshc.2006.018093

Bonner, A., Castle, N., Men, A., & Handler, S. M. (2009). Certified nursing assistants' perceptions of nursing home patient safety culture: Is there a relationship to clinical outcomes? *Journal of the American Medical Directors Association, 10*(1), 11–20. https://doi.org/10.1016/j.jamda.2008.06.004

Borkowski, N. (2016). *Organizational behavior, theory, and design in health care* (2nd ed.). Jones & Bartlett Learning.

Burns, J. M. (1978). *Leadership*. Harper & Row.

Cameron, K. S., & Quinn, R. E. (1999). *Diagnosing and changing organizational culture: Based on the competing values framework*. Addison-Welsey.

Castle, N. G., & Decker, F. H. (2011). Top management leadership style and quality of care in nursing homes. *Gerontologist, 51*(5), 630–642. https://doi.org/10.1093/geront/gnr064

Centers for Medicare & Medicaid Services. (2023, September 6). *Quality safety & oversight—Guidance to laws and regulations*. https://www.cms.gov/medicare/health-safety-standards/guidance-for-laws-regulations

Chopra, P. K., & Kanji, G. K. (2010). Emotional intelligence: A catalyst for inspirational leadership and management excellence. *Total Quality Management & Business Excellence, 21*(10), 971–1004. https://doi.org/10.1080/14783363.2010.487704

Dewar, B., Barrie, K., Sharp, C., & Meyer, J. (2019). Implementation of a complex intervention to support leadership development in nursing homes: A multimethod participatory study. *Journal of Applied Gerontology, 38*(7), 931–958. https://doi.org/10.1177/0733464817705957

Digman, J. M. (1990). Personality structure: Emergence of the five-factor model. *Annual Review of Psychology, 41*, 417–440. https://doi.org/10.1146/annurev.ps.41.020190.002221

DiMartino, L. D., Birken, S. A., Hanson, L. C., Trogdon, J. G., Clary, A. S., Weinberger, M., Reeder-Hayes, K., & Weiner, B. J. (2018). The influence of formal and informal policies and practices on health care innovation implementation: A mixed-methods analysis. *Health Care Management Review, 43*(3), 249–260. https://doi.org/10.1097/HMR.0000000000000193

Engle, R. L., Gillespie, C., Clark, V. A., McDannold, S. E., Kazi, L. E., & Hartmann, C. W. (2023). Factors differentiating nursing homes with strong resident safety climate: A qualitative study of leadership and staff perspectives. *Journal of Gerontological Nursing, 49*(2), 13–17. https://doi.org/10.3928/00989134-20230106-03

Glisson, C. (2015). The role of organizational culture and climate in innovation and effectiveness. *Human Services Organizations, Leadership, and Governance, 39*(4), 245–250. https://doi.org/10.1080/23303131.2015.1087770

Lawrence, P. R., & Lorsch, J. W. (1967). *Organization and environment: Managing differentiation and integration*. Harvard University.

McCain, N., Ferguson, T., Hultquist, T. B., Wahl, C., & Struwe, L. (2023). Influencing a culture of quality and safety through huddles. *Journal of Nursing Care Quality, 38*(1), 26–32. https://doi.org/10.1097/NCQ.0000000000000642

McKinney, S. H., Corazzini, K., Anderson, R. A., Sloane, R., & Castle, N. G. (2016). Nursing home director of nursing leadership style and director of nursing-sensitive survey deficiencies. *Health Care Management Review, 41*(3), 224–232. https://doi.org/10.1097/HMR.0000000000000072

Morgan, G. (2006). *Images of organization*. Sage Library of Social Research. (Original work published 1986)

Pfeffer, J., & Salancik, G. R. (1978). *The external control of organizations*. Harper & Row.

Poels, J., Veshueren, M., Millsen, K., & Vlaeyen, E. (2020). Leadership styles and leadership outcomes in nursing homes: A cross-sectional analysis. *BMC Health Services Research, 20*, 1009–1018. https://doi.org/10.1186/s12913-020-05854-7

Ree, E., & Wiig, S. (2019). Linking transformational leadership, patient safety culture and work engagement in home care services. *Nursing Open, 7*(1), 256–264. https://doi.org/10.1002/nop2.386

Roberts, B., Holloway-Kew, K., Pretorius, T., Hosking, S., Kennedy, A., & Armstrong, K. (2020). Does 20-min rounding reduce falls in an aged care setting? A pilot intervention study. *Geriatric Nursing, 41*, 579–584. https://doi.org/10.1016/j.gerinurse.2020.03.003

Scales, K. (2022). Transforming direct care jobs, reimagining long-term services and supports. *Journal of the American Medical Directors Association, 23*(2), 207–213. https://doi.org/10.1016/j.jamda.2021.12.005

Scott, T., Mannion, R., Davies, H., & Marshall, M. (2003). The quantitative measurement of organizational culture in health care. *Health Services Research, 38*(3), 923–945. https://doi.org/10.1111/1475-6773.00154

Scott, W. R., & Davis, G. F. (2006). *Organizations and organizing: Rational, natural, and open system perspectives*. Routledge.

Scott-Cawiezell, J., Jones, K., Moore, L., & Vojir, C. (2005). Nursing home culture: A critical component in sustained improvement. *Journal of Nursing Care Quality, 20*(4), 341–348. https://doi.org/10.1097/00001786-200510000-00010

Shen, K., McGarry, B. E., & Gandhi, A. D. (2023). Health care staff turnover and quality of care of nursing homes. *JAMA Internal Medicine, 183*(11), 1247–1254. https://doi.org/10.1001/jamainternmed.2023.5225

Siegel, E. O., & Young, H. M. (2021). Assuring quality in nursing homes: The black box of administrative and clinical leadership—A scoping review. *Gerontologist, 61*(4), e147–e162. https://doi.org/10.1093/geront/gnaa175

Song, Y., Hoben, M., Norton, P., & Estabrooks, C. A. (2020). Association of work environment with missed and rushed care tasks among care aides in nursing homes. *JAMA Network Open, 3*(1), e1920092. https://doi.org/10.1001/jamanetworkopen.2019.20092

Vaughan, V. M., Saint, S., Krein, S. L., Forman, J. H., Meddings, J., Ameling, J., Winter, S., Townsend, W., & Chopra, V. (2019). Characteristics of healthcare organisations struggling to improve quality: Results from a systematic review of qualitative studies. *BMJ Journal of Quality and Safety, 28*, 74–84. https://doi.org/10.1136/bmjqs-2017-007573

Vindrola-Padros, C., Pape, T., Utley, M., & Fulop, N. J. (2017). The role of embedded research in quality improvement: A narrative review. *BMJ Journal of Quality and Safety, 26*, 70–80. https://doi.org/10.1136/bmjqs-2015-004877

Vogelsmeier, A. A., Farrah, S. J., Roam, A., & Ott, L. (2010). Evaluation of a leadership development academy for RNs in long-term care. *Nursing Administration Quarterly, 34*(2), 122–129. https://doi.org/10.1097/NAQ.0b013e3181d91778

Werner, R. M., Templeton, Z., Apathy, N., Skira, M. M., & Tamara Konetzka, R. (2021). Trends in post-acute care in US nursing homes: 2001–2017. *Journal of the American Medical Directors Association, 22*(12), 2491–2495. https://doi.org/10.1016/j.jamda.2021.06.015

Zubkoff, L., Neily, J., King, B., Morgan, S., Young-Xu, Y., Boar, S., & Mills, P. (2017). Preventing pressure ulcers in the Veterans Health Administration using a virtual breakthrough series collaborative. *Journal of Nursing Care Quality, 32*(4), 301–308. https://doi.org/10.1097/NCQ.0000000000000242

CHAPTER 13

LEVERAGING TECHNOLOGY AND INNOVATION TO ENHANCE LONG-TERM CARE DELIVERY

David G. Wolf and Darren Liu

Learning Objectives

After completing this chapter, each learner will be able to:

- Understand the difference between technology, innovation, and information technology.
- Understand how assistive robotics and automated medication dispensing systems can streamline daily tasks and medication management workflows in long-term care (LTC) settings.
- Explore how the integration of technology, including robotics and automation, can foster a more interconnected and resident-centered care environment in LTC.
- Gain knowledge about the benefits and challenges of implementing different technologies, including electronic health records, robotics, and automated medication systems, in LTC.
- Learn about the benefits and disadvantages of different technologies and become aware of the ethical implications of using robots and other technologies in LTC.

INTRODUCTION

The trajectory of technology within long-term care (LTC) or postacute care (PAC) has been marked by notable milestones, reflecting a journey from early assistive technology to transformative shifts in care practices. In LTC's infancy, pioneering technological innovations aimed at enhancing resident care emerged, spanning from basic medical equipment (Agree et al., 2005) to the adoption of rudimentary communication systems (Wakefield et al., 2004). These foundational advancements laid the groundwork for subsequent progressions in supporting resident well-being.

As LTC facilities adapted to evolving healthcare dynamics and the needs of residents, technology underwent a metamorphosis, transitioning from simple tools to sophisticated systems designed to address complex care challenges. This evolution reflects an enduring commitment to enhancing care quality, safety, and resident outcomes within LTC settings. As technology continues to advance, the potential for further innovation and improvement in LTC remains vast.

Throughout LTC history, pivotal innovation milestones have reshaped care delivery practices, influencing how care is administered and experienced by consumers and care providers alike. Key advances include the integration of electronic health records (EHRs), telehealth services, assistive technologies, and remote monitoring devices, revolutionizing resident care and fostering personalized and proactive healthcare approaches. These innovative technologies have profoundly impacted care delivery practices by facilitating improvements in medication management (Black et al., 2024), enhancing caregiver–resident communication (R. Wilson et al., 2020), and ultimately leading to better outcomes and experiences for all stakeholders.

The landscape of LTC is undergoing rapid transformation through the integration of various technological and innovative advancements, enhancing care quality, streamlining operations, and boosting resident outcomes. This chapter aims to explore the transformative role of technology, innovation, and information technology (IT) in LTC settings. It emphasizes how modern advancements such as EHRs, telehealth, and artificial intelligence (AI) are not only revolutionizing resident care but also optimizing operational efficiencies and improving resident health outcomes.

TECHNOLOGIES, INNOVATIONS, AND INFORMATION TECHNOLOGIES: THE DEFINITIONS

Understanding the fundamental principles is crucial for healthcare providers to navigate the evolving healthcare landscape and meet the increasing demands of resident care within LTC settings. To facilitate comprehensive discussions, it is essential to grasp the nuanced distinctions between technology, innovation, and IT.

Technology refers to the application of scientific knowledge, tools, and techniques to solve practical problems or achieve specific objectives, encompassing *tangible* products, processes, and systems designed to enhance efficiency or create new opportunities. IT specifically involves the use of computers, software, and telecommunications equipment to *store, retrieve, transmit,* and *manipulate* data, playing a pivotal role in managing and processing information efficiently within organizations. *Innovation,* on the other hand, is a broader concept encompassing the creation, development, and implementation of *novel* ideas, methods, or approaches to tackle existing challenges or seize emerging opportunities.

While innovation often utilizes technology, it extends beyond it to encompass organizational strategies, business models, and creative thinking processes aimed at driving positive change and gaining competitive advantages. Table 13.1 provides a comparative overview of these concepts, highlighting their distinct characteristics and implications.

In LTC settings, technology plays an indispensable role in enhancing resident care and optimizing operational processes. It encompasses a diverse range of tools, systems, and methodologies designed to meet the unique needs of both residents and care providers. Drawing upon

TABLE 13.1 Technology Versus Innovation Versus Information Technology

	TECHNOLOGY	INNOVATION	INFORMATION TECHNOLOGY
Definition	New machinery and equipment that has been developed using scientific knowledge or processes (A tool for human creativity)	A *novel* idea, design, product, etc. (The application of new process or device to improve procedures)	The science and activity of *using computers and software* to store and send information (The use of computers and telecommunications to process, *store, and transmit* information/data)
Tangibility	Tangible	Can be intangible	Tangible
Relationship to Innovation	Can be used to implement innovation	Driven by innovation	Facilitates innovation
Purpose	Making lives easier	Solving problems	Processing and transmitting information *efficiently*
Development Path	Typically follows a linear path	Can happen in any direction	N/A (Not applicable, as it is a subset of technology)
Example	• Assistive devices that support daily activities • Robot	• Development of a new medical procedure	• Implementation of telemedicine platforms • EHRs • MDS

EHRs, electronic health records; MDS, Minimum Data Set.

scientific knowledge, LTC facilities develop an array of medical devices, diagnostic tools, communication systems, and software applications tailored to their specific requirements. These technological advancements, spanning from specialized wheelchairs (Labbé et al., 2020) to virtual reality programs (Chaze et al., 2022), are designed to foster resident independence, elevate quality of life, and alleviate caregiver burden. Through the strategic integration of technology, LTC facilities can deliver safer, more efficient, and more personalized care to residents, leading to improved overall outcomes and satisfaction.

Innovation in LTC involves the development and implementation of novel approaches to address existing challenges or seize emerging opportunities in resident care. For instance, introducing a groundbreaking medical procedure to improve treatment outcomes for residents with chronic conditions such as pressure ulcers or diabetes exemplifies innovative thinking. This may involve adopting advanced medical technologies to enhance resident care (Perri et al., 2020; Verbeek et al., 2020), integrating evidence-based care protocols, or implementing interdisciplinary care models. Leading institutions such as the Centers for Medicare & Medicaid Services (CMS) Innovation Center spearhead the creation of pioneering healthcare payment models aimed at curbing rising costs, enhancing care quality, and boosting efficiency (Kaiser Family Foundation [KFF], 2018). Innovation profoundly impacts LTC delivery by streamlining workflows (Lapp et al., 2022), reducing errors (Garland et al., 2021), and empowering residents to actively participate in their care (Buist et al., 2018). Moreover, it fosters collaboration among healthcare stakeholders, promotes knowledge sharing, and drives continuous improvement initiatives.

IT plays a pivotal role in LTC by optimizing the processing, storage, and transmission of resident-related data and information. This enables electronic documentation and monitoring of residents' medical histories, treatment plans, and medication administration records, ultimately enhancing care coordination and patient safety. For example, EHRs, digital communication platforms, and automated reporting systems streamline workflow efficiency and accuracy, enhancing overall operational effectiveness. Moreover, IT and innovation streamline administrative tasks such as documentation, scheduling, and billing, reducing paperwork and freeing up staff time for more critical responsibilities, thus optimizing resource allocation within LTC facilities. By automating workflows and enhancing communication, these advancements enable staff to prioritize direct resident care and ensure efficient resource utilization. Innovative technologies further aid LTC facilities in resource optimization by providing real-time data insights and predictive analytics, thereby facilitating staffing management, inventory control, and financial planning. This ensures that resources are allocated where they are most needed to meet resident needs and facility goals.

In the subsequent sections, we introduce specific examples of technology and innovation in LTC settings, exploring their applications, advancements, and challenges. A comprehensive understanding of these concepts empowers LTC stakeholders to leverage technology effectively, ultimately leading to superior care experiences and positive outcomes for residents.

THE APPLICATIONS OF TECHNOLOGIES AND INNOVATIONS IN LONG-TERM CARE

In an era marked by an aging population and increasing healthcare demands, technology offers indispensable tools for managing complex medical conditions, promoting wellness, and optimizing resource allocation (Schulz et al., 2015). Technology-driven innovations hold the potential to address long-standing challenges in LTC, such as medication management, care coordination, and communication barriers. Within LTC contexts, innovation encompasses a broad spectrum of initiatives ranging from process improvements to the introduction of disruptive technologies. At its essence, innovation involves the introduction of new approaches, processes, or solutions that challenge conventional practices and bring about positive change. By fostering a culture of innovation, LTC facilities or systems can continuously adapt to evolving healthcare landscapes and deliver services that align with best practices and emerging trends.

TABLE 13.2 Technology Applications to Important Life Domains

TECHNOLOGY FUNCTIONS	LIFE DOMAINS				
	PHYSICAL AND MENTAL HEALTH	MOBILITY	SOCIAL CONNECTEDNESS	SAFETY	EVERYDAY ACTIVITIES AND LEISURE
Monitoring/ measurement (person, environment)	Physiologic functioning (e.g., heart rate, blood pressure, and oximetry), affect, health behaviors	Speed and variability of gait, distance covered, vestibular functioning, driving behavior, daily exercise	Frequency and duration of mobile and fixed communication device uses; frequency and duration of time in direct communication with other humans; frequency and time spent in social settings	Frequency of falls, location, driving ability	Frequency, accuracy, and speed of daily task performance; frequency and duration of leisure activities
Diagnosis, screening	Clinical conditions, risk status for clinical conditions	Risk of falling; ambulatory ability, adequacy of daily physical exercise	Social isolation, social integration	Emergency situation, being lost, at risk for driving accidents	Critical cognitive functioning, critical ADL/ IADL status
Treatment, intervention (compensation, prevention, enhancement)	Remote behavioral treatment, chronic disease management, prevention and wellness interventions, clinical decision support	Guidance assistance, risk mitigation (e.g., risk of falling), encouragement, and support for exercise	Enhanced social integration, connectivity through computers/ communication technologies	Emergency response systems, computerized driving assistance, alert systems	Task assistance or training, entertainment, education

ADL, activities of daily living; IADL, instrumental activities of daily living.

Source: Adapted from Schulz, R., Wahl, H.-W., Matthews, J. T., De Vito Dabbs, A., Beach, S. R., & Czaja, S. J. (2015). Advancing the aging and technology agenda in gerontology (Table 1). *The Gerontologist*, *55*(5), 724–734. https://doi.org/10.1093/geront/gnu071

Table 13.2 represents the various life domains and how technology can influence them for resident quality and safety, as identified by Schulz et al. (2015). They have pinpointed five fundamental life domains crucial for technological research in aging. These areas have been primary focal points for technological advancement thus far and are anticipated to remain central to future development efforts. These domains encompass: "(a) physical and mental health, (b) mobility, (c) social connectedness, (d) safety, and (e) daily activities and leisure" (Schulz et al., 2015, p. 726). It is important to note that these categories are not mutually exclusive; enhancements in one area, such as augmenting social connectedness and safety, are likely to have positive repercussions on health and overall well-being. This study stresses the importance of gerontologists' role in optimizing the development process of technologies aimed at benefiting the older population.

DIGITIZING RESIDENT ASSESSMENTS AS HEALTH INFORMATION TECHNOLOGY

The Minimum Data Set (MDS) resident assessment instrument (RAI) for nursing home residents can be considered a form of health information technology (HIT; Liu, 2009). The MDS is a standardized assessment tool mandated by the CMS that collects comprehensive data on residents' health, functional status, and care needs.

Nursing homes are required to submit MDS information electronically to receive reimbursement. This digital submission process exemplifies the use of technology to manage health information efficiently. The MDS provides a standardized format for assessing and recording resident data, which enhances interoperability between different healthcare systems and providers. This standardization is a key component of effective HIT.

Originally introduced in the late 1980s as part of the Nursing Home Reform Act, the MDS has continuously evolved to meet changing healthcare standards and regulations (Zimmerman, 2003). Today, the MDS 3.0 RAI plays a pivotal role in conducting comprehensive evaluations and developing personalized care plans for nursing home residents (CMS, 2024a). Beyond its primary function in care provision, the MDS serves various purposes, including reimbursement determination and the generation of quality indicators used in initiatives such as Care Compare (see Chapter 6).

Assisted living and skilled nursing facilities (SNFs) utilize assessment tools similar to the MDS to capture residents' healthcare needs and preferences. For instance, assisted living facilities employ the RAI or state-specific assessments to evaluate residents' functional abilities, cognitive status, and care needs. Similarly, home health agencies integrate the outcome and assessment information set (OASIS) into their assessments, transmitting quality data to the CMS. OASIS measures a range of activities crucial for self-care including eating, bathing, dressing, mobility, continence, and toileting, as well as more complex tasks such as using the phone, shopping, meal preparation, medication management, house cleaning, transportation, and bill payment (CMS, 2024b). The digitization of the assessment tools such as MDS and OASIS enhances care delivery efficiency, data accuracy, and communication among healthcare providers in LTC and home health services.

As the landscape of LTC evolves, technological innovations are reshaping its trajectory and anticipating future trends in the industry. These advancements, depicted in Figure 13.1, span a spectrum of forms, ranging from EHR systems to telemedicine platforms, empowering caregivers with actionable insights and facilitating remote consultations with healthcare professionals. Additionally, assistive robotics and automated medication dispensing systems are streamlining daily tasks and medication management workflows, ensuring resident safety and staff productivity. As LTC continues to progress, the integration of these technologies will increasingly define its future, fostering a more interconnected and resident-centered care environment. In the subsequent sections, we delve into the prevalent technologies, innovations, or information technologies shaping today's LTC landscape.

CURRENT AND EMERGING INNOVATIONS IN LONG-TERM CARE

Health Information Technology

HIT is pivotal in modern healthcare, streamlining the management of health and medical information through electronic means. This includes a range of tools such as computer systems, software, and internet-based platforms, all geared toward enhancing communication and decision-making within healthcare settings. HIT, as defined by Thompson and Brailer (2004), spans various applications for storing, retrieving, sharing, and utilizing healthcare data. Initiatives such as the Office of the National Coordinator on Health Information Technology (ONC), catalyzed by President Bush's *Executive Order 13335* in April 2004, signify a concerted push toward interoperable HIT systems over the past decade (Exec. Order No. 13335, 2004). This commitment reflects a collective endeavor to improve healthcare quality and reduce errors through HIT implementation. In LTC settings, HIT has transformed resident care and operational efficiency. Through advanced medical devices, telehealth services, and innovative treatments, LTC facilities now offer personalized and streamlined care. HIT digitizes patient records, facilitating seamless data sharing across care settings, thereby improving healthcare delivery. It also enhances resident outcomes and boosts satisfaction levels, ultimately elevating LTC quality.

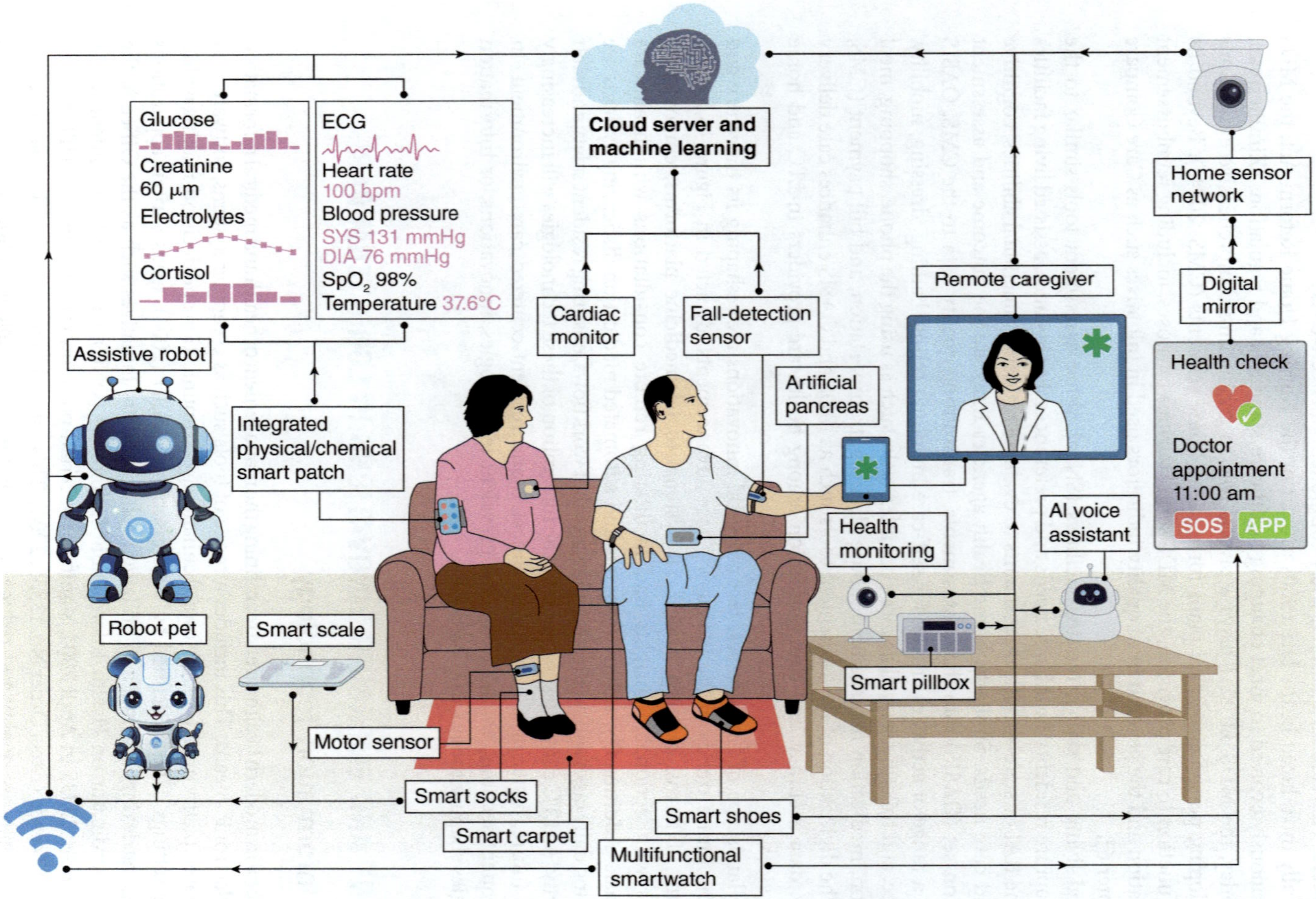

FIGURE 13.1. The future of geriatric healthcare in the home setting.

AI, artificial intelligence; BPM, beats per minute; DIA, diastolic; SYS, systolic.

Source: Adapted from Chen, C., Ding, S., & Wang, J. (2023). Digital health for aging populations. *Nature Medicine*, *29*(7), 1623–1630. https://doi.org/10.1038/s41591-023-02391-8

Electronic Health Records

EHRs are a central component of HIT systems. Serving as comprehensive repositories, EHRs store essential details including medications, treatment plans, and past care outcomes, empowering healthcare professionals to make informed decisions and deliver personalized care seamlessly. EHRs can integrate with other HIT systems, such as electronic prescribing systems, laboratory information systems, and patient portals, to further improve coordination of care and patient engagement. The widespread adoption of EHRs in LTC facilities, particularly by SNFs with an impressive 84% adoption rate in 2018 (Dougherty et al., 2023, p. 6), has significantly elevated care quality, ensured data interoperability, and streamlined processes. Integration of EHRs with MDS data further enhances clinical decision-making, care planning, and regulatory compliance. However, achieving seamless *interoperability*[1] requires robust measures such as staff training and stringent data security protocols (Dore et al., 2022; Vest et al., 2019).

Telemedicine and Telehealth

Telemedicine and telehealth services in LTC revolutionize healthcare delivery by offering medical consultations, therapy sessions, and health monitoring remotely, enabling residents to access care without leaving their facilities. For example, a resident in a rural nursing home can consult with a specialist in a distant city via videoconferencing, receiving expert advice and treatment without the burden of travel. This approach not only extends healthcare access to underserved areas but also enhances convenience for residents. The COVID-19 pandemic has underscored the significance of these remote healthcare delivery methods in ensuring the safety and accessibility of care for LTC residents (Walter et al., 2022).

Wearable Technology

Wearable technology encompasses devices or sensors worn or attached to the body, which are capable of monitoring various health-related data, including vital signs, falls, and sleep patterns. In LTC settings, examples of wearable technologies include fitness trackers and health monitoring devices, which are increasingly utilized. These devices enable continuous tracking of residents' vital signs, physical activity, and overall health status, offering valuable insights for both residents and healthcare providers. Residents benefit from actively engaging in their health management, while healthcare providers can leverage the data for informed decision-making and early detection of health issues (Baig et al., 2019; Bassi et al., 2024).

Robot Technology

Robot technology is rapidly gaining traction in LTC settings and among aging populations, reshaping the way care is provided and received (Shishehgar et al., 2018). Expected to drive significant advancements, robotics and automation offer a range of benefits in LTC settings such as streamlining workflows, reducing manual labor, and enhancing resident independence. Moreover, they have the potential to augment LTC staff capabilities and elevate overall care quality. Equipped with advanced sensors, AI, and interactive features, these sophisticated machines provide a diverse array of services, including mobility assistance, medication management (Liang et al., 2023), companionship (Hudson et al., 2020), and cognitive stimulation (Khan, 2023). As they integrate into LTC facilities and homes, robots not only enhance efficiency and effectiveness but also foster independence, social engagement, and overall well-being among older adults.

---

[1] *Interoperability* is the ability of different IT systems and software applications to communicate, exchange data, and use the exchanged information.

Population Health Management

Population health management (PHM) entails employing various strategies, including HIT utilization, EHR-based risk stratification, and model performance evaluation, to enhance the health outcomes of specific population groups (Kharrazi et al., 2023). In the context of LTC facilities, PHM focuses on enhancing the overall health and well-being of residents while also addressing the unique challenges and needs of this population. PHM can be considered a groundbreaking innovation leveraging data-driven approaches and advanced technologies to proactively optimize residents' health. For instance, amid the heightened risks posed by the COVID-19 pandemic, effective PHM has become paramount in LTC. Utilizing digital solutions for remote monitoring and communication, LTC facilities enhance infection control efforts (Rayan et al., 2021). By harnessing technology and employing big data analytics, facilities can prevent, detect, and manage outbreaks more effectively, ensuring resident safety and well-being. This data-driven approach empowers LTC facilities to implement targeted strategies and make informed decisions, showcasing the innovative potential of PHM in LTC (Dore et al., 2022).

Artificial Intelligence

Anticipated advancements in AI and machine learning (ML) hold immense promise for revolutionizing LTC settings. AI, a branch of computer technology, involves creating systems that can perform tasks that typically require huge human intelligence. In LTC, AI can be utilized in various ways to enhance resident care (Fear & Gleber, 2023). For example, AI-driven predictive analytics leverage complex algorithms to analyze vast amounts of resident data, enabling the forecasting of health outcomes and identification of individuals at risk of specific conditions or adverse events (Czaja & Ceruso, 2022). This allows for early intervention and the development of personalized care plans tailored to individual needs and preferences. Moreover, AI-powered decision support systems assist healthcare providers in diagnosing conditions and optimizing treatment plans, ensuring that residents receive the most effective care. By integrating AI into LTC settings, facilities can improve care quality, enhance operational efficiency, and foster proactive intervention strategies, ultimately benefiting both residents and caregivers.

ENHANCING DIRECT CARE: THE TRANSFORMATIVE IMPACT OF TECHNOLOGY IN HEALTHCARE

As we will discuss further in Chapter 14, direct care workers (DCWs)—including nurse aides, home health aides, and personal care aides—are the cornerstone of hands-on care for over 13 million older adults and Americans with disabilities. Predominantly women of color, home health aides dedicate extensive hours to caring for patients with serious conditions such as heart failure, diabetes, and dementia. Their responsibilities span essential personal and medical care, logistical support for healthcare needs such as doctor visits, medication management, dietary monitoring, vital signs tracking, and personalized meal preparation to meet nutritional requirements (Khatutsky et al., 2011).

The integration of technology into direct care work presents a pivotal opportunity to significantly enhance patient outcomes, elevate job satisfaction among workers, and optimize healthcare resource utilization. For instance, rugged mobile devices are revolutionizing home healthcare by digitizing workflows, reducing errors, and facilitating real-time access to comprehensive patient records through robust connectivity and integrated cameras. These devices empower aides during home visits to capture detailed images of medical conditions, including wounds or rashes, enabling accurate and thorough reporting to the care team.

The emergence of 5G technology further expedites healthcare transformation by enabling swift data transmission, thereby catalyzing the adoption of telemedicine and internet of things (IoT) for real-time monitoring of vital health metrics such as heart rate and blood pressure (Gupta et al., 2021). DCWs can also use wearables and smart devices for ongoing data collection, providing holistic insights into patients' health. Environmental sensors contribute by tracking home conditions, while centralized data integration and advanced analytics offer predictive insights and personalized care plans.

Given their pivotal role, DCWs stand to gain substantially from these technological advancements. Online training modules offer continuous education and updates on best practices (Gaugler et al., 2016; Yeh et al., 2023), while collaborative tools enhance communication among care team members (Fabius et al., 2023). Hands-free devices such as Apple Siri, Amazon Alexa, or other interactive voice assistants (IVAs) such as the recently released GPT-4o[2] have the potential to streamline task management and information access, optimizing workflow and facilitating personalized care (Bartle et al., 2022).

Despite their potential, these technologies are presently underutilized in healthcare. Advocating for their widespread adoption could revolutionize direct care work, thereby improving both the quality of care and the working conditions of caregivers. By enhancing home safety, streamlining communication, automating operational tasks, and enabling better data collection and analysis, technology can lead to improved patient outcomes and more effective policy decisions, ultimately elevating the overall quality of home health services.

ADOPTING INNOVATION IN LONG-TERM CARE: CHALLENGES AND OPPORTUNITIES

Notably, LTC facilities have been facing common challenges such as managing chronic health conditions, ensuring effective medication administration, maintaining adequate staffing levels, coordinating care among multiple providers, addressing communication barriers, and enhancing the overall quality of life for residents. Overcoming these challenges is essential to shape the future of care delivery. LTC facilities are actively embracing innovative technologies to address specific challenges and enhance the experiences of residents under their care. However, implementing advanced technologies comes with its own set of challenges and considerations that must be addressed to ensure successful adoption and integration (Dugstad et al., 2019; Grigorovich et al., 2021). For example, Cherry et al. (2008) identified key barriers to adopting EHRs in LTC facilities including costs, training needs, and cultural change. Primary facilitators included training programs, well-defined implementation plans, government assistance, evidence of improved care outcomes, and regulatory support. Overall, the pursuit of innovation spans both organizational and systemic levels:

Organizational Level

At the organizational level, many LTC facilities have successfully integrated cutting-edge technologies, ranging from advanced monitoring systems to EHRs, leading to tangible improvements in resident outcomes and operational efficiency. Moreover, AI-driven assistants, such as ChatGPT, stand poised to significantly contribute to technological advancement within LTC facilities. One of the primary barriers to adopting new technologies in LTC is *financial constraints*. LTC facilities often operate on limited budgets, making it challenging to invest in expensive technology infrastructure and equipment. Additionally, ongoing maintenance and support costs can further strain budgets, hindering the adoption of innovative technologies.

Staff training and resistance to change represent another significant challenge. Introducing new technologies requires staff members to undergo training to effectively use these tools (M. G. Wilson et al., 2022). However, resistance to change and reluctance to learn new systems can impede the successful implementation of technology initiatives. Addressing staff concerns, providing comprehensive training programs, and fostering a culture of innovation are essential to overcoming these barriers.

[2] Released on May 13, 2024, GPT-4o is an efficient variant of GPT-4 designed for high-quality performance. It excels in applications such as IVAs, which involve converting text responses into natural speech. This integration ensures quick, accurate, and conversational real-time interactions. GPT-4o's advanced capabilities make it ideal for enhancing user experiences in voice-based applications (OpenAI, 2024).

Ethical and legal implications accompany the adoption of technology in LTC. While technology advances care delivery, it also raises pertinent ethical and legal considerations. Privacy concerns regarding the handling of resident health information loom large, necessitating strict adherence to regulations such as the Health Insurance Portability and Accountability Act (HIPAA) to safeguard resident confidentiality and prevent unauthorized access to sensitive data. LTC facilities must prioritize the implementation of robust security measures and protocols to uphold resident privacy while harnessing the benefits of technology (Ho, 2020).

International organizations such as the United Nations (UN) and World Health Organization (WHO) play a vital role in shaping AI governance in healthcare, ensuring *alignment with global norms* for safety, security, and trust. Recent UN resolutions stress effective governance and human rights in AI systems (UN General Assembly, 2024). Likewise, the WHO provides guidance on AI ethics and governance, highlighting its potential in improving healthcare outcomes, including through large multimodal models (LMMs; WHO, 2021). These efforts are crucial in navigating the ethical and legal terrain of technology adoption in LTC, promoting responsible innovation for residents and caregivers.

Ensuring equity in access to and use of technology is a crucial ethical consideration in LTC, as socioeconomic disparities and digital divides may prevent some residents from fully benefiting from technological advancements (Cid et al., 2020; Hung et al., 2022). LTC facilities must address these disparities by providing equitable access to technology, supporting residents who face barriers to adoption, and ensuring that technology solutions are inclusive and accessible to residents with disabilities. Digital health equity is vital for HIT adoption in LTC, as it ensures fair access to digital health tools regardless of residents' backgrounds or circumstances, thereby overcoming barriers to widespread HIT adoption and leading to better healthcare outcomes and experiences for LTC residents (Rodriguez et al., 2020).

While technologies such as assistive technology, e-learning, and information and communication technology (ICT) offer potential for enhancing home care services, their adoption remains limited due to challenges such as restricted availability, inadequate research and development investment, and complex regulatory processes. Additionally, concerns about liability risks, prolonged approval timelines, and limited accessibility exacerbate the situation. Low wages, insufficient resources, and privacy issues further hinder adoption. Clear guidelines and ethical frameworks are essential for navigating these challenges and ensuring quality service amid technological advancements (Scales, 2019; Scales et al., 2019).

Systemic Level

On a systemic level, adopting new innovations encompasses various innovative care models. Programs such as the *Green House* and Programs of All-Inclusive Care for the Elderly (PACE) have demonstrated promising results in shaping LTC delivery. These efforts underscore the transformative potential of innovations in redefining care delivery in LTC settings. However, systemic challenges remain, including integrating these models and technologies into existing healthcare frameworks, securing sustainable funding, addressing regulatory and policy constraints, and fostering collaboration among stakeholders to ensure the widespread adoption and scalability of successful approaches.

To fully harness the potential of HIT, such as EHRs, a reevaluation of efforts toward HIT adoption is essential. The journey toward HIT adoption is mapped across three distinct phases in Figure 13.2—preparation, transition (or implementation), and integration—each presenting its own set of challenges and opportunities (Liu, 2009, p. 94).

Preparation involves the collaborative development of essential tools and standards by stakeholders, while transition focuses on refining these tools and addressing challenges such as interoperability and usability. Integration aims for the establishment of a comprehensive national health information infrastructure (NHII), facilitating seamless data exchange across all levels of care (Lumpkin & Richards, 2002). Despite the national push for HIT adoption since the early 2000s, progress remains between the preparation and transition phases, indicating ongoing

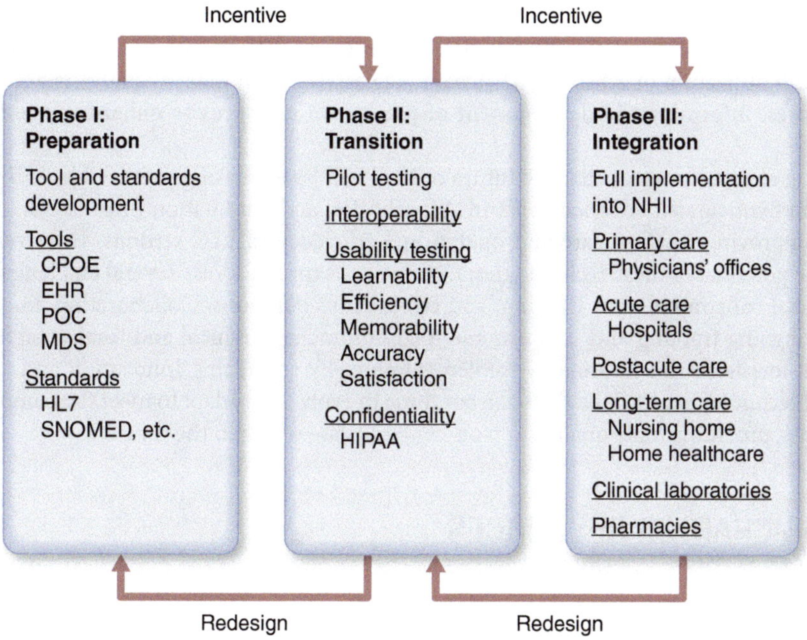

FIGURE 13.2. The three phases for HIT adoption

CPOE, computerized physician order entry; EHR, electronic health record; HIPAA, Health Insurance Portability and Accountability Act; HIT, health information technology MDS, Minimum Data Set; NHII, National Health Information Infrastructure; POC, point of care.

Source: Adapted from Liu, D. (2009). *Health information technology and nursing homes* (p. 94, Figure 1). Doctoral dissertation, University of Pittsburgh, PA. ProQuest Dissertations Publishing.

efforts toward comprehensive adoption. Challenges persist, particularly in the implementation of HIT in nursing homes, as highlighted by Kistler et al. (2021) across six key domains: data transfer, communication, regulatory compliance, quality improvement, structured clinical documentation, and medication use processes.

The lack of *incentive programs* has been cited as a significant barrier to optimal HIT adoption in LTC.[3] However, the latest *2024–2030 Federal Health IT Strategic Plan* offers hope by aiming to "expand health IT use beyond hospitals and physician offices [to include] providers in behavioral health, long-term and post-acute care, and home health settings" (ONC, 2024, p. 14). Nevertheless, various initiatives are already underway to introduce HIT into LTC domains, aimed at enhancing healthcare quality, optimizing patient transfers, and minimizing hospitalizations from nursing homes. Interventions such as COVID-19 apps and ML modeling showcase the potential of technology in predicting hospital readmissions and improving care delivery (Echeverría et al., 2020; Howard et al., 2021). Decision support tools, templates, and systems further complement these efforts, aiding healthcare professionals in making informed decisions and enhancing overall patient care.

SUMMARY

This chapter delineates the evolution of technological innovations in LTC, beginning with basic medical equipment and rudimentary communication systems aimed at enhancing resident care. Subsequent advancements, such as the integration of EHRs, telehealth services, and remote

[3] Incentive programs (or promoting interoperability programs) do not include LTC/PAC. "In 2011, the Centers for Medicare and Medicaid Services (CMS) established the Medicare and Medicaid Electronic Health Record (EHR) Incentive Programs to encourage eligible professionals (EPs), eligible hospitals, and critical access hospitals (CAHs) to adopt, implement, upgrade, and demonstrate meaningful use of certified electronic health record technology (CEHRT)" (CMS, 2024, para. 1).

monitoring devices, have significantly transformed and revolutionized resident care delivery. The chapter explores the vast potential for future innovation in LTC settings, particularly through the utilization of AI tools. AI-driven data analysis can identify patterns and trends in health issues, informing the development of preventive measures to enhance resident health outcomes.

Looking ahead, it is clear that the future of LTC will be increasingly shaped by technological innovation. Anticipated advancements in AI, robotics, and automation offer exciting possibilities for improving resident care and operational efficiency in LTC settings. However, to fully realize the potential of these technologies, LTC facilities must address several challenges, including financial constraints, staff training, and ethical considerations. Collaboration among stakeholders, ongoing training and support, and a commitment to ethical and legal compliance will be crucial for successful technology implementation. By embracing innovation and leveraging emerging technologies, LTC facilities can continue to evolve and adapt to meet the complex needs of residents, providing high-quality, person-centered care well into the future.

END-OF-CHAPTER RESOURCES

DISCUSSION QUESTIONS

1. In what ways can assistive robotics and automated medication dispensing systems streamline daily tasks and medication management workflows?
2. How can the integration of technology in LTC foster a more interconnected and resident-centered care environment?
3. How can the utilization of AI personal assistant technologies such as ChatGPT effectively contribute to innovative customized care planning and decision-making processes, enhancing the resident experience?
4. How can the use of telemedicine technology improve access to healthcare for residents in LTC facilities?

SPRINGER PUBLISHING CONNECT™ | A robust set of instructor resources designed to supplement this text is located at http://connect.springerpub.com/content/book/978-0-8261-4935-0. Qualifying instructors may request access by emailing textbook@springerpub.com.

REFERENCES

Agree, E. M., Freedman, V. A., Cornman, J. C., Wolf, D. A., & Marcotte, J. E. (2005). Reconsidering substitution in long-term care: When does assistive technology take the place of personal care? *The Journals of Gerontology Series B: Psychological Sciences and Social Sciences*, *60*(5), S272–S280. https://doi.org/10.1093/geronb/60.5.s272

Baig, M. M., Afifi, S., GholamHosseini, H., & Mirza, F. (2019). A systematic review of wearable sensors and IoT-based monitoring applications for older adults—a focus on ageing population and independent living. *Journal of Medical Systems*, *43*, 233. https://doi.org/10.1007/s10916-019-1365-7

Bartle, V., Lyu, J., El Shabazz-Thompson, F., Oh, Y., Chen, A. A., Chang, Y.-J., Holstein, K., & Dell, N. (2022, April 28). "A second voice": Investigating opportunities and challenges for interactive voice assistants to support home health aides. In S. Barbosa & C. Lampe, *Proceedings of the 2022 CHI Conference on Human Factors in Computing Systems* (pp. 1–17). Association for Computing Machinery. https://doi.org/10.1145/3491102.3517683

Bassi, E., Santomauro, I., Basso, I., Maoret, R., & Dal Molin, A. (2024). Wearable technology use in long-term care facilities for older adults: A scoping review protocol. *JBI Evidence Synthesis, 22*(2), 325–334. https://doi.org/10.11124/JBIES-23-00079

Black, A., Tribble, D., Strumpf, J., Fitzgibbons, S., Dumitru, D., Lucaci, J., Jung, M., & Ramudhin, A. (2024). Impact of automated dispensing solutions in long-term care facilities and closed-door pharmacies: A mixed methods study of medication management. *Journal of the American Pharmacists Association, 64*(3), 102065. https://doi.org/10.1016/j.japh.2024.102065

Buist, Y., Verbeek, H., de Boer, B., & de Bruin, S. R. (2018). Innovating dementia care; implementing characteristics of green care farms in other long-term care settings. *International Psychogeriatrics, 30*(7), 1057–1068. https://doi.org/10.1017/S1041610217002848

Centers for Medicare & Medicaid Services. (2024a, January 12). *Minimum Data Set (MDS) 3.0 resident assessment instrument (RAI) manual.* Retrieved May 15, 2024, from https://www.cms.gov/medicare/quality/nursing-home-improvement/resident-assessment-instrument-manual

Centers for Medicare & Medicaid Services. (2024b, May 3). *OASIS data sets.* Retrieved May 15, 2024, from https://www.cms.gov/medicare/quality/home-health/oasis-data-sets

Centers for Medicare & Medicaid Services. (2024, September 10). *Promoting interoperability programs.* Retrieved May 10, 2024, from https://www.cms.gov/medicare/regulations-guidance/promoting-interoperability-programs

Chaze, F., Hayden, L., Azevedo, A., Kamath, A., Bucko, D., Kashlan, Y., Dube, M., De Paula, J., Jackson, A., Reyna, C., Dupuis, K., & Tsotsos, L. (2022). Virtual reality and well-being in older adults: Results from a pilot implementation of virtual reality in long-term care. *Journal of Rehabilitation and Assistive Technologies Engineering, 9*, 20556683211072384. https://doi.org/10.1177/20556683211072384

Cherry, B., Carter, M., Owen, D., & Lockhart, C. (2008). Factors affecting electronic health record adoption in long-term care facilities. *Journal for Healthcare Quality, 30*(2), 37–47. https://doi.org/10.1111/j.1945-1474.2008.tb01133.x

Cid, A., Sotelo, R., Leguisamo, M., & Ramírez-Michelena, M. (2020). Tablets for deeply disadvantaged older adults: Challenges in long-term care facilities. *International Journal of Human-Computer Studies, 144*, 102504. https://doi.org/10.1016/j.ijhcs.2020.102504

Czaja, S. J., & Ceruso, M. (2022). The promise of artificial intelligence in supporting an aging population. *Journal of Cognitive Engineering and Decision Making, 16*(4), 182–193. https://doi.org/10.1177/15553434221129914

Dore, D. D., Myles, L., Recker, A., Burns, D., Murray, C. R., Gifford, D., & Mor, V. (2022). The long-term care data cooperative: The next generation of data integration. *Journal of the American Medical Directors Association, 23*(12), 2031–2033. https://doi.org/10.1016/j.jamda.2022.09.006

Dougherty, M., McGavin, R., Richardson, J. E., Wines, R. C., & Horvath, M. (2023, December 5). *Health information technology adoption and utilization in long-term and post-acute care settings.* U.S. Department of Health & Human Services, Office of the Assistant Secretary for Planning and Evaluation, Office of Behavioral Health, Disability, and Aging Policy. https://aspe.hhs.gov/sites/default/files/documents/c39b80481327bb3136a07f2c0afd0f65/hit-adoption-utilization-ltpac-settings.pdf

Dugstad, J., Eide, T., Nilsen, E. R., & Eide, H. (2019). Towards successful digital transformation through co-creation: A longitudinal study of a four-year implementation of digital monitoring technology in residential care for persons with dementia. *BMC Health Services Research, 19*, 366. https://doi.org/10.1186/s12913-019-4191-1

Echeverría, P., Bergas, M. A. M., Puig, J., Isnard, M., Massot, M., Vedia, C., Peiró, R., Ordorica, Y., Pablo, S., Ulldemolins, M., Iruela, M., Balart, D., Ruiz, J. M., Herms, J., Clotet Sala, B., & Negredo, E. (2020). COVIDApp as an innovative strategy for the management and follow-up of COVID-19 cases in long-term care facilities in Catalonia: Implementation study. *JMIR Public Health and Surveillance, 6*(3), e21163. https://doi.org/10.2196/21163

Exec. Order No. 13335. (2004, April 27). *Incentives for the use of health information technology and establishing the position of the national health information technology coordinator.* https://www.federalregister.gov/documents/2004/04/30/04-10024/incentives-for-the-use-of-health-information-technology-and-establishing-the-position-of-the

Fabius, C. D., Wec, A., Saylor, M. A., Smith, J. M., Gallo, J. J., & Wolff, J. L. (2023). "Caregiving is teamwork…" Information sharing in home care for older adults with disabilities living in the community. *Geriatric Nursing, 54*, 171–177. https://doi.org/10.1016/j.gerinurse.2023.09.001

Fear, K., & Gleber, C. (2023, September 13). Shaping the future of older adult care: ChatGPT, advanced AI, and the transformation of clinical practice. *JMIR Aging, 6*, e51776. https://doi.org/10.2196/51776

Garland, C. T., Guénette, L., Kröger, E., Carmichael, P. H., Rouleau, R., & Sirois, C. (2021). A new care model reduces polypharmacy and potentially inappropriate medications in long-term care. *Journal of the American Medical Directors Association, 22*(1), 141–147. https://doi.org/10.1016/j.jamda.2020.09.039

Gaugler, J. E., Hobday, J. V., Robbins, J. C., & Barclay, M. P. (2016). Direct care worker training to respond to the behavior of individuals with dementia: The CARES® dementia-related behavior™ online program. *Gerontology and Geriatric Medicine, 2*. https://doi.org/10.1177/2333721415626888

Grigorovich, A., Kulandaivelu, Y., Newman, K., Bianchi, A., Khan, S. S., Iaboni, A., & McMurray, J. (2021). Factors affecting the implementation, use, and adoption of real-time location system technology for persons living with cognitive disabilities in long-term care homes: Systematic review. *Journal of Medical Internet Research, 23*(1), e22831. https://doi.org/10.2196/22831

Gupta, N., Juneja, P. K., Sharma, S., & Garg, U. (2021, May). Future aspect of 5G-IoT architecture in smart healthcare system. In *2021 5th International Conference on Intelligent Computing and Control Systems (ICICCS)* (pp. 406–411). IEEE. https://ieeexplore.ieee.org/document/9432082

Ho, A. (2020). Are we ready for artificial intelligence health monitoring in elder care? *BMC Geriatrics, 20*(1), 358. https://doi.org/10.1186/s12877-020-01764-9

Howard, E. P., Morris, J. N., Schachter, E., Schwarzkopf, R., Shepard, N., & Buchanan, E. R. (2021). Machine-learning modeling to predict hospital readmission following discharge to post-acute care. *Journal of the American Medical Directors Association, 22*(5), 1067–1072. https://doi.org/10.1016/j.jamda.2020.12.017

Hudson, J., Ungar, R., Albright, L., Tkatch, R., Schaeffer, J., & Wicker, E. R. (2020). Robotic pet use among community-dwelling older adults. *Journals of Gerontology: Series B, 75*(9), 2018–2028. https://doi.org/10.1093/geronb/gbaa119

Hung, L., Mann, J., Perry, J., Berndt, A., & Wong, J. (2022). Technological risks and ethical implications of using robots in long-term care. *Journal of Rehabilitation and Assistive Technologies Engineering, 9*, 20556683221106917. https://doi.org/10.1177/20556683221106917

Kaiser Family Foundation. (2018, February 27). *"What is CMMI?" and 11 other FAQs about the CMS Innovation Center*. https://www.kff.org/medicare/fact-sheet/what-is-cmmi-and-11-other-faqs-about-the-cms-innovation-center/

Kharrazi, H., Horrocks, D., & Weiner, J. (2023). Use of health information exchanges for value-based care delivery and population health management: A case study of Maryland's health information exchange. *Health Information Exchange*, 523–542. https://doi.org/10.1016/b978-0-323-90802-3.00011-3

Khan, A. A. (2023). Humanoid robots administering cognitive stimulation therapy to help improve cognition and reduce neuropsychiatric disorders. *Alzheimer's & Dementia, 19*, e082197. https://doi.org/10.1002/alz.082197

Khatutsky, G., Wiener, J., Anderson, W., Akhmerova, V., Jessup, E. A., & Squillace, M. R. (2011, March). *Understanding direct care workers: A snapshot of two of America's most important jobs: Certified nursing assistants and home health aides*. U.S. Department of Health & Human Services. https://aspe.hhs.gov/sites/default/files/private/pdf/76186/CNAchart.pdf

Kistler, C. E., Zimmerman, S., & Khairat, S. (2021). Health information technology challenges and innovations in long-term care. *Journal of the American Medical Directors Association, 22*(5), 981–983. https://doi.org/10.1016/j.jamda.2021.03.017

Labbé, D., Mortenson, W. B., Rushton, P. W., Demers, L., & Miller, W. C. (2020). Mobility and participation among ageing powered wheelchair users: Using a lifecourse approach. *Ageing & Society, 40*(3), 626–642. https://doi.org/10.1017/S0144686X18001228

Lapp, L., Egan, K., McCann, L., Mackenzie, M., Wales, A., & Maguire, R. (2022). Decision support tools in adult long-term care facilities: Scoping review. *Journal of Medical Internet Research, 24*(9), e39681. https://doi.org/10.2196/39681

Liang, F., Su, Z., Sheng, W., Bishop, A., & Carlson, B. (2023). Medication adherence management for in-home geriatric care with a companion robot and a wearable device. *Smart Health, 30*, 100434. https://doi.org/10.1016/j.smhl.2023.100434

Liu, D. (2009). *Health information technology and nursing homes*. Doctoral dissertation, University of Pittsburgh, PA. ProQuest Dissertations Publishing.

Lumpkin, J. R., & Richards, M. S. (2002). Transforming the public health information infrastructure. *Health Affairs, 21*(6), 45–56. https://doi.org/10.1377/hlthaff.21.6.45

Office of the National Coordinator for Health Information Technology. (2024, March). *2024–2030 Federal health IT strategic plan: Draft for public comment*. https://www.healthit.gov/sites/default/files/facas/2024-05-16_Draft_2024%E2%80%932030_Federal_Health_IT_Strategic_Plan_Presentation.pdf

OpenAI. (2024). *Hello GPT-4o*. https://openai.com/index/hello-gpt-4o

Perri, G. A., Abdel-Malek, N., Bandali, A., Grosbein, H., & Gardner, S. (2020). Early integration of palliative care in a long-term care home: A telemedicine feasibility pilot study. *Palliative & Supportive Care, 18*(4), 460–467. https://doi.org/10.1017/S1478951520000012

Rayan, R. A., Zafar, I., & Tsagkaris, C. (2021). Artificial intelligence and big data solutions for COVID-19. In M. Niranjanamurthy, S. Bhattacharyya, & N. Kumar (Eds.), *Intelligent data analysis for COVID-19 pandemic* (pp. 115–127). Springer Nature. https://doi.org/10.1007/978-981-16-1574-0_6

Rodriguez, J. A., Clark, C. R., & Bates, D. W. (2020). Digital health equity as a necessity in the 21st century cures act era. *Journal of American Medical Association, 323*(23), 2381–2382. https://doi.org/10.1001/jama.2020.7858

Scales, K. (2019). Leveraging technology to support—not supplant—the home care workforce. *Health Affairs Forefront*. https://doi.org/10.1377/forefront.20190805.54553

Scales, K., Sturgeon, J. M., Espinoza, R., Campbell, S., & Cook, A. (2019). *Envisioning the future of home care: Trends and opportunities in workforce policy and practice*. PHI. https://www.phinational.org/resource/envisioning-the-future-of-home-care-trends-and-opportunities-in-workforce-policy-and-practice

Schulz, R., Wahl, H.-W., Matthews, J. T., De Vito Dabbs, A., Beach, S. R., & Czaja, S. J. (2015). Advancing the aging and technology agenda in gerontology. *The Gerontologist, 55*(5), 724–734. https://doi.org/10.1093/geront/gnu071

Shishehgar, M., Kerr, D., & Blake, J. (2018). A systematic review of research into how robotic technology can help older people. *Smart Health, 7*, 1–18. https://doi.org/10.1016/j.smhl.2018.03.002

Thompson, T. G., & Brailer, D. J. (2004, July 21). *The decade of health information technology: Delivering consumer-centric and information-rich health care*. U.S. Department of Health & Human Services. https://www.govinfo.gov/content/pkg/GOVPUB-HE-PURL-gpo800/pdf/GOVPUB-HE-PURL-gpo800.pdf

United Nations General Assembly. (2024, April 1). *Seizing the opportunities of safe, secure and trustworthy artificial intelligence systems for sustainable development*. https://digitallibrary.un.org/record/4043244/files/A_RES_78_265-EN.pdf?ln=en

Verbeek, H., Zwakhalen, S. M. G., Schols, J. M. G. A., Kempen, G. I. J. M., & Hamers, J. P. H. (2020). The living lab in ageing and long-term care: A sustainable model for translational research improving quality of life, quality of care and quality of work. *Journal of Nutrition, Health and Aging, 24*(1), 43–47. https://doi.org/10.1007/s12603-019-1288-5

Vest, J. R., Jung, H.-Y., Wiley, K., Jr., Kooreman, H., Pettit, L., & Unruh, M. A. (2019). Adoption of health information technology among US nursing facilities. *Journal of the American Medical Directors Association, 20*(8), 995–1000. https://doi.org/10.1016/j.jamda.2018.11.002

Wakefield, B. J., Buresh, K. A., Flanagan, J. R., & Kienzle, M. G. (2004). Interactive video specialty consultations in long-term care. *Journal of the American Geriatrics Society, 52*(5), 789–793. https://doi.org/10.1111/j.1532-5415.2004.52220.x

Walter, J. R., Kim, D.-H., Myers, D., Hill, M., Snoll, B., Lee, J. Y., Kulikova, E., Fagan, K., Cauinian, R., Nguyen, L., Shapiro, M., Heitor, F., O'Brien, K. T., & Xu, S. (2022). Pilot and feasibility deployment of an advanced remote monitoring platform for COVID-19 in long-term care facilities. *Journal of the American Geriatrics Society, 70*(4), 9680–971. https://doi.org/10.1111/jgs.17673

Wilson, R., Cochrane, D., Mihailidis, A., & Small, J. (2020). Mobile apps to support caregiver-resident communication in long-term care: Systematic search and content analysis. *JMIR Aging, 3*(1), e17136. https://doi.org/10.2196/17136

Wilson, M. G., Gauvin, F. P., DeMaio, P., Alam, S., Drakos, A., Soueidan, S., Costa, A., Reid, R., Simeonov, D., Sixsmith, A., Sveistrup, H., & Lavis, J. N. (2022, September). Enhancing the use of technology in the long-term care sector in Canada: Insights from citizen panels and a national stakeholder dialogue. *Healthcare Management Forum, 35*(5), 310–317. https://doi.org/10.1177/08404704221108466

World Health Organization. (2021). *Ethics and governance of artificial intelligence for health*. https://www.who.int/publications/i/item/9789240029200

Yeh, J., Beld, M., Pond, B., Neri, M., Martinez, S., Hollister, B., Garcia, A., Mauricio, J., Mata-Pacheco, J., Emelle, M., Castaneda, M., Eldridge, C., & Ross, L. (2023). Innovation in direct care worker training: Preparing a workforce to provide in-home care to older adults living with Alzheimer's disease and related dementias. *Alzheimer's & Dementia, 19*, e082768. https://doi.org/10.1002/alz.082768

Zimmerman, D. R. (2003). Improving nursing home quality of care through outcomes data: The MDS quality indicators. *International Journal of Geriatric Psychiatry, 18*(3), 250–257. https://doi.org/10.1002/gps.820

PART IV

SHAPING THE FUTURE

CHAPTER 14

ENHANCING THE LONG-TERM CARE WORKFORCE

Clare Luz

Learning Objectives

After completing this chapter, each learner will be able to:

- Discuss the context of long-term care (LTC) workforce shortages: history, extent, and impact.
- Identify the reasons for the direct care worker (DCW) shortage.
- Understand the crucial link between the LTC workforce and ensuring quality and safety in care delivery.
- Give examples of best practices and key, evidence-based strategies for addressing the DCW shortage.
- Examine a framework for effective statewide leadership aimed at addressing DCW shortages.
- Determine strategies that may be relevant and achievable in an individual state or organization.

INTRODUCTION

The long-term care (LTC) workforce shortage is not new. In 2008, the Institute of Medicine's (IOM) Committee on the Future Health Care Workforce for Older Americans was tasked with examining how prepared the nation was to care for a rapidly aging population. They conducted extensive research including citing major prescient reports dating back 30 years that predicted massive shortages in part due to little interest in geriatric professions despite a vast, growing need. Their report, *Retooling for an Aging America* (IOM, 2008), projected dire workforce shortages if the health status and healthcare utilization of older adults remained stable or increased and no proactive action was taken to address reasons for the shortage. Even then, among the existing physicians, nurses, pharmacists, physician assistants, and social workers, only 1% to 4% had specialized aging-related training or certification.

The IOM report outlined 14 recommendations: one overall recommendation and 13 specific ones focused on increasing the size, competence, and flexibility of the eldercare workforce. It stressed that immediate and drastic steps would need to be taken and substantial progress made by 2030, when all Baby Boomers reach age 65, to avert an eldercare workforce shortage crisis. The recommendations focused on (a) boosting the size of the workforce with recruitment and retention strategies for a broad range of geriatric specialists, including direct care workers (DCWs) and family caregivers; (b) enhancing the competency of this workforce; and (c) redesigning and implementing innovative care models including expanding provider roles for greater flexibility.

In 2020, Foley and Luz revisited the IOM report to review progress made in fulfilling the 14 recommendations, focusing primarily on physicians and DCWs (Foley & Luz, 2021). Their study found that only one of the recommendations had been fully met, continued funding for geriatric academic career awards and geriatrics workforce enhancement programs. Four recommendations had not been met at all, including increased pay and benefits for DCWs through setting wage floors, establishing minimum percentages of service rates directed to direct care labor costs, and other measures. Some progress had been made on the remaining recommendations, but with much more work to be done. In addition, the healthcare status and healthcare utilization among older adults had not changed substantially or declined enough to deflect the 2008 predictions. Rather than grow in numbers, healthcare providers with specialized training in the care of older adults were dwindling. The number of geriatricians had dropped nationwide, with a dramatic deficit predicted by 2025 and equally disturbing downward trends in geriatric psychiatry, nursing, social work, and other specialties (National Center for Health Workforce Analysis, 2017).

UNDERSTANDING THE SCALE OF THE WORKFORCE CRISIS

DCWs provide hands-on care to older adults and persons with disabilities, have also been severely impacted by shortages. Home health aides and unlicensed personal care aides account for approximately 80% of paid care provided (Seavey, 2011). The Bureau of Labor Statistics estimates that these categories of DCWs are in the top five fastest job growth occupations in the United States. A 34% increase in demand is anticipated between 2015 and 2030 (National Center for Health Workforce Analysis, 2018), a demand that will most assuredly not be met. Although there are approximately 4.5 million DCWs across the United States, in private homes, residential care homes, nursing facilities, and other settings such as hospitals, the number is insufficient. Estimates of an expected shortfall of DCWs by 2030 range from 151,000 (Osterman, 2017) to approximately 336,000, more than any other health profession (Foley & Luz, 2021).

The magnitude of this problem is exacerbated by high turnover rates among DCWs (Figure 14.1). The national annual turnover rate is estimated to be between 40% and 60%, with home care agencies reporting even higher rates, from 65% to 89% (Farrell, 2018; Roman et al., 2022). In 2019, Holly reported that the median turnover rate among DCWs was 82%, a 15% increase from 2017 (Holly, 2019). These astronomical turnover rates disrupt continuity of care, destabilize the workforce, and incur substantial costs. For example, in Michigan in 2020, turnover rates could cost employers as

Jennifer Lugo says, "Person-centered care always revolves around the client and their wishes, *not mine*." She believes the role of a DCW is pivotal, explaining, "A few seconds can be the difference between life and death for a person." She also expresses concern about the impact of turnover on her clients: "I can't imagine what that would be like. In the morning, you have one DCW, at night you have another, and the next day, yet another."

Jennifer speaks passionately about the need for standardized training, insurance coverage for home care workers, and higher wages. Having just completed her associate degree, she is currently writing a book and actively advocates for DCWs as skilled professionals.

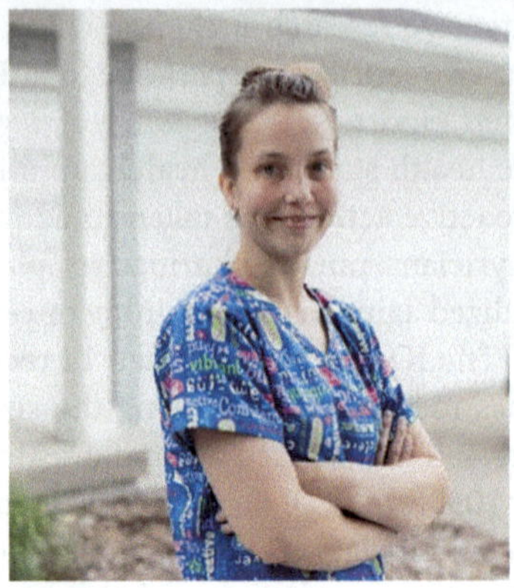

Jennifer Lugo, Kent City, Michigan

FIGURE 14.1. Certified nursing assistant on turnover.

DCW, direct care worker.

Source: Photo by Khalid Ibrahim, Eat Pomegranate Photography.

much as $7,000 to replace a single DCW in home care when including both direct and indirect costs (Public Sector Consultants, 2021). The increasing need for DCWs, coupled with high turnover rate and fewer new workers, threatens to escalate the shortage if this workforce is not stabilized. This situation is further complicated by a decrease in informal and family caregivers (Flinn, 2018) and the COVID-19 pandemic, which brought these issues to the forefront. States are struggling to meet critical services provided through behavioral health, community mental health, and LTC systems to support individuals with disabilities and older adults in a range of settings including their own homes. The impact of this shortage goes well beyond LTC. It affects everyone, individually and collectively. It has an impact on the economy, workforce and economic development, health systems, housing, nonhealthcare businesses, and most other corners of society. Employers are now shuttering their doors, cutting back services, and turning individuals away, which is putting peoples' lives at risk. Without a direct care workforce, there is no well-functioning LTC system.

By 2030, the oldest members of Generation X will reach age 65, joining over 70 million other aging adults in America. Their healthcare needs will demand far more from our existing health systems. As forewarned in the 2008 IOM report, the healthcare workforce is unprepared to manage these escalating demands in the coming decade unless aggressive measures are implemented immediately. The original framework of the 2008 IOM recommendations, emphasizing policy and system reforms across three areas—workforce size, competency, and new care models—remains highly relevant. Individual states are making promising progress in each of these strategy areas (Roman et al., 2022; Stepick, 2023; Twomey, 2019; Ward et al., 2021; Winters et al., 2021). However, states continue to wrestle with effectively addressing debilitating LTC workforce shortages. A wide range of approaches are limited by availability of evidence-based data, challenges in stakeholder coordination, and varying wage scales and collective bargaining acceptance.

MICHIGAN: A CASE EXAMPLE

In Michigan, a statewide, coordinated strategy is emerging, specifically focused on the shortage of DCWs, which is leading to unprecedented progress. The valuable lessons learned can be applied in any state and across all healthcare specialties. This example is offered to give not only concrete recommendations to healthcare administrators, providers, state governments, advocates, and any others who care about the quality and safety of LTC, but also hope that change is possible.

Michigan leadership is taking the approach that expanding and stabilizing the direct care workforce requires a commitment to two fundamental concepts: economic security and respect for all DCWs. All strategies need to lead to these two outcomes. For a deeper understanding of why this is important, it is helpful to understand why there is a shortage.

Roots of the Direct Care Workforce Shortage

There are decades of evidence that repeatedly point to several key reasons for the direct care workforce shortage, all of which lead to a lack of economic security. Over 20 years ago, Mickus et al. (2004) conducted one of the first statewide studies of DCWs examining factors associated with entry into direct care work, retention, and reasons for leaving this field, including caseload, wages, supervisory style, and job satisfaction (Mickus et al., 2004). They surveyed 1,100 DCWs in Michigan. Sadly, their findings are almost identical to recently published study results both in Michigan and across the country.

Low wages and benefits top the list of reasons to consider leaving the field (Figure 14.2). The median wage for DCWs was just $15.43 per hour in 2022 (Scales & Stepick, 2023). However, the wage range was wide, with workers in home care making far less than those in hospitals or nursing homes, and a large portion making minimum wage. Wages also vary by race, ethnicity, and number of persons in the household, with Latinx DCWs earning the lowest wages of any group (Hartmann & Hayes, 2017). Due to the low wages, DCWs often need to work multiple part-time jobs, across settings, programs, and payors. Part-time employment rarely provides

Mare Martell, who worked as a DCW for 3 years, shares, "it makes me *blissfully happy* to be able to serve others." She adds, "I would do it for free, but unfortunately, free doesn't pay the bills." She loves animals, has a menagerie of pets including a house chicken, and is an artist and published author. Like many DCWs, Mare has trouble making ends meet in part due to part-time split hours, some that require driving long distances. "It is intense and exhausting . . . to go to one client in the morning and one in the evening, and sometimes have a third shift." A lack of guaranteed hours or injuries compounds the situation. Mare recently injured her shoulder while transferring a client, so she is currently not working as a DCW.

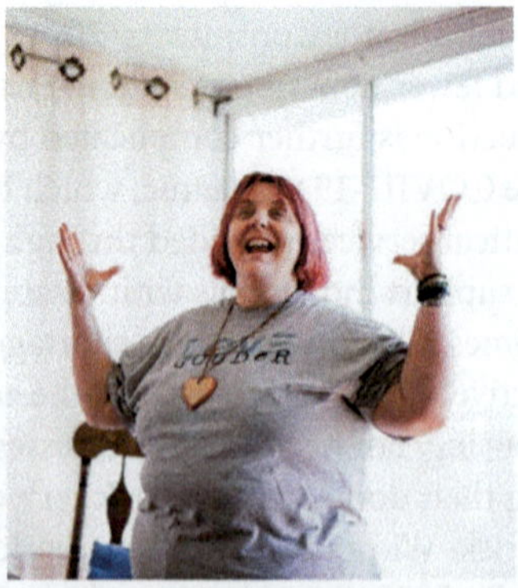

Mare Martell, Grand Rapids, Michigan

FIGURE 14.2. Former DCW on low wages.

DCW, direct care worker.

Source: Photo by Khalid Ibrahim, Eat Pomegranate Photography.

employer-based healthcare or paid sick time, putting many workers at risk of financial hardship if illness or an injury occurs (Campbell et al., 2021). Poverty status plays a major role in the retention of DCWs. Nearly half live at or below the poverty line and 47% qualify for publicly funded programs such as Medicaid (Paraprofessional Healthcare Institute [PHI], 2021b). Others have income just above the Medicaid eligibility limits and cannot afford exchange-based health insurance (Farrington, 2021). A whopping 84% of DCWs do not have access to an employer-based retirement benefit (Weller et al., 2020). Workers from poorer households are significantly more likely to leave direct care than those with higher incomes, meaning that poverty is also a major determinant of job turnover.

A second reason for the shortage is lack of training (Figure 14.3). While the federal government requires just 75 hours of basic mandated training for DCWs, few states require more than that. As a results, DCWs often feel unprepared for the tasks they are asked to perform (PHI, n.d.-a). Certified nursing assistants (CNAs) in nursing homes have federally mandated training requirements but most home care workers do not, leaving them without the necessary skill to provide adequate care. Further, few states require DCWs to participate in continuing education that would increase their skill sets over time, and there are limited opportunities for professional advancement. Most DCWs do not have official credentials (Figure 14.4). They report that even with credentials, experience, and training they are often unable to garner higher wages and their achievements are not portable or transferable if they change jobs (Roman & Crumley, 2021).

There is clear evidence that training increases skills and job satisfaction, which reduces turnover. Luz and Hanson's research, which was part of a federally funded six-state demonstration project, found that skills, employability, and job satisfaction significantly improved among participants in a comprehensive, person-centered DCW training program titled, "Building Training . . . Building Quality™." Study findings also indicated that "intent to stay" was associated with increased confidence in ability to do the job (Luz & Hanson, 2015a). PHI, a national organization working on behalf of DCWs, calls for overhauling DCW training curricula to reflect the full set of skills needed for this work and establishing a national standard for direct care competencies (Campbell et al., 2021; PHI, n.d.-b, 2020).

Other compounding factors include DCWs struggling with being given little information about the backgrounds, preferences, and evolving care needs of the individuals they are supporting (Kemper et al., 2008; Roman & Crumley, 2021). They feel a lack of respect and control from their immediate supervisors but also from a society that demonstrates limited value placed on

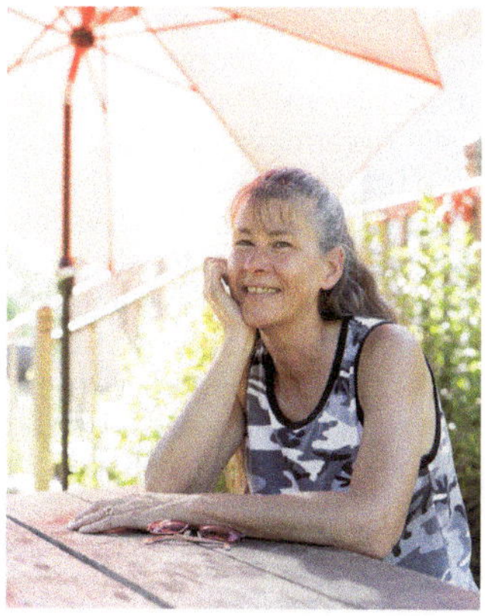

Ann Bilyeu, Grayling, Michigan

Ann Bilyeu, mother of eight, began as a DCW 18 years ago at an eight-bed adult foster care home for persons with mental illness. While the beginning was challenging, she viewed it as an adventure. Ann describes the job as both demanding and a significant responsibility. "It involves feces, urine, vomit, turning people that are three times bigger than you are, changing a bed with the client in it, cooking, cleaning, helping someone who's at end of life and trying to do your best to take care of the person with family there asking questions, and making life or death decisions. There's so much expected of you." Despite these responsibilities, her job title is "homemaker," which she detests. She prefers to call herself a "very hardworking caregiver." When asked how to recruit and retain more DCWs, Ann stresses the importance of "training, training, and more training." She has clear recommendations for agencies and policy makers: Test for critical thinking in common situations that DCWs face, provide *higher pay*, offer *more respect*, and improve management *training and support*. To young people considering PCA work as a profession, Ann advises, "Talk to others. Find out the worst of it, the best of it. Give quality, compassionate care and demand respect." Ann now prefers one-on-one home care and says she will never give it up. In her off hours, she loves gardening, being in her home deep in the woods with her animals and family, and stargazing.

FIGURE 14.3. DCW on the need for training.

DCW, direct care worker; PCA, personal care aide.

Source: Photo by Khalid Ibrahim, Eat Pomegranate Photography.

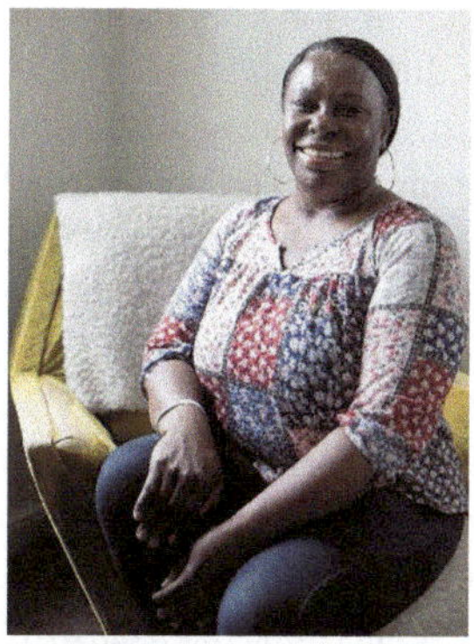

Henrietta Ivey, Detroit, Michigan

Henrietta Ivey started out as a licensed pharmacy technician. After becoming a family caregiver, her paid work as a DCW grew by word-of-mouth. For her, it is all about the love and compassion she gives, the relationships she develops with her clients, and knowing she's made someone's life better. She hopes someone will be compassionate enough to help her out one day.

Henrietta takes pride in doing her job well and refers to herself as a home care professional. She bristles at being called "the maid" or a "glorified butt wiper" and points out that home care and certified nursing work are similar. Yet, she feels CNAs don't get called derogatory names because they have recognized credentials, work in institutional settings, and typically make more money.

Henrietta has become a staunch activist, fighting for home care workers' rights to a living wage, benefits, and more respect. She has been told by policymakers, "This is not a real job that you do. Get a real job." to which she responds, "We're part of the healthcare system, so it would be nice for someone to finally recognize that these are real workers. We should not have to be ridiculed or disrespected because of the choices we make in our efforts to help other people."

FIGURE 14.4. Licensed pharmacy technician on the need for credentials.

CNAs, certified nursing assistants; DCW, direct care worker.

Source: Photo by Khalid Ibrahim, Eat Pomegranate Photography.

Vernette Mahone graduated from high school and wanted to become a computer technician but, it was challenging as a teen mom. Then, when her mother became ill, Vernette was determined to take care of her. She has worked in direct care ever since and says, "It's not a job; It's a lifestyle." Like many DCWs, she's not in it for the money, but feels the impact of what she describes as "*horrible*" working conditions. "To be told you're insignificant because you care about people . . . to not be recognized as a professional, that's heartbreaking. How can you be expected to make a decision on buying your kids some shoes or putting food on the table?" Vernette has become an activist. "We are the champions . . . we will continue to let it be known that home care workers are important. If you don't recognize home care workers now, then who's gonna take care of you?"

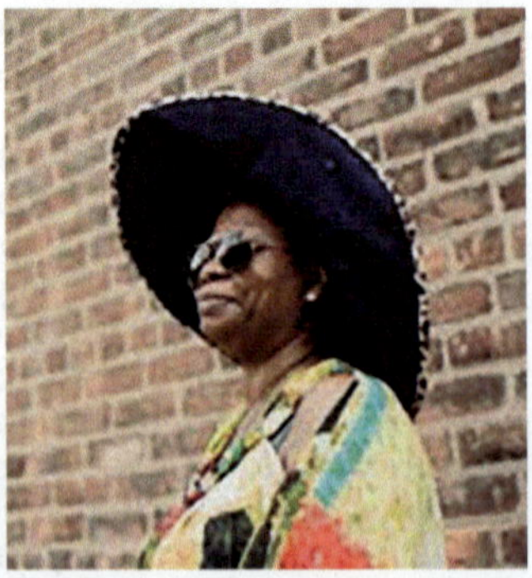

Vernette Mahone, Detroit, Michigan

FIGURE 14.5. Personal care aide on the undervalued role of direct care work.

DCW, direct care worker.

Source: Photo by Khalid Ibrahim, Eat Pomegranate Photography.

the work (FrameWorks Institute, 2021; Figure 14.5). A host of other job characteristics have been cited as being important and potentially influential but not necessarily predictive of job tenure. These include isolation from peers, unclear lines of authority, possible unsafe working conditions, no allowance for travel or training time, and high work-related injury rates (Luz, 2001; Mickus et al., 2003; Turnham & Dawson, 2003). Many factors that exist today, including low wages, few if any benefits, and a lack of guaranteed hours and respect, are grounded in long-standing cultural, societal, and economic values and norms that support such negative job conditions, which makes them particularly challenging to dismantle.

DCW job conditions can be thought of as symptoms of much more deeply rooted reasons for the shortage, which are entrenched in historical and institutional racism, sexism, ageism, and discrimination against immigrants and persons with disabilities. They are steeped in a belief that families should "take care of their own" and traditional gender roles, which typically designates women as the caregivers. These beliefs persist despite the rapid growth of women in the paid workforce and a growing shortage of family caregivers. They are the backdrop for the fact that DCWs are mostly women, disproportionately women of color, and foreign-born (McCall & Scales, 2022; PHI, 2021a). McCall and Scales (2022) reported that the percentage of workers who are women of color increased from 45% to 53% between 2009 and 2019—growing from 1.4 to 2.4 million workers. Poor job quality both reflects and perpetuates the long-standing societal disadvantages facing women, people of color, and other marginalized populations. For decades, certain government decisions (e.g., anti-immigrant policies, changes to Medicaid, and workforce protections not applying to direct care) have harmed the health and financial security of all DCWs, particularly workers of color (PHI, 2022b). If the ultimate goal really is to have an ample, stable, and qualified direct care workforce, then a transformative light needs to shine on these underlying causes of economic instability and a lack of respect while simultaneously laying low the symptoms themselves.

MAJOR STRATEGIES FOR ADDRESSING THE DIRECT CARE WORKER SHORTAGE

Just as the main reasons for the DCW shortage are known, so are key solutions. Study after study makes it clear that addressing the shortage must include raising wages and benefits; professionalizing this workforce by establishing quality standards; providing comprehensive training for DCWs, trainers, and managers; issuing competency-based credentials; and providing career pathways and support. It is also clear that success requires culture change such that society places a higher value on this workforce, and a strategic, coordinated, statewide plan that considers all these solutions simultaneously. These strategies are known to reduce turnover and lead to higher quality care with better outcomes. Simply making one change to enhance opportunities for DCWs, such as raising wages or requiring more training hours, is not enough. It is a Band-Aid approach that will not lead to large-scale, successful, and sustainable change. Most everyone agrees that DCWs need to be paid higher, living wages. Most everyone likely also agrees that it is not a good idea to pay workers substantially higher rates if they are incompetent and could bring great harm to the people they are paid to support. Likewise, it will not help to champion training without paying competent workers higher wages. Having highly competent workers will not matter if they cannot find a job with a living wage, afford a car or gas for the car they have, or overcome serious challenges to economic security.

In 2020, important steps were taken in Michigan to address the DCW shortage. These steps became game-changers. The first notable catalyst was the formation of a statewide Direct Care Workforce Advisory Committee, distinguished from prior committees in several ways. It was initiated by the Michigan Department of Health & Human Services (MDHHS) Aging and Adult Services Agency. Rather than include only people from within state government, which is often done, a clear goal was to engage a broad range of both internal and external stakeholders comprised of representatives from all LTC settings, programs, payors, and populations served. Still functioning, it also includes MDHHS leadership, regulatory agents, DCWs, advocates, and others with a vested interest in working together to expand, stabilize, and support this workforce. The Advisory Committee is co-chaired by an external organization, the Integrated Model for Personal Assistant Research and Training (IMPART) Alliance, whose institutional home is in the College of Osteopathic Medicine at Michigan State University, which serves as a neutral convener. IMPART's leadership has a deep knowledge of key direct care workforce issues and a long history of community-based research and projects, often in partnership with state government and multiple collaborators across the state.

Early on, the Advisory Committee members agreed on three primary groups of strategies for addressing the shortage that are consistent across much of the literature and being used in other states (Roman & Crumley, 2021; Winters et al., 2021). These were (a) raising wages and benefits, (b) professionalization of this workforce, and (c) societal-cultural change to increase the value placed on direct care work. Further, they agreed that these groups of strategies are interdependent, must be addressed simultaneously, and must focus on achieving economic security, respect, and equity for all DCWs versus individual segments of this workforce. These goals rested on a mutual understanding that success requires evidence-based state-level leadership and action, collaboration, and coordination of strategies within and across state agencies, governance and external sectors, organizations, and stakeholders. Reaching consensus on each of these principles started with one initial strategy: Committee members talking to each other, with cautious hope that by doing so, they might be able to successfully address their shared distress over the workforce shortage.

Historically, many of the members had been siloed in their own agencies, working on parallel, often redundant projects without any knowledge of what was happening in other sectors. For example, members from the aging and disability communities rarely crossed paths despite overlapping needs and potential for partnership to affect change benefitting both groups. However, as the shortage became more severe, members realized a different approach was needed, and that all the recruitment and retention strategies in the world would not succeed without state-level system reforms. Once started, Committee members began to develop relationships, learn about each other, partner through workgroups, build a strong network based on respect and trust, and be encouraged by several victories. The Committee has been meeting virtually every month for over 3 years and, remarkably, attendance has not waned, members have found common ground, and momentum continues to grow.

One of the many successes was the development of 14 key recommendations for addressing the shortage, which were based on 2 years of in-depth work by the Committee's State Policy Recommendations Workgroup and which were recently endorsed by the full Committee and submitted to MDHHS leadership for consideration of adoption. The Committee's experience has made clear the power and necessity of strategic, coordinated statewide leadership. As a result, the recommendations made to the state are divided into four primary sets of strategies instead of three, the first being state leadership. The argument is that success within the other three (increased wages and benefits, professionalization of this workforce, and societal-cultural change, as previously noted) is dependent on the first. Recommendations in all four categories require a combination of strategic actions or levers available to state-level leadership, including (a) legislation; (b) administrative oversight or assistance, regulations, or executive orders; (c) funding through general funds, Medicaid rate-setting, federal/state matches, supplemental funds, or special federal funds such as from the American Rescue Plan Act (ARPA); (d) funded research and data structure; and (e) stakeholder advocacy. The following explores the four major categories of strategies for addressing the workforce shortage, with particular attention on state leadership and professionalization.

EFFECTIVE STATEWIDE LEADERSHIP

During the Advisory Committee's tenure, there have been many key lessons learned that are crucial to the ability to maintain cohesion and forward movement (Box 14.1). Lessons have come through commissioned studies, experiences in other states, and a commitment to taking the time to wrestle through tough challenges.

Most of these lessons have already been touched upon. There are two additional ones to which attention should be drawn. The Committee learned early on that the wide diversity of members necessitated determining a shared language. An excellent example of this was the need to reach some level of consensus on what is meant by the term *direct care worker*. DCWs go by many names including *direct support professional, personal care aide,* and *home health aide,* just to name a few. The names vary across settings, programs, payors, and populations served. They vary in the general public and among persons receiving support. Further complicating the matter, the range of DCW roles is vast and may include a job coach in a vocational community services setting to DCWs that provide 24/7 assistance with all activities of daily living (ADLs) and personal hands-on care in a nursing home or hospice setting, and everyone in between. In general, there is no commonly agreed upon terminology. In fact, what are appropriate terms has been debated for decades, with some people taking hardline positions such that it can get contentious, just as there is little consensus on the "appropriate" term for older adults. Some people cringe at terms such as *senior citizens* or *elders,* while others prefer to apply these terms to themselves as they denote wisdom, in their view. It is futile to attempt to be too prescriptive, especially when there is currently a strong push for "person-centered thinking," which prescribes to honoring individual preferences.

BOX 14.1 Lessons Learned: Key Components of Success

- Statewide leadership that cuts across sectors, programs, settings, payors, populations served
- Coordination inclusive of all stakeholders
- Building relationships based on respect, transparency, trust, and collaboration versus competition
- Recognition of the interrelatedness of solutions
- Finding common ground and goals
- A shared definition of DCWs
- Advocacy on behalf of *all* DCWs
- A neutral convener
- Commitment, passion, patience, and persistence

However, some common terminology must be agreed upon, if only for the sake of succeeding in affecting change through policy reforms. It is counterproductive when one group approaches policy makers referring to DCWs by one term, and asking for something framed a certain way, and another group approaches the same policy maker referring to DCWs using another term, and perhaps asking for the same help, or slightly different help, framed in a very different way. This results in a confused policy maker and the two groups undermining each other's efforts. Recognizing this, a Committee workgroup developed a common definition for a DCW that everyone on the Committee can live with (Box 14.2). It took close to 2 years to arrive at the final definition, which is meant to be as inclusive as possible, and which indicates what a difficult undertaking it was. Even still, it is described as a living definition, subject to future modifications. This achievement has meant that when members approach legislators, they are all using the same term, defined in the same way. The definition has been distributed to legislators in an effort to raise their awareness of who DCWs are, what they do, the critical value of this workforce, and its importance to any discussion or decisions related to LTC.

Another notable lesson learned is the need for the Committee to work on behalf of all DCWs versus one subset or another. Similar to different language used among members, there is wide variance on what their primary goals are, rightfully driven by the needs of their individual constituents. Historically, they have fought for advances in wages, higher reimbursement rates, less regulatory restrictions, and so forth, within their sector. The literature indicates, as does anecdotal evidence, that gains in one segment of DCWs can put other segments at a disadvantage, thereby jeopardizing the potential for successfully addressing the direct care workforce shortage crisis that is affecting all sectors (Roman et al., 2022). One example of this is when legislators in Michigan voted to give one subset of DCWs a small wage increase and several months later, when another group of advocates petitioned for a wage increase for all DCWs, they were told by a legislator that raises had already been given. The legislator was shocked to learn that the previous raise only covered a fraction of the direct care workforce in Michigan. Since the advent of the Advisory Committee, members still advocate for their constituents, but any policy action recommended by the Committee is done on behalf of all DCWs.

A second step was taken in 2020 that has also been critical to success. PHI received funding from the Kellogg Foundation to work with three states to advocate on behalf of DCWs through policy reforms in three areas: "(1) addressing LTC financing and DCW compensation; (2) investing

BOX 14.2 A Shared Definition of Direct Care Workers

- DCWs provide essential services through behavioral health, community mental health, and LTC systems to support older adults and individuals with long-term disabilities or postacute care needs in a range of settings including private homes, group homes, assisted living facilities, nursing homes, and community living support settings.
- DCWs go by many titles including, but not limited to, certified nursing assistants, home health aides, home help providers, hospice aides, personal care assistants, direct support professionals, self-directed home care workers, and home care companions.
- DCWs are distinguished by core tasks shared by most DCWs that generally include assisting with hands-on personal care, ADLs, instrumental activities of daily living (IADLs), vocational assistance, rehabilitation, and community living supports.
- DCWs are paid primarily through Medicaid but may also be covered by private insurance, the Older Americans Act funds, Medicare, directly by individuals, or other funding sources.

in recruitment, training, career advancement, and other workforce innovations; and (3) improving data and research to inform efforts to strengthen the direct care workforce" (Scales, 2023, p. 3). They chose North Carolina, New Mexico, and Michigan and an anchor organization in each of the states: IMPART Alliance in Michigan. One of the goals for each state was to establish a statewide coalition, referred to as the Essential Jobs, Essential Care™ (EJEC™) Coalition. Michigan's Coalition has grown from approximately 50 to over 1,000 members in just 3 years, which indicates the deep need individuals and organizations feel to learn about the efforts of others, connect with them, stay on top of what is happening across the state, and to join forces. It has provided hope, if for no other reason than learning that they are not alone. They are not struggling in a vacuum, believing that no one cares, and nothing is being done to provide help.

However, the Coalition has proven to be much more powerful than this. A Coalition of this size provides the opportunity to mobilize people quickly, all with the same message, for specific policy actions. For example, during the pandemic, many states voted to give DCWs an hourly pay increase, sometimes referred to as premium pay. In Michigan, most DCWs initially received $2.00 per hour in addition to their regular pay rate, a rate that was raised to $2.35 soon after. As the peak impact of COVID-19 lessened, states began to discontinue the additional pay. In anticipation of this potentially happening in Michigan, an action alert went out to all Coalition members who were encouraged to contact their legislators and ask that the wage increase be made permanent. Specific text was provided, which members could modify but it ensured that the messaging would be consistent. Legislators were barraged with an unprecedented outpouring from their constituents. As a result, Michigan was the only state that voted in favor of continuing the added pay (PHI, 2022a) and has since raised it another 85 cents. For states considering their options, having both a statewide Advisory Committee devoted exclusively to the direct care workforce and using all levers available to statewide leadership, coupled with a statewide Coalition, is a powerful combination. Excerpts of other strategies in the leadership category that are included in the 14 recommendations submitted to the MDHHS are noted in Table 14.1.

TABLE 14.1 Recommendations for Statewide Leadership
1. Establish a state-level, internal/external DCW Recommendations Action Team, with a dedicated staff, that will oversee implementation of all 14 recommendations in partnership with state government and existing/emerging advocacy groups for cross-collaboration. The focus will be on DCW economic security and value, equitable worker experiences, and participant outcomes.
2. Sustain the MDHHS DCW Advisory Committee and Workgroups with representatives from both state and external advocates and regional stakeholders to advise the Action/Implementation Team and champion all endorsed plans with the MDHHS, legislators, and other decision-makers.
3. Sustain the Essential Jobs, Essential Care™ DCW Coalition so that it continues to provide a venue for large-scale participation in advocacy.
4. Adopt an existing shared definition of DCW and scope of work for each DCW category to increase equity and efficiency and lower costs.
5. Establish a plan to increase the number and quality of DCWs and improve recruitment/retention rates through a focus on economic security for all DCWs; attention to regional, local, and current data on wages, turnover rates, challenges to success, and so forth; policy changes for flexible, innovative, nontraditional benefits; development of creative career success models; and engagement in societal-cultural change initiatives.
6. Address irreconcilable training and credentialing systems by developing a streamlined system with standardized requirements to increase career options, quick entry into workforce, continuity of care, portability, reciprocity, administrative efficiencies, and cost-containment.
7. Develop a data structure to support all recommendations, evidence-based decisions, resource allocation, accountability, and determination of worthiness for further investment.

DCW, direct care worker; MDHHS, Michigan Department of Health & Human Services.

As a result of this coordinated state leadership, multiple other goals have been achieved including adopting statewide DCW competency guidelines, progress on developing curricula and credentials that map to these competencies, development of a novel career success model that will soon be piloted, expanding career pathways through consideration of four new categories of DCWs, and development of the Michigan Care Career online platform to match employers with individuals seeking direct care work employment. These efforts have led to multiple, substantial grants through the Michigan Department of Labor and Economic Development (LEO), the state general fund, and ARPA funds designated for support of home and community-based services. The ARPA funds are now being used to establish a statewide Direct Care Career Center for comprehensive, coordinated training, credentialing, and advocacy. IMPART Alliance is again serving as the convener to manage these grants and accomplish identified recommendations and goals through extensive partnerships across the state. This all underscores the dramatic progress that has been made in Michigan and the current, unprecedented opportunity to change the future of direct care work in the state. It is an opportunity that is not taken for granted and rests on sustaining the statewide leadership so that important gains can be made related to the key sets of strategies for successfully addressing the direct care workforce shortage: wages and benefits, professionalization, and societal-cultural change.

WAGES AND BENEFITS

In this category of strategies, there are multiple options that can be considered. Advocates often focus solely on one strategy, raising the Medicaid reimbursement rate, and bemoan the fact that this is a complex and difficult goal that may feel unreachable, as it is. However, it is a worthy goal and needs to be pursued if the rate is too low, but Medicaid is not the only available resource. While pursuing this goal, other options should be considered. In Michigan, various mechanisms are being explored, piloted, or in development. Excerpts of strategies in the wages and benefits category that are included in the 14 recommendations submitted to the MDHHS are noted in Table 14.2.

TABLE 14.2 Recommendations for Wages and Benefits
1. Prioritize livable, functional wages/benefits for all categories of DCWs and immediate supervisors.
2. Use Benefits Cliff Calculator to avoid negative impact of higher wages on ability to secure benefits.
3. Earmark portion of Medicaid reimbursement or "set-aside" for wages, benefits, or training.
4. Raise Medicaid reimbursement rates high enough to cover employer costs.
5. Advocate for higher benefits, COLAs, paid sick leave, paid vacation, health insurance, and so forth.
6. Cover/streamline administration of wage/benefit increases.
7. Use designated Medicaid skilled nursing facility workforce support funds for DCW wages/benefits.
8. Work for federal level policy reforms to incentivize hiring full-time employees with benefits versus part-time.
9. Tie contracts, including rate increases and incentive payments, to DCW-related quality measures.
10. Provide equitable funding for family caregivers, self-determined individuals, providers, and businesses.
11. Explore DCW-led models of care and foster partnerships with small business development centers.
12. Establish occupational codes for all categories of DCWs.

COLAs, cost-of-living adjustments; DCW, direct care worker.

PROFESSIONALIZING THE DIRECT CARE WORKFORCE

Professionalizing this workforce means establishing the hallmarks of any profession: competency, professionalism, and ethical standards; training requirements; credentials; career pathways; career success models; and, typically, a professional association. Achieving professional status should lead to higher wages and economic security, which leads to a more stable workforce. Most DCW stakeholders, including employers, want a qualified workforce. What they understandably do not want are unfunded training mandates or training that leads to unaffordable wage increases. Again, reforms need to recognize the interrelatedness of all factors contributing to the shortage, the impact of change in one area on other areas, the need to diversify ways in which to fund a better direct care and LTC system, and the economic argument for professionalization. A qualified, stable workforce is far cheaper than no workforce, the constant struggle to recruit and retain workers, and unsustainable turnover rates.

Several years ago, IMPART Alliance convened a group of DCWs who were interested in establishing a Direct Care Worker Professional Association. They agreed that the first step would be to develop a set of competency guidelines. Over the course of a year, they proceeded to systematically collect, study, and synthesize nationally known lists of related guidelines from sources such as the federal Centers for Medicare & Medicaid Services (CMS) and the National Association of Direct Support Professionals (NADSP). Based on this research, they drafted a set of 15 competencies that are specific to direct care work and submitted them to the Advisory Committee. An Advisory Committee Competency Workgroup vetted, expanded, and edited the list based on consultation with a wide range of stakeholders to ensure that it was inclusive of all types of DCWs, working across all populations served. It was then submitted to the full Committee, which unanimously endorsed it in late 2020, after which it was submitted to the director of the MDHHS. A turnover in directors delayed its review, but in early 2022 the new director issued a statement of support such that Michigan now has standardized Direct Care Worker Competency Guidelines. Since then, the Committee has disseminated the guidelines widely, through the Coalition and other networks; held multiple webinars to raise awareness of the guidelines among employers, trainers, and others affected by them; and developed and distributed a list of frequently asked questions. Currently, the guidelines are not mandatory, but they represent an important first step for progress in other areas. It is very difficult to develop training programs when the competencies needed to be a DCW are not known or well defined. Standardized training programs and credentials can now be wrapped around this set of endorsed competencies.

Standardized training programs are under development as part of the grant received by Michigan's Department of Labor and Economic Opportunity (LEO) through the Michigan Industry Cluster Approach (MICA) program. This initiative is designed to support employer-led collaboratives focused on addressing shared workforce challenges. The goal is to bring a cluster of employers, along with key partners, to solve talent needs based on local demands with leadership driven by the industry itself. The solutions are focused on workforce development, specifically in training and skill-building that leads to industry-recognized credentials, defined career paths, and employment opportunities, ultimately positioning workers for higher wages. MICA grants require that the employers collaborate with Michigan's workforce development system, educational institutions, and allied organizations to ensure training solutions are tailored to both industry needs and local workforce priorities.

Development of training programs has also been supported by a major grant through the 2023 Michigan general budget to build a statewide training and credentialing infrastructure (TCI). The overall goal of both projects is to increase the number of qualified DCWs in Michigan who have economic security by increasing the state's capacity to provide opportunities for affordable, accessible training; credentialing; career paths; and career success. The vision for the TCI includes three main components: a central administrative structure for efficiencies, a training arm, and a credentialing arm with a firewall between the two arms. The goal is to increase the capacity for training to be delivered at the local level using existing infrastructures such as community colleges, area agencies on aging, senior centers, high schools, and so forth. As mentioned, the MICA grant engages employers, workforce development agencies, educational institutions and other partners. The TCI project works to bring in all voices—employers, DCWs, businesses, people receiving support, a wide array of allies, and others—to work jointly on reaching goals for training, credentialing, and expanding career paths, but also on developing the infrastructure through which these new options can be delivered. Both projects share a Training and Credentialing Workgroup that works closely with the DCW Advisory Committee's Education Workgroup. Both groups have engaged in deep research over the course of the past 2 years, trying to determine the best training strategies for Michigan to pursue, and there have been many lessons learned that may help inform others interested in going down this path.

Determining the best training model requires an understanding of the current training system including what training requirements currently exist. The group was interested in how well requirements and existing curricula mapped to the 15 competency guidelines adopted by the state. Several possible outcomes were proposed including developing one standardized curriculum that could be used by all employers and trainers. Another was to develop a system of vetting existing curricula to determine how well-aligned they were with the state competency guidelines, which would make it possible to make recommendations for curricular improvements. It is important to note that this process focused mainly on topics covered in training requirements and curricula. It did not address other factors that contribute to high-quality training such as the delivery model (in-person, virtual, hybrid, and prerecorded) and the quality of the instructors.

However, what the group discovered was that the current system is so complex and fragmented that these types of proposals were not feasible, perhaps even impossible, and would not serve Michigan well even if achieved. The group concluded that the current training needs and requirements across types of DCWs, settings, programs, payors, and populations served are so wildly different that trying to reconcile them and design one-size-fits-all standards is futile. For example, there are DCWs who never provide hands-on personal care. Training requirements in one program are extensive but do not lead to a credential. Requirements in another program are nearly nonexistent even though the DCWs may support individuals who need complex, skilled care. Some requirements are not based on competency but rather payment models. This all leads, in Michigan, to multiple training requirements, inefficient administrative costs, and poorer outcomes with little chance for developing efficiencies such as a strategic, coordinated, standardized system of required competencies and training across settings and programs upon which portable credentials, test-out procedures, and a wide range of affordable options and career pathways can be built.

As a result, the workgroup decided to identify the most important, underlying desired outcome that should drive training and credentialing reforms and came to the following conclusion. A long-term goal that everyone should be able to agree on is simply for DCWs to be competent in the skills needed to provide the supports and services they are assigned to do. Further, if they can demonstrate these skills, they should receive a credential that is recognized across programs, settings, and payors. If the main objective is competency relevant to the job, then variables such as population served, setting, payor, job title, and other factors should not matter. This shift in thinking means that all training and all credentials must be competency based.

Adhering to these guiding principles, a new framework and plan began to emerge, with both short- and long-term goals that can lead to training and credentialing options that are more portable, efficient, and cost-effective with better outcomes. Reaching the goal of competency-based training and credentials that are universally recognized is clearly a long-term, complex undertaking. As ways in which to achieve this long-term goal are explored, short-term goals and strategies are being developed and piloted. The following is a brief summary of several of these initiatives.

The Advisory Committee's and grant project's Training and Credentialing Workgroups agreed that an important starting point is to develop new categories of DCWs with competency requirements that map to all the new 15 competency guidelines, as no such category, curricula, or credentials currently exist. There are now four stackable categories with associated competencies under consideration. They are:

1. *Direct care foundations (certificate),* which include competencies that every DCW should have before they start work, regardless of the setting they work in or the population served. The certificate covers topics such as person-centered thinking, ethical guidelines, Health Insurance Portability and Accountability Act (HIPAA) rules, professional boundaries, communication and listening skills, critical thinking, basic body mechanics, self-care, and diversity and cultural awareness. One advantage to having such a certificate is that it allows for increasing the number of DCWs without sacrificing quality. DCWs, with at least basic competence, can enter the field quickly and begin to meet the immediate need for a competent workforce. It also allows for workers themselves to get experience and decide if they want to build a direct care career by achieving additional credentials.
2. *Direct care associate,* which goes into the same topics in more depth as well as introductory classes on other topics such as dementia; mental illness; intellectual and developmental disabilities; trauma; and grief, loss, and end of life.
3. *Home and direct care specialist,* which adds in IADLs, particularly when supports are provided in a home setting.
4. *Certified DCW,* which adds in all the ADLs including personal hands-on care and in-depth content on all earlier topics.

In addition to these levels, specialty certificates will be developed to cover other individualized competencies needed to work in specific settings, with specific populations, or to meet special regulatory requirements.

These new categories will not replace or supersede existing categories. The goal is to increase training and credentialing options, not reduce them. Each of the levels will have an associated competency-based credential that is not linked to training but to demonstration of the competencies. Competency assessments will allow for the opportunity to test-out of training. All these features will make joining the field more expedient, which should increase the number of people joining as well as the number preparing for advanced credentials. An initial focus on virtual training will make training more accessible and affordable. Another project goal is to stay committed to comprehensive, high-quality teaching that is predominantly live and interactive via Zoom for a richer learning experience than what prerecorded, asynchronous education can provide. Eventually, when the system is more resourced, classes that are all in-person will be offered.

A common question is why not just train everyone as a CNA. The value that this new approach and the new categories add includes:

1. They are based on person-centered principles versus the traditional medical model that many CNA programs are rooted in.
2. The first level covers baseline competencies that all DCWs should have.
3. The third level covers skills needed to provide high-quality support in home settings. Most current CNA programs have no home care or IADL component even though most people prefer to remain in their own homes. Additionally, it is very different to provide support in a home setting versus an institutional setting such as a nursing home, as the DCW is typically alone with no back-up staff to call on for help. They must have the ability to make independent, competent, and sometimes very critical decisions.
4. It establishes credentials that don't currently exist and that recognize the important skills and work of entry-level DCWs who provide non-IADL or ADL support as well as for those who provide invaluable IADL support in home settings.

5. The competency-based credentials align with all the new state-supported DCW competency guidelines.
6. These categories and credentials will exist in addition to current categories with credentials such as CNAs, which increases career options.
7. They provide a system foundation for eventually being able to recognize all currently noncertified DCWs.
8. Most of the classes in these levels have been developed and piloted. The next step is to scale up by developing the system for delivering classes and competency assessments through local, existing organizations. The process of developing credentials associated with each of these levels is in progress. The project team is working with a national corporation specializing in helping organizations develop sound credentials, and experts in developing psychometric assessments, to determine competence. Processes for assessing competence on a largescale are being explored. By the end of the current grant, a recognized credential will exist for at least level one competencies; by the end of the forthcoming grant, there will be a credential for all four levels.

As presented, professionalization includes expansion of opportunities for career development. For maximum increases in recruitment and retention, it also makes career success resources available, especially for individuals for whom obstacles to success exist. It is not enough to train someone or even help them secure a job. For many potential or incumbent DCWs, it is a leaky pipeline if they do not receive resources and support from the moment an interest in direct care work is sparked. Luz and Hanson (2015b) examined why students in a DCW training program dropped out. None of the reasons related to the training program itself. All the reasons related to social determinants of outcomes such as a lack of transportation and child or elder care, and insufficient income to be able to miss work. The literature and logic suggest that a comprehensive recruitment and retention plan must include a career success component that meets people where they are. In Michigan, a model is being developed and piloted that begins with recruitment into an orientation program in which potential DCWs learn what it means to be a DCW. Such orientations have been shown to dramatically cut rates of attrition from training programs, which reduces a time and resource drain on both the programs and the individuals. It does not make sense to go through costly training programs only to learn that direct care work was not the right career choice.

The proposed model helps a person navigate through the whole career development process, starting with career counseling, determining what type of direct care work is preferred, what training and competencies will be needed, what challenges have to be overcome such as the need for tuition assistance, how to overcome these obstacles, job search preparation, job matching, and even possibly continuing to provide support to both the new employee and the employer during the initial job period. Employer support may include management or supervisory training to deter one of the major reasons DCWs leave the field, as discussed earlier. A prototype of the early phases of such a model are currently being piloted in Michigan's Upper Peninsula by the Caregiver Incentive Project through a grant from the Michigan Health Endowment Fund. Lessons learned from "The Caregiver Career Pipeline" project will provide a foundation for development of a career success model that can be tested, then scaled up statewide, using allocated ARPA funds.

SUMMARY

It is an exciting time with unprecedented potential to advance DCWs if the pressure can stay on to build momentum for system changes through policy reforms. It is crucial for all who are involved in this endeavor to understand the context of the LTC workforce shortages, the reasons for the shortage, and the link between the LTC workforce and ensuring quality and safety in care delivery. Michigan's example can help shed light on how to move forward and achieve workforce goals. The key lessons learned, including components for success, can be modified to meet the unique needs of individual states and organizations, as can the examples that have been offered on a framework for effective state leadership and best practices and evidence-based strategies for addressing the shortage. As healthcare administrators, providers, state governments, advocates, and others who care about the quality of LTC wrestle with tough workforce questions, it is necessary to stay focused on the end goals, the shared goals, and the strategies that are most relevant and feasible within the individual system. Whatever plans are developed, there should be both a call for breaking the plan down into manageable steps as well as simultaneously recognizing and having a sense of urgency. The opportunities that are available at this rare moment in time need to be seized and leveraged. They will likely not be available indefinitely and, to use a variation on a well-known quote, "If not us, then who? If not now, when?"

Take-Home Points

- The primary reasons driving the DCW shortage include low wages and benefits, lack of competency and training standards, career paths, and respect.
- Strategies for addressing the shortage must tackle historical and institutional sexism, racism, ageism, and discrimination against immigrants and persons with disabilities.
- Four key categories of strategies are organized, coordinated, statewide leadership; raising wages and benefits; professionalizing the workforce; and societal-cultural change, all of which must be undertaken simultaneously.
- Coordinated statewide leadership is essential; inclusive of all stakeholders; and based on respect, transparency, trust, and collaboration.
- Building relationships across stakeholders, recognizing interrelated solutions, and advocating on behalf of all DCWs are imperative.
- A neutral convener can facilitate communication and serve as a catalyst for ongoing movement forward, breaking the process down into manageable steps and fostering commitment, passion, patience, persistence, and hope for change.

END-OF-CHAPTER RESOURCES

DISCUSSION QUESTIONS

1. Provide a high-level overview of your organization or state. Include defining features such as the political strengths and challenges that exist, the sociocultural history and milieu, the economic forecast, and other factors that might influence the feasibility of strategies to address the direct care workforce shortage.
2. What is the status of DCWs? How do you define direct care work and workers? How many workers currently exist? What are the projected shortages and by when? What is their economic status, demographic make-up, and distribution across settings and populations served? What are the training requirements for each type of DCW? It is important to conduct this type of landscape and gap analyses.
3. What direct care workforce initiatives or research efforts are already being undertaken?
4. What statewide, standardized competency, training, credentialing, and career pathways exist or are in development?
5. What are the federal, state, and local programs that are having an impact currently on the local direct care workforce?
6. What levers are available for use such as legislation, regulatory changes, or funding?
7. Are there champions that exist or could be cultivated within the state legislature?

8. Are there existing coalitions, advocates, or member organizations outside of state government that could be marshaled from a range of constituencies including aging services, behavioral health, intellectual and developmental disability communities, and others?
9. Who could serve as a neutral convener?
10. What are the most pressing problems related to the direct care shortage that need immediate attention?
11. Describe promising ideas and innovations that are exciting in the state or elsewhere around the country such as training models, permanently raising wages, effective registries, and strategies for retention. Is there any empirical evidence to support the positive impact of these ideas?
12. What data and measures are available to mark progress and impact?

TOOLS FOR FURTHER LEARNING

- Lessons learned in Michigan could be applied in other states and settings.
- Promising strategies are being tried across the country, including:
  - *Direct Care Workforce Policy and Action Guide* (Roman et al., 2022)
  - National Governors Association report on state strategies for retention of the direct care health workforce (Winters et al., 2021)
  - Kaiser Family Foundation (KFF) report on payment rates for Medicaid home- and community-based services detailing states' responses to workforce challenges (Burns et al., 2023)
- Key finding: Most states are increasing Medicaid's payment rates to expand worker opportunities.
- Growing body of literature and evidence on the impact of state actions on health workforce challenges:
  - Ziemann's study on governor directives changing health workforce flexibility (Ziemann et al., 2023)
  - Evidence on state options for wise investments in the direct care workforce for planning and policy reforms (Twomey, 2019)
- The CMS provides invaluable tools and reading materials on:
  - Person-centered practice (CMS, 2021)
  - Coordinating care across systems and settings (CMS, 2021)
  - Professional development (CMS, 2021)
  - Pay for performance (CMS, 2021)
  - Self-directed care (CMS, n.d.)
  - Direct service workforce learning collaboratives (CMS & Lewin Group, 2023)
  - Core competencies (CMS, 2014)
- National efforts to address the direct care workforce shortage include:
  - American Rescue Plan Act funds increasing Michigan's ability to establish a statewide Direct Care Career Center
  - President Biden's executive order (April 2023) to increase access to high-quality care and support caregivers (Biden, 2023)
  - PHI reports on national nursing home staffing standards (PHI, 2023a)
  - Summary of the timeliness of the Home- and Community-Based Services Relief Act (PHI, 2023b)
  - PHI website (phinational.org) as an important resource for the direct care workforce shortage
- Recommended readings provide a good starting point for developing a better understanding of the issues and potential options for states and organizations moving forward.

SPRINGER PUBLISHING CONNECT™ | A robust set of instructor resources designed to supplement this text is located at http://connect.springerpub.com/content/book/978-0-8261-4935-0. Qualifying instructors may request access by emailing textbook@springerpub.com.

REFERENCES

Biden, J. (2023, April 18). *Executive order on increasing access to high-quality care and supporting caregivers*. The White House. https://www.whitehouse.gov/briefing-room/presidential-actions/2023/04/18/executive-order-on-increasing-access-to-high-quality-care-and-supporting-caregivers/

Burns, A., Mohamed, M., & O'Malley Watts, M. (2023, October 24). *Payment rates for Medicaid home- and community-based services: States' responses to workforce challenges*. KFF. https://www.kff.org/medicaid/issue-brief/payment-rates-for-medicaid-home-and-community-based-services-states-responses-to-workforce-challenges/

Campbell, S., Del Rio Drake, A., Espinoza, R., & Scales, K. (2021). *Caring for the future: The power and potential of America's direct care workforce*. Paraprofessional Healthcare Institute. http://phinational.org/wp-content/uploads/2021/01/Caring-for-the-Future-2021-PHI.pdf

Centers for Medicare and Medicaid Services. (n.d.). *Direct care workforce resources*. Retrieved September 27, 2024, from https://www.medicaid.gov/medicaid/long-term-services-supports/workforce-initiative/overviews-of-workforce-challenges-and-effective-improvement-strategies/index.html

Centers for Medicare and Medicaid Services. (2014). *The DSW core competency project*. https://www.medicaid.gov/medicaid/long-term-services-supports/direct-care-workforce/dsw-core-competency-project/index.html

Centers for Medicare and Medicaid Services. (2021, April). *Summary report: HCBS direct service workforce intensive*. https://www.nahc.org/wp-content/uploads/2021/04/DSW_Intensive_Summary_Report_508.pdf

Centers for Medicare and Medicaid Services, & Lewin Group. (2023). *Direct service workforce learning collaborative summary report*. http://www.medicaid.gov/medicaid/long-term-services-supports/downloads/hcbs-learning-collaborative-summary.pdf

Farrell, C. (2018, April 18). *The shortage of home care workers: Worse than you think*. Forbes. https://www.forbes.com/sites/nextavenue/2018/04/18/the-shortage-of-home-care-workers-worse-than-you-think

Farrington, R. (2021, December 10). *The benefits cliff: When a higher minimum wage results in lost benefits*. Forbes. https://www.forbes.com/sites/robertfarrington/2021/04/05/the-benefits-cliff-when-a-higher-minimum-wage-results-in-lost-benefits

Flinn, B. (2018, May). *Millennials: The emerging generation of family caregivers*. AARP Public Policy Institute. https://www.aarp.org/content/dam/aarp/ppi/2018/05/millennial-family-caregivers.pdf

Foley, K., & Luz, C. (2021). Retooling the health care workforce for an aging America: A current perspective. *The Gerontologist, 61*(4), 487–496. https://doi.org/10.1093/geront/gnaa163

FrameWorks Institute. (2021, April). *Public thinking about care work in a time of social upheaval: Preliminary findings from the culture change project*. https://www.frameworksinstitute.org/wp-content/uploads/2021/05/Care-work-culture-change-report_PDF-PROOF_5-6-21.pdf

Hartmann, H., & Hayes, J. (2017). The growing need for home care workers: Improving a low-paid, female-dominated occupation and the conditions of its immigrant workers. *Public Policy & Aging Report, 27*(3), 88–95. https://doi.org/10.1093/ppar/prx017

Holly, R. (2019, May 8). *Home care industry turnover reaches all-time high of 82%*. Home Health Care News. https://homehealthcarenews.com/2019/05/home-care-industry-turnover-reaches-all-time-high-of-82

Institute of Medicine. (2008). *Retooling for an aging America: Building the health care workforce*. National Academies Press. https://doi.org/10.17226/12089

Kemper, P., Heier, B., Barry, T., Brannon, D., Angelelli, J., Vasey, J., & Anderson-Knott, M. (2008). What do direct care workers say would improve their jobs? *The Gerontologist, 48*(Suppl. 1), 17–25. https://doi.org/10.1093/geront/48.Supplement_1.17

Luz, C. (2001). *Self-employed caregivers: Their motivations, labor conditions, and patterns of decision making related to work selection and tenure*. Unpublished dissertation, University of Wisconsin-Milwaukee.

Luz, C., & Hanson, K. (2015a). Filling the care gap: Personal home care worker training improves job skills, status and satisfaction. *Home Health Care Management & Practice, 27*(4), 230–237. https://doi.org/10.1177/1084822315584316

Luz, C., & Hanson, K. (2015b). Training the personal and homecare aide workforce: Challenges and solutions. *Home Health Care Management & Practice, 27*(3), 150–153. https://doi.org/10.1177/1084822314566301

McCall, S., & Scales, K. (2022, February 8). *Direct care worker disparities: Key trends and challenges.* Paraprofessional Healthcare Institute. https://phinational.org/resource/direct-care-worker-disparities-key-trends-and-challenges

Mickus, M., Luz, C., & Hogan, A. (2004, April 22). *Voices from the front: Recruitment and retention of direct care workers in long-term care across Michigan.* https://www.phinational.org/wp-content/uploads/legacy/clearinghouse/MI_vocices_from_the_front.pdf

National Center for Health Workforce Analysis. (2017, April). *National and regional projections of supply and demand for geriatricians: 2013–2025.* U.S. Department of Health & Human Services, Health Resources and Services Administration, Bureau of Health Workforce. https://bhw.hrsa.gov/sites/default/files/bureau-health-workforce/data-research/geriatrics-report-51817.pdf

National Center for Health Workforce Analysis. (2018, March). *Long-term services and supports: Direct care worker demand projections, 2015–2030.* U.S. Department of Health & Human Services, Health Resources and Services Administration, Bureau of Health Workforce. https://bhw.hrsa.gov/sites/default/files/bureau-health-workforce/data-research/hrsa-ltts-direct-care-worker-report.pdf

Osterman, P. (2017). *Who will care for us? Long-term care and the long-term workforce.* Russell Sage Foundation.

Paraprofessional Healthcare Institute. (n.d.-a). *Home health aide training requirements by state.* Retrieved November 4, 2023, from https://www.phinational.org/advocacy/home-health-aide-training-requirements-state-2016

Paraprofessional Healthcare Institute. (n.d.-b). *Strengthen training standards and delivery systems for direct care workers.* Retrieved November 4, 2023, from https://phinational.org/issue/data-collection-quality

Paraprofessional Healthcare Institute. (2020, July 14). *Inconsistent and outdated training standards limit direct care workers.* https://www.phinational.org/resource/inconsistent-and-outdated-training-standards-limit-direct-care-workers

Paraprofessional Healthcare Institute. (2021a, September 7). *Direct care workers in the United States—Key facts.* https://phinational.org/resource/direct-care-workers-in-the-united-states-key-facts-2

Paraprofessional Healthcare Institute. (2021b, August 13). *The economic case for improving direct care jobs.* https://phinational.org/the-economic-case-for-improving-direct-care-jobs

Paraprofessional Healthcare Institute. (2022a, November 29). *How Michigan permanently increased wages for direct care workers.* https://www.phinational.org/news/how-michigan-permanently-increased-wages-for-direct-care-workers

Paraprofessional Healthcare Institute. (2022b, February 8). *PHI launches institute to address inequities in the direct care workforce* [Press release]. http://www.phinational.org/news/phi-launches-institute-to-address-inequities-in-the-direct-care-workforce

Paraprofessional Healthcare Institute. (2023a, September 19). *Nursing home staffing standards are finally becoming a reality.* https://www.phinational.org/nursing-home-staffing-standards-are-finally-becoming-a-reality

Paraprofessional Healthcare Institute. (2023b, November 8). *The HCBS Relief Act: A timely response to America's caregiving crisis.* https://www.phinational.org/the-hcbs-relief-act-a-timely-response-to-americas-caregiving-crisis

Public Sector Consultants. (2021, August). *Michigan's direct care workforce: Living wage and cost turnover analysis.* https://www.chcs.org/media/Michigans-Direct-Care-Workforce-Living-Wage-and-Turnover-Cost-Analysis.pdf

Roman, C., & Crumley, D. (2021, December). *Forging a path forward to strengthen Michigan's direct care workforce.* Center for Health Care Strategies. https://www.chcs.org/media/Forging-a-Path-Forward-to-Strengthen-Michigans-Direct-Care-Workforce.pdf

Roman, C., Luz, C., Graham, C., Joseph, N., & McEvoy, K. (2022, May 18). *Direct care workforce policy and action guide.* Milbank Memorial Fund. https://www.milbank.org/publications/direct-care-workforce-policy-and-action-guide

Scales, K. (2023, July 27). *Building the direct care workforce movement: The essential jobs, essential care multi-state initiative final report.* Paraprofessional Healthcare Institute. https://www.phinational.org/resource/building-the-direct-care-workforce-movement-the-essential-jobs-essential-care-multi-state-initiative-final-report

Scales, K., & Stepick, L. (2023). *Understanding the direct care workforce.* Paraprofessional Healthcare Institute. http://phinational.org/policy-research/key-facts-faq

Seavey, D. (2011). Caregivers on the front line: Building a better direct-care workforce. *Generations Journal, 34*(4), 27–35. https://www.proquest.com/docview/858457970?sourcetype=Scholarly%20Journals

Stepick, L. (2023, February 7). *Direct care workforce state index maps out progress and potential.* Generations. https://generations.asaging.org/direct-care-workforce-state-index-maps-progress

Turnham, H., & Dawson, S. (2003, April). *Michigan's care gap: Our emerging direct care workforce crisis.* Paraprofessional Healthcare Institute. https://www.phinational.org/wp-content/uploads/legacy/clearinghouse/MI%20Care%20Gap%20Publicn.pdf

Twomey, M. (2019, April 10). *State options for making wise investments in the direct care workforce.* Center for American Progress. https://www.americanprogress.org/article/state-options-making-wise-investments-direct-care-workforce

Ward, H., Ralls, M., Roman, C., & Crumley, D. (2021, December). *Strengthening the direct care workforce: Scan of state strategies.* Center for Health Care Strategies. https://www.chcs.org/media/Strengthening-the-Direct-Care-Workforce-Scan-of-State-Strategies.pdf

Weller, C., Almeida, B., Cohen, M., & Stone, R. (2020). *Making care work pay: How paying at least a living wage to direct care workers could benefit care recipients, workers, and communities.* Leading Age. https://www.ltsscenter.org/wp-content/uploads/2020/09/Making-Care-Work-Pay-Report-FINAL.pdf

Winters, A., Block, L., Maxey, H., Medlock, C., Ruane, K., & Hockenberry, S. (2021, September). *State strategies for sector growth and retention for the direct care health workforce.* National Governors Association Center for Best Practices. https://www.nga.org/wp-content/uploads/2021/10/NGA_SectorGrowth-DirectCare_report.pdf

Ziemann, M., Strasser, J., Krips, M., Yang, T., & Pittman, P. (2023). How governor directives changed health workforce flexibility in response to the COVID-19 pandemic. *Public Health Reports, 138*(Suppl. 1), 78S–89S. https://doi.org/10.1177/00333549221132534

CHAPTER 15

FUTURE TRENDS AND CAREERS IN LONG-TERM CARE

Darren Liu and Nicholas G. Castle

"I wish as I age I can still enjoy the things I did when I was younger, like how I enjoy playing badminton, chess, singing, and reading books. Just like the busy bees in the hive who continue working and enjoying their tasks, I hope to stay active and happy. Whether it's playing games, singing songs, or diving into a good book, I want to keep these joys in my life forever."

Dora Liu, McMurray Elementary School, Class of 2031

Learning Objectives

After completing this chapter, each learner will be able to:

- Understand the challenges and opportunities in the long-term care (LTC) industry and how they may impact future developments.
- Explore the interdisciplinary nature of LTC and how students can be better prepared to pursue careers in this field.
- Gain insights into the perspectives of experts in the LTC industry, as presented in their research and chapter contributions.
- Learn about potential career paths in LTC and the advice offered by experienced educators and mentors.
- Envision a future where aging is approached with peace of mind and confidence, guided by principles of quality and safety.

STUDENT: "HOW DO QUALITY AND SAFETY IN LONG-TERM CARE SHAPE THE FUTURE OF AGING FOR OLDER ADULTS?"

Quality and safety are crucial elements in the realm of long-term care (LTC), profoundly influencing the trajectory of aging for older adults. They serve as the foundation for ensuring their well-being and autonomy as they navigate this phase of life. In the dynamic landscape of LTC, where challenges and opportunities coexist, embracing innovation becomes imperative. By integrating innovative strategies and fresh perspectives, we can address current challenges and pave the way for a future where aging is met with optimism and vitality. Thus, the significance of quality and safety in LTC extends far beyond the present moment, profoundly influencing the trajectory of aging for generations to come.

Innovation does not always necessitate starting from scratch. Established concepts such as aging-in-place, home- and community-based services (HCBS), and patient-centered care retain their relevance. These strategies are pivotal in promoting active aging and prioritizing continual support and services to support the health, happiness, and independence of older adults.

At the core of active aging lies the preservation of seniors' autonomy and their active engagement in community life. This emphasizes the importance of maintaining physical and mental well-being while nurturing social connections. Prioritizing quality and safety in LTC constructs environments that empower older adults to live fulfilling and independent lives as they age.

Looking ahead, the concept of active living and the prioritization of quality and safety are shaping the future trends in LTC. There will be a greater emphasis on creating environments and services that promote physical activity, mental stimulation, and social engagement. Technological advancements, such as telehealth and wearable health devices, will support these goals by enabling continuous health monitoring and personalized care. HCBS will expand, providing more opportunities for older adults to receive care in familiar and comfortable settings. Additionally, innovations in patient-centered care models will ensure that the unique needs and preferences of each individual are met.

As we develop these innovations, several principles need to be kept in mind. It is essential to maintain a person-centered approach, ensuring that care is tailored to the individual's preferences and needs. Ensuring accessibility and inclusivity is crucial, so all older adults can benefit from advancements in care. Finally, fostering collaboration among caregivers, healthcare professionals, and community resources will be vital in creating a cohesive and supportive network for aging adults.

These future trends, driven by the principles of active living and a steadfast commitment to quality and safety, promise to enhance the well-being and independence of older adults, allowing them to age with dignity and vitality.

STUDENT: "PROFESSOR, YOU'VE DISCUSSED ACTIVE AGING TO REFRAME OUR UNDERSTANDING OF AGING, BUT WHAT ABOUT THE CONCEPT OF SUCCESSFUL AGING? HOW DOES IT FIT INTO THIS NARRATIVE?"

In their groundbreaking 1987 paper titled "Human Aging: Usual and Successful," John W. Rowe and Robert L. Kahn challenged conventional beliefs surrounding aging. They argued against the notion that age-associated cognitive and physiologic deficits were solely attributable to the aging process itself. Instead, they emphasized the significant influence of *extrinsic factors* such as lifestyle choices, habits, diet, and psychosocial elements in shaping how individuals age (Rowe & Kahn, 1987). This seminal work laid the foundation for what later became known as the *MacArthur model* of successful aging, a paradigm shift that redirected the focus from decline and disease to health and growth.

In the MacArthur model, two distinct categories of aging emerge: *usual aging* and *successful aging*. Usual aging, a subcategory of normal aging, is characterized by the *negative* impact of extrinsic factors on age-related declines. In contrast, successful aging represents another facet of normal aging, where extrinsic factors play a *neutral or even positive* role, facilitating a transition from usual to successful aging. This nuanced distinction challenges the prevailing notion that aging follows a uniform trajectory for everyone, emphasizing instead the dynamic interplay between intrinsic and extrinsic factors in shaping the aging process.

In essence, Rowe and Kahn's work not only revolutionized our understanding of aging but also paved the way for a more holistic approach to gerontology, one that recognizes the multifaceted nature of the aging process and the potential for individuals to age successfully through proactive engagement with their environment and lifestyle choices.

STUDENT: "CAN YOU TELL ME MORE ABOUT THE 'MACARTHUR MODEL'?"

The MacArthur model, introduced in the late 1980s through the MacArthur Studies of Successful Aging, represents a pioneering approach to understanding the complexities of aging. Spearheaded by a diverse team of interdisciplinary scholars, including sociologists, psychologists, and medical researchers, these studies aimed to transcend traditional biomedical models by examining the intricate interplay of psychosocial factors in determining successful aging outcomes (Rowe & Kahn, 1987).

Figure 15.1 encapsulates the essence of the MacArthur model, illustrating its three primary components:

1. *Low risk of disease and disease-related disability:* This component underscores the importance of maintaining optimal physical health and minimizing the risk of chronic diseases and disabilities commonly associated with aging.
2. *Maintenance of high mental and physical function:* This facet highlights the critical role of preserving cognitive function, emotional well-being, and physical capabilities. It advocates for implementing strategies to sustain mental sharpness, emotional resilience, and physical fitness throughout the aging process.
3. *Continued engagement with life:* This component highlights the intrinsic value of maintaining social connections and actively participating in meaningful activities. It emphasizes the significance of nurturing relationships, engaging in community or volunteer endeavors, and pursuing personal passions and aspirations to foster a fulfilling and purposeful life as one ages.

The extensive longitudinal research conducted as part of the MacArthur Studies examined diverse cohorts of older adults to unravel the complex interactions among these factors and their influence on aging outcomes. Findings from these studies have yielded invaluable insights into the multifaceted nature of successful aging, informing interventions and policies aimed at promoting healthy aging across the lifespan (Rowe & Kahn, 1987, 1997, 2015).

Rowe and Kahn's seminal contributions sparked a paradigm shift in gerontology, reshaping our understanding of aging as a dynamic journey influenced by both *intrinsic* and *extrinsic* factors. While the MacArthur model has been praised for its comprehensive approach, it has also faced critiques for its perceived limitations, including its narrow focus and potential

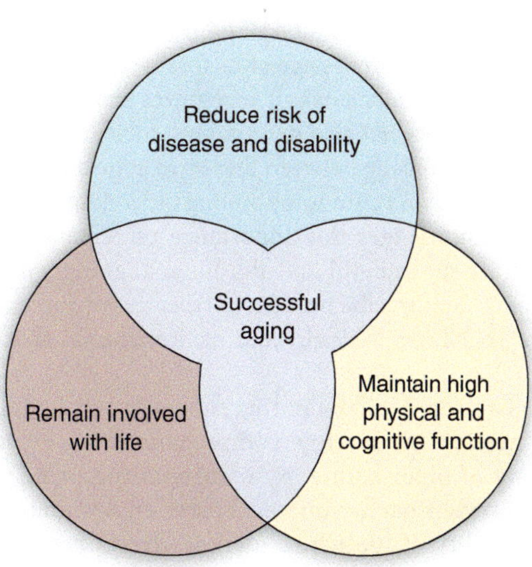

FIGURE 15.1. A model of successful aging.

Source: Data from Rowe, J. W., & Kahn, R. L. (1997). Successful aging. *The Gerontologist, 37*(4), 433–440. https://doi.org/10.1093/geront/37.4.433

stigmatization of those not aging well (Calasanti, 2016; Katz & Calasanti, 2015; Martin et al., 2015; Martinson & Berridge, 2015).

In response to these critiques, Rowe and Kahn (2015) introduced Successful Aging 2.0, a revised framework that embraces a more holistic perspective on aging in the 21st century. This updated model acknowledges the pivotal role of *social factors*, adopts a *subjective* definition of successful aging, and incorporates a life-course perspective, recognizing the cumulative impact of life experiences on aging outcomes. Furthermore, Successful Aging 2.0 emphasizes *cultural diversity*, highlighting the importance of *person-centered care* and *culturally sensitive* approaches in promoting successful aging across different populations.

STUDENT: "THANK YOU, PROFESSOR! NOW THAT I UNDERSTAND WHAT 'SUCCESSFUL AGING 2.0' ENTAILS, IT SEEMS LIKE IT ALIGNS WITH SEVERAL SOCIAL PERSPECTIVES WE HAVE EXPLORED IN CHAPTERS 9 AND 10. BUT HOW DOES IT RELATE TO THE CONCEPT OF 'ACTIVE AGING'?"

Active aging emerged from international dialogues on aging policy, particularly stemming from the World Health Organization's (WHO's) discussions in the late 20th century. Introduced during the 1982 World Assembly on Aging (United Nations, 1982), it gained prominence in the 1990s and was later defined in the WHO 2002 active aging policy framework (WHO, 2002). This framework outlined strategies for promoting active aging at various levels, reflecting a global shift toward valuing older adults' contributions and fostering healthy and engaged lifestyles in later years. It emphasized remaining actively engaged in life and participating in meaningful activities as individuals age. It promotes the idea that older adults can continue to contribute to society, pursue personal interests, and lead fulfilling lives well into their later years. By encouraging ongoing engagement and autonomy, active aging empowers older adults to lead fulfilling lives while contributing to their communities. As a guiding principle, active aging not only influences individual well-being but also informs policies and initiatives aimed at supporting aging populations worldwide.

Successful Aging 2.0 and active aging are interconnected concepts that share common goals and principles but approach aging from slightly different perspectives. Table 15.1 shows the differences between the two concepts. Successful Aging 2.0 expands upon traditional notions of successful aging by incorporating a broader range of factors beyond physical health, such as social, psychologic, and environmental dimensions. It recognizes that aging successfully involves not only avoiding disease and disability but also maintaining social connections, cognitive function, and overall well-being. The relationship between these two concepts lies in their mutual emphasis on promoting holistic well-being and autonomy among older adults.

Successful Aging 2.0 acknowledges the importance of remaining socially connected and engaged in activities that are meaningful and fulfilling, aligning with the principles of active aging. Similarly, active aging supports the broader perspective of Successful Aging 2.0 by emphasizing the importance of social, psychologic, and environmental factors in shaping the aging experience.

As future LTC administrators, understanding these concepts equips you with the knowledge and perspective needed to develop comprehensive care plans that prioritize the well-being and autonomy of older adults. By incorporating principles of active aging and successful aging into your approach, you can create environments that promote healthy aging and enhance the quality of life for residents. Always keep these principles in mind when brainstorming innovations; ensuring that your strategies are grounded in fostering physical, mental, and social well-being; and supporting older adults in living fulfilling and independent lives.

TABLE 15.1 Active Aging Versus Successful Aging 2.0

ASPECT	ACTIVE AGING	SUCCESSFUL AGING 2.0
Definition	Process of optimizing opportunities for health, participation, and security to enhance quality of life as people age	Focuses on promoting positive outcomes and quality of life in later years
Emphasis	Maintaining physical, social, and mental well-being	Enhancing overall well-being and autonomy
Activities	Staying engaged physically and mentally	Participating in meaningful activities
Social Connections	Emphasized as a key aspect of active engagement	Recognized as important for overall well-being
Adaptability	Emphasizes adaptability and flexibility to changes	Acknowledges the diversity of aging experiences
Inclusivity	Promotes inclusivity regardless of abilities	May inadvertently overlook individuals with limitations
Perspective	Encourages individuals to lead fulfilling lives	Recognizes the potential for growth and thriving

STUDENT: "WHICH CARRIES MORE WEIGHT FOR HEALTHCARE ADMINISTRATION AND PUBLIC HEALTH—ACTIVE AGING OR SUCCESSFUL AGING 2.0—AND WHY?"

This is an excellent question because it helps us understand the broader implications of these aging concepts and prepares us to apply them effectively in our future roles. By examining the practical applications and impacts of active aging and Successful Aging 2.0, we can better tailor our approaches to meet the diverse needs of older adults, ensuring we prioritize their well-being and autonomy in all aspects of LTC.

Both active aging and Successful Aging 2.0 hold significant relevance for healthcare administration and public health, particularly for students working as public health practitioners in HCBS. However, the importance of these concepts may vary depending on the specific context and goals of healthcare systems and public health initiatives.

Active aging plays a crucial role in public health efforts aimed at promoting healthy aging and preventing age-related disabilities and chronic diseases. By encouraging individuals to remain physically, socially, and mentally active, active aging can help mitigate healthcare costs associated with age-related illnesses and enhance overall population health outcomes (Walker, 2002). For students working in HCBS promoting active aging may involve developing and implementing community-based programs and policies that support older adults in staying active and engaged in their communities (Hooker et al., 2005).

In contrast, Successful Aging 2.0 emphasizes the importance of fostering positive outcomes and quality of life for older adults, regardless of their health status or functional abilities. This concept recognizes the diverse needs and preferences of older adults and underscores the significance of person-centered care approaches that prioritize individual well-being and autonomy. For students working in healthcare administration, Successful Aging 2.0 may inform the development of age-friendly healthcare services and policies that support older adults in leading fulfilling and independent lives as they age (Lundy et al., 2021; Pohnert et al., 2023).

Ultimately, both active aging and Successful Aging 2.0 contribute to promoting healthy and fulfilling aging experiences for older adults. The relative importance of each concept in healthcare administration and public health may depend on factors such as population demographics, healthcare priorities, and available resources in a given context. Integrating both concepts into healthcare policies and programs can help address the multifaceted needs of aging populations and improve overall health outcomes for older adults.

STUDENT: "BEING A GEN Y OR Z, WHY SHOULD I CARE ABOUT PLANNING FOR LONG-TERM CARE?"

The intricacies of the LTC system highlight the widespread challenge of fragmentation, which arises from a multitude of factors. These include the presence of numerous providers, varied funding sources, intricate regulations, care continuity issues, and siloed healthcare delivery systems. Consequently, disparities persist in accessing and receiving quality care, alongside inefficiencies and less-than-optimal outcomes. Addressing this complex issue necessitates comprehensive efforts aimed at streamlining services, enhancing coordination, and advocating for integrated care models, ultimately bolstering care quality and continuity.

Moreover, it is essential to recognize that LTC is not governed solely by one-size-fits-all solutions. Rather, it is deeply influenced by various factors, including individual preferences, socioeconomic backgrounds, and geographic locations. Innovation emerges as a crucial tool in meeting the diverse needs of individuals within this complex landscape. This realization prompts us to reflect on our individual aging journeys and the evolving nature of LTC provision. Whether in the United States or elsewhere, actively engaging with this dynamic landscape becomes imperative for you as members of Gen Y and Gen Z.

To begin, assessing the suitability of current living environments for aging in place is paramount. This involves evaluating factors such as accessibility, safety features, and proximity to services. Establishing a robust support network comprising family, friends, and healthcare professionals is indispensable. Additionally, researching local community resources and support services for aging in place, reviewing financial situations, and exploring funding options such as LTC insurance and government assistance are vital steps. Proactively planning for aging in place paves the way for a more comfortable, independent, and fulfilling lifestyle as individuals age.

Navigating these steps may appear daunting, especially for those without a background in higher education. However, there are avenues for contribution, such as brainstorming innovations to facilitate the preparation process. This may include endeavors to reduce search times, conduct evidence-based research, or engage in volunteer work. As policymakers, distributing resources to aid individuals in planning for or accessing LTC is essential. By addressing these aspects collectively, we can work toward a future where aging is met with confidence and preparedness.

STUDENT: "SO, PROFESSOR, HOW DO I POSITION MYSELF AS A KEY PLAYER IN THE LONG-TERM CARE FIELD?"

To position oneself as a key player in the LTC field, the authors of the book offer insightful strategies that encompass various aspects of career development and industry engagement. These strategies are designed to empower individuals with the knowledge, skills, and experiences necessary to thrive in this dynamic and vital sector of healthcare. Here are some effective strategies to consider:

Education and training: Invest in relevant education and professional training beyond college. Pursuing degrees in healthcare administration, nursing, or social work provides essential foundational knowledge for understanding the complexities of LTC.

Advanced education in long-term care: Similarly, obtaining certifications such as licensed nursing home administrator (LNHA) or certified assisted living administrator (CALA) enhances your credentials and demonstrates expertise in the field. For example, completing a master of health administration (MHA) program with a concentration in LTC management prepares students for executive leadership roles within healthcare organizations.

Hands-on and leadership experience: Embark on a journey of practical learning by gaining hands-on experience through internships, volunteer programs, or entry-level positions within LTC settings such as Genesis HealthCare, Brookdale Senior Living, or local care facilities, which offer invaluable opportunities for mentorship and career advancement. These experiences enable the development of essential skills and insights into industry operations, while early leadership engagement within student organizations, volunteer groups, or part-time roles demonstrates initiative and potential for future success. Serving as officers of healthcare-focused student clubs, for instance, showcases leadership skills and organizational abilities, setting you apart in the competitive job market and illuminating your path toward professional triumphs.

Stay informed: Staying informed about industry trends involves engaging with relevant publications, attending webinars, and participating in discussions with industry experts. Organizations such as the American Health Care Association (AHCA; www.ahcancal.org), Vision Centre (www.visioncentre.org), or the National Association of Long Term Care Administrator Boards (NAB; www.nabweb.org) offer valuable insights into regulatory changes and best practices. For example, attending a webinar on the implementation of telehealth in LTC facilities can offer crucial insights into emerging trends and technologies shaping the industry. By actively engaging with these resources, individuals can remain informed and position themselves for success in the ever-evolving landscape of LTC.

Achieving and maintaining cultural competence: As the aging population becomes increasingly diverse, LTC providers and administrators must develop and sustain an awareness of and sensitivity to the varied preferences, traditions, and needs of the individuals they serve. This requires ongoing education, active engagement with different cultural communities, and the implementation of inclusive policies and practices that respect and honor the diverse cultures and backgrounds of residents. By fostering an environment of cultural competence, providers and administrators can ensure more personalized, respectful, and effective care for all individuals under their supervision.

STUDENT: "YOU KEEP REMINDING US ABOUT THE IMPORTANCE OF 'INNOVATIONS'. CAN YOU DISCUSS THE DRIVING FACTORS BEHIND GROUNDBREAKING INNOVATIONS?"

Innovation is a cornerstone of progress, particularly within the American context. As we have learned in Chapter 13, innovations often emerge in response to pressing needs or problems that demand solutions. Take, for instance, the printing press, which revolutionized book replication during the Renaissance to meet the growing demand for knowledge dissemination. Similarly, the internet was born out of the necessity for faster and more efficient communication across vast distances.

Furthermore, groundbreaking innovations typically build upon existing technologies or ideas. Gutenberg's printing press, drawing from earlier printing methods from Asia and Europe, significantly improved book replication with movable type. Likewise, the internet evolved from earlier networking technologies to become the global network we know today.

Contemporary research highlights that groundbreaking innovations often stem from a combination of factors. Rogers (2003) outlines four main elements in the diffusion of innovations. First, an innovation is defined by individuals or groups as a new idea, practice, or project perceived as such. Uncertainty about an innovation's consequences can hinder adoption, making it crucial to inform individuals about its pros and cons. Second, communication channels play a vital role, with interpersonal channels being more potent in influencing attitudes due to their social nature. Channels can be local or cosmopolite, each significant at different stages of the innovation–decision process. Third, time is an essential but often overlooked aspect of diffusion research. Including time in the study of innovation helps understand the innovation–diffusion process, adopter categorization, and rate of adoptions. Fourth, the social system, defined as a set of units working toward a common goal (see "Systems Thinking" in Chapter 12), influences the diffusion process. Social structure (see "social stratification" in Chapter 9), or the patterned arrangements within the system, affects individuals' innovativeness, a key criterion for categorizing adopters.

Understanding these elements sheds light on how innovations spread and are adopted within society. It is important to note that innovation is not confined to technologies but extends to creative solutions from various sources.

STUDENT: "HOW CAN INNOVATIONS ADDRESS PRESSING ISSUES LIKE HEALTHCARE QUALITY, STAFFING SHORTAGES, AND THE DEMAND FOR MORE HOMELIKE, LONG-TERM CARE OPTIONS? COULD YOU SHARE SPECIFIC EXAMPLES OF HOW INNOVATION IS RESHAPING LONG-TERM CARE?"

Certainly! In light of these pressing challenges, there has been a notable surge in both interest and investment in innovative strategies for long-term services and supports. The goal is to seamlessly integrate these services and amenities into the fabric of communities, enhancing accessibility, quality, and overall satisfaction for individuals requiring LTC. Importantly, this trend is not confined to the United States alone. Let us explore international perspectives on LTC to deepen our understanding and ignite inspiration for innovative solutions on a global scale.

Taiwan

Taiwan has taken proactive steps to implement technology-driven solutions aimed at supporting active aging, while placing a strong emphasis on maintaining quality and safety standards. Taiwan's *Long-Term Care 2.0* policy is centered on community-based care and aims to establish a comprehensive system catering to older adults and individuals with disabilities, prioritizing top-notch quality and safety standards (Chen & Fu, 2020). This strategy entails expanding HCBS, elevating care quality, and fostering active aging through initiatives such as home care, day centers, respite care, and assistive technology. The policy also entails the establishment of *community-based long-term care stations* (社區關懷據點), offering diverse support services, health screenings, exercise programs, and caregiver assistance to uphold rigorous quality and safety standards. Having a strong community-based network in mind, these measures reflect Taiwan's dedication to ensuring the well-being and independence of its aging population while providing robust support for caregivers. Figure 15.2 spotlights Taiwan's innovative practices, showcased alongside those from four countries, with a focus on enhancing visibility and awareness of caregiver issues (International Alliance of Carer Organizations, 2020). These practices effectively address caregivers' needs through integrated health and social care approaches.

Netherlands

De Hogeweyk, known as the "Dementia Village" in Weesp, Netherlands, stands as a pioneering model of care globally (Glass, 2014). Originating from a traditional LTC facility, its inception in 1993 was driven by staff recognizing the need for a more humane approach. With a focus on "life as usual," significant improvements were made, leading to enhanced satisfaction among residents, family, and staff. Subsequently funded with $22.5 million, De Hogeweyk opened its doors in 2008, offering a unique living experience for its 152 residents with severe dementia. The village

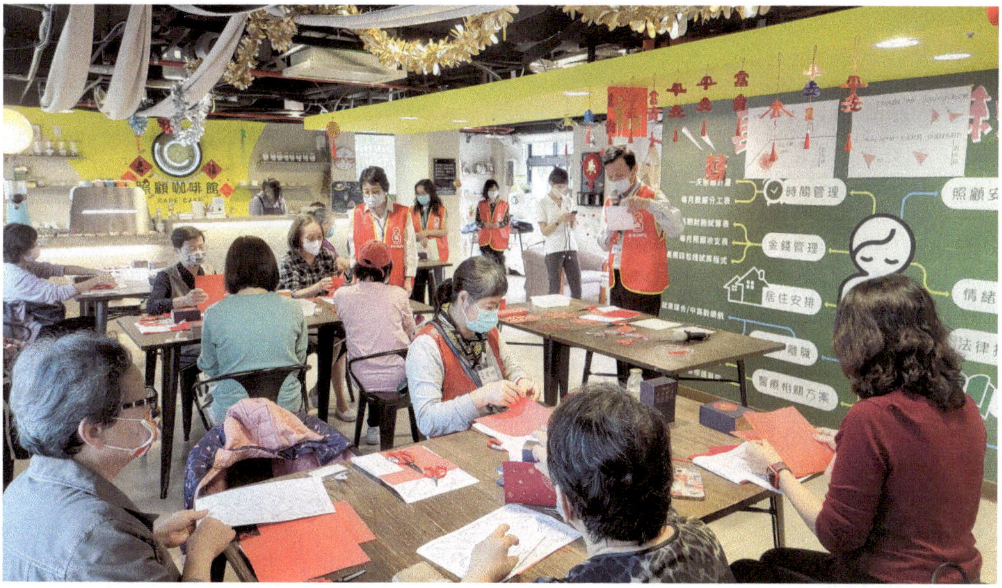

FIGURE 15.2. Care Café in Taipei City, Taiwan.

Note: The Taiwan Association of Family Caregivers innovates with its *Care Café* (照顧咖啡館) program, utilizing local resources to support caregivers. Through trust-building activities and respite programs, the initiative fosters innovation in caregiver support, aiming for nationwide recognition and contributing to LTC development for healthier communities.

comprises 23 small houses intentionally designed to foster a sense of community and safety while preserving the residents' dignity. Each house accommodates six to seven residents who share similar lifestyles, ensuring personalized care and meaningful interactions. Nonetheless, more research is needed to confirm the positive impact of small-scale homelike living (SSHL) facilities on older adults' physical functioning, social participation, and quality of life compared to conventional nursing homes (Krier et al., 2023).

The Netherlands has pioneered innovative approaches to eldercare, including the concept of *green care farms*. These farms offer older adults the opportunity to engage in meaningful activities such as gardening, animal care, and agricultural work, all within a natural and therapeutic setting. By promoting physical activity, social interaction, and a sense of purpose, green care farms contribute to the overall well-being and vitality of older participants (de Boer et al., 2017; Nowak et al., 2015).

Another notable innovation is *Buurtzorg*, meaning "neighborhood care" in Dutch. This community-based nursing model prioritizes holistic and personalized care for clients in their own homes (Gray et al., 2015). Buurtzorg revolutionizes healthcare delivery by organizing self-managed teams of nurses, typically consisting of 10 to 12 members, to provide comprehensive home care. This approach marks a departure from traditional *hierarchical* structures, empowering teams to make collective decisions regarding patient care, scheduling, and management without middle managers or supervisors. Collaboration is central to the Buurtzorg model, with nurses working closely together and with other healthcare professionals to ensure tailored and effective care. Supported by coaches who facilitate rather than dictate, Buurtzorg teams foster a culture of innovation, encouraging experimentation and the sharing of best practices.

Australia

Australia has implemented various *intergenerational programs* that bring together older adults and younger generations to foster mutual support, learning, and social connections. For example, "grandparent storytelling" programs involve older adults sharing their life experiences with schoolchildren, while initiatives such as "senior tech club" provide older adults with opportunities to learn about technology from younger mentors (MacCallum et al., 2010). These programs promote intergenerational understanding and cooperation while combating social isolation. However, further research is pivotal to discern the factors influencing older adults' engagement in intergenerational programs (Krisnan et al., 2023).

United States

The *age-friendly cities* initiative, launched by the WHO and AARP, has gained traction in various cities across the United States. This initiative aims to create urban environments that are accessible and inclusive for people of all ages, with a particular focus on older adults. Participating cities implement policies and infrastructure improvements to promote active aging, such as accessible transportation, pedestrian-friendly streets, and affordable housing options (Jeste et al., 2016). Key factors for successful age-friendly community development encompass robust leadership and governance, resource optimization, adherence to the age-friendly framework, collaboration across multiple sectors, rigorous monitoring and reporting of evaluation results, comprehensive summation, dissemination plans, and active engagement of older adults (Black & Oh, 2022).

The *Program of All-Inclusive Care for the Elderly* (PACE) is a comprehensive managed care program in the United States that provides medical, social, and LTC services to older adults who are eligible for nursing home care but prefer to live in the community (Hirth et al., 2009). PACE programs coordinate all aspects of care, including primary and specialty medical care, medications, and supportive services. However, the evidence on the effectiveness of PACE compared to other care programs for older adults is limited and inconclusive. While certain studies indicate superior outcomes for PACE participants, others show mixed results or no significant differences (Arku et al., 2022). Hence, there is a pressing need for more high-quality comparative effectiveness studies to gain a clearer understanding of which care models effectively meet the functional needs of older adults residing in U.S. communities.

The Green House Project (GHP) revolutionizes senior care with its intimate, homelike environment catering to those needing daily assistance. Diverging from conventional nursing homes or assisted living facilities, GHP fosters close-knit communities of 10 to 12 residents where meaningful relationships between residents and staff flourish. These homes mirror traditional residences with private rooms and shared spaces, promoting social interaction and a familial atmosphere (The Green House Project, n.d.). Rooted in person-centered care, the *Shahbaz* (plural: Shahbazim; i.e., caregivers) provide holistic, relationship-based support, prioritizing individual preferences and autonomy. Green House emphasizes overall wellness, offering tailored nutrition, social engagement, and meaningful activities, empowering residents to control their routines and care decisions. With a flat staffing model, direct care staff collaborate closely with residents and families, fostering transparency and trust, making Green House a compassionate and empowering alternative in senior care (Waters, 2021).

CAPABLE (**C**ommunity **A**ging in **P**lace—**A**dvancing **B**etter **L**iving for **E**lders) is a 10-session, home-based program involving an occupational therapist, nurse, and handyworker. It targets older adults' self-identified functional goals, enhancing their capacity and home environment (Szanton et al., 2011). By addressing basic and instrumental activities of daily living, fall efficacy, depression, pain management, and cost savings, CAPABLE aims to reduce disability and improve crucial outcomes. Successfully replicated in various settings, its innovation lies in tailoring services to individuals' needs, then delivering interprofessional care at home. This holistic approach prevents hospitalizations, relocations, or nursing home placements, resulting in significant cost savings (Szanton et al., 2021).

Papa (www.papa.com) is one of the emerging tech solutions designed to address societal isolation among seniors, a problem that has worsened due to the pandemic (Kotwal et al., 2021; National Academies of Sciences, Engineering and Medicine, 2020). It pairs older adults with vetted and trained companions known as "Papa pals." These companions provide a range of non-medical assistance that promotes overall well-being, including technology help, meal preparation, light housework, transportation, and social interaction. Recognizing the importance of accessible transportation, Papa has also partnered with Uber Health to ensure that seniors can attend doctor visits and engage in meaningful social activities without transportation barriers. The healthcare sector, including insurers, is increasingly recognizing the merit of innovative approaches such as Papa. Research has demonstrated its potential in lowering medical costs, increasing cancer screening rates, reducing readmissions, and cutting overall healthcare expenses (Papa, n.d.).

There exists a myriad of innovative technologies waiting to be introduced and explored further. From advanced artificial intelligence (AI)-driven diagnostics to groundbreaking telemedicine platforms, the landscape of healthcare innovation is vast and continually evolving. Additionally, wearable health monitoring devices, personalized medicine solutions, and virtual reality therapies are just a glimpse into the transformative potential of modern technology in healthcare. As we continue to push the boundaries of what's possible, these innovations promise to revolutionize our future patient care, enhance treatment outcomes, and reshape the LTC landscape for the better.

STUDENT: "THAT IS FANTASTIC! HOW DO I AS A COLLEGE STUDENT MAKE A DIFFERENCE IN LONG-TERM CARE?"

Regardless of your major, you possess unique skills and passions that can shape the future of LTC. For instance, if you are studying language studies, your expertise in linguistics offers numerous opportunities. From facilitating cross-cultural communication and providing translation services to offering cultural competence training and conducting research, your language proficiency can profoundly impact the quality of care for older adults. Similarly, if you are majoring in computer science, your technical knowledge can revolutionize LTC through innovative solutions. You can develop systems for managing healthcare data, enhance communication between healthcare professionals, or design assistive technologies tailored to the needs of older adults (O'Brien et al., 2020).

There are countless avenues for making a meaningful contribution to LTC. Embrace your skills and interests, and explore how you can leverage them to improve the lives of older adults. Your background is a valuable asset that can drive positive change in the LTC industry. To learn more about planning your career in LTC, refer to Case Study15.1.

Case Study 15.1 The Contribution of Language Study Background to Long-Term Care System Development

Dora, a linguistics graduate, joined a LTC facility as a language access coordinator. She implemented language proficiency assessments for staff members, developed multilingual communication materials, and organized cultural competence training workshops. Dora also established partnerships with local immigrant advocacy groups to provide additional support services for non–English-speaking residents. Through her efforts, the facility improved communication and cultural responsiveness, leading to enhanced resident satisfaction and better health outcomes.

Background

Language study encompasses a broad range of disciplines, including linguistics, language acquisition, translation, and cultural studies. While traditionally not associated with healthcare, individuals with a background in language study bring unique skills and perspectives that can significantly contribute to the development of the LTC system.

(*continued*)

Case Study 15.1 The Contribution of Language Study Background to Long-Term Care System Development (*continued*)

Contribution Areas

Cross-Cultural Communication

Individuals with a language study background possess proficiency in multiple languages and cultural awareness. In the context of LTC, they can facilitate communication between diverse groups of residents, caregivers, and healthcare professionals. Effective communication is essential for ensuring that the needs and preferences of older adults are understood and respected, ultimately improving the quality of care.

Translation and Interpretation Services

Language study experts are adept at translating complex medical terminology and interpreting for non–English-speaking residents. By providing accurate and culturally sensitive translation services, they bridge language barriers and ensure that older adults receive comprehensive care and information about their health status and treatment options.

Cultural Competence Training

Language study professionals can develop and deliver cultural competence training programs for LTC staff. These programs educate caregivers about cultural norms, values, and communication styles, enabling them to provide culturally competent care to diverse populations. By promoting cultural sensitivity and awareness, these initiatives foster a more inclusive and respectful care environment.

Literature and Research

Language study scholars can conduct research on language barriers and cultural factors affecting access to LTC services. Their findings can inform policy development and service delivery strategies aimed at addressing linguistic and cultural disparities in care. Additionally, they can contribute to the development of educational materials and resources tailored to diverse linguistic and cultural backgrounds.

Case Study Discussion Questions

1. What are some of the key challenges associated with providing high-quality care to LTC residents from diverse linguistic and cultural backgrounds? How can caregivers overcome these challenges to ensure that all residents receive culturally sensitive and appropriate care?
2. Why do you think individuals with a language study background are uniquely positioned to make an impact in the LTC system? Are there any other types of educational backgrounds or experiences that could be similarly beneficial in this context?
3. Can you think of any experiences or skills from your own background (educational or otherwise) that could be useful in the context of LTC? How do you think you could apply these skills to improve the quality of care for residents?

RECENT CHANGES TO THE OLDER AMERICANS ACT WARRANT ATTENTION FOR THEIR SIGNIFICANT IMPLICATIONS

In Chapter 2, the authors underscore the pivotal role of the Older Americans Act (OAA) in supporting community well-being, adapting to shifting healthcare contexts, and fostering inclusive environments for individuals of all ages as aging populations evolve.

BOX 15.1 Changes Made in the 2024 OAA Updates

- Part 1321: Grants to State and Community Programs on Aging—Title III of the OAA
- Part 1322: Grants to Indian Tribes and Native Hawaiian Grantees for Supportive, Nutrition, and Caregiver Services—Title VI of the OAA
- Part 1323: State Long-Term Care Ombudsman Program, Prevention of Elder Abuse, Neglect, and Exploitation, and State Legal Assistance Development—Title VII of the OAA
- Part 1324: Allotments for Vulnerable Elder Rights Protection Activities—Title VII of the OAA

OAA, Older Americans Act.

Source: Administration for Community Living. (2024, February 14). *Older Americans Act Regulations; Final Rule* [Federal Register, 89 FR 11566]. Department of Health & Human Services. https://www.govinfo.gov/content/pkg/FR-2024-02-14/pdf/2024-01913.pdf

However, it is crucial to note that the Administration for Community Living (ACL) recently issued a final rule on February 6, 2024, updating the regulations governing its OAA programs for the first time since 1988 (ACL, 2024; Box 15.1). This long-awaited update responds to the changing landscape of aging demographics and their associated needs. Effective as of March 15, 2024, with a compliance deadline for regulated entities set for October 1, 2025, these revisions aim to fortify the national aging network delivering OAA services and streamline program implementation.

The comprehensive overhaul reflects extensive collaboration across ACL teams to ensure clarity and support, particularly for underserved populations, drawing on insights gleaned from the challenges posed by the COVID-19 pandemic.

The final rule reaffirms existing requirements while introducing new provisions pertaining to fiscal policies, emergency flexibilities, and specific programs such as the family caregiver support program. Notable highlights of the 2024 OAA final rule include (ACL, 2024):

- clarifying requirements for state and area plans on aging,
- improving consistency between state and tribal OAA programs, and
- strengthening provisions for prioritizing individuals with the greatest social and economic needs.

These updates herald a new chapter in the delivery of OAA services, poised to better meet the evolving needs of older adults, enabling them to maintain independence and thrive within their homes and communities.

STUDENT: "PROFESSOR, HOW DO THE CHANGES TO THE OLDER AMERICANS ACT RELATE TO QUALITY AND SAFETY IN LONG-TERM CARE? IS THERE ANYTHING ELSE YOU'D LIKE TO REMIND ME?"

The recent changes to the OAA have indeed ushered in significant improvements in the standards of quality and safety within LTC facilities. These updates introduce stricter oversight measures, including more frequent inspections and robust reporting protocols, all aimed at ensuring strict compliance with safety standards. Notably, Part 1323 of the amended rule reinforces the State Long-Term Care Ombudsman Program, which serves as a vital advocate for the rights and well-being of residents in nursing homes and other LTC facilities. Moreover, there is a heightened focus on preventing elder abuse, neglect, and exploitation through enhanced programs, underscoring the commitment to safeguarding vulnerable older adults and upholding their dignity.

Furthermore, the updated regulations place a strong emphasis on caregiver training and support, recognizing the indispensable role they play in delivering high-quality care while adhering to safety standards. By fostering better coordination among various services, the revisions aim to streamline care delivery processes, thereby reducing the likelihood of errors and ultimately enhancing overall care quality. These collective enhancements significantly contribute to elevating the quality and safety of care provided to older adults in LTC settings.

In addition to enhancing quality and safety standards, the revised regulations underscore a broader commitment to addressing disparities in care. Notably, there is a robust emphasis on serving individuals with the greatest social and economic needs, including low-income minority older adults, those with limited English proficiency, and those residing in rural areas. It is crucial to consider the impact of these factors on access to and quality of care. Thorough review of the provisions outlined in Titles III, VI, and VII is essential, as they provide detailed insights into the various programs and services affected by these updates, facilitating a comprehensive understanding necessary for continued study and work in the field.

SUMMARY

This chapter commences by highlighting the paramount importance of quality and safety in LTC, emphasizing their profound influence on the well-being of older adults and the impetus for innovation within the field. It proceeds to explore a range of innovative and established strategies aimed at elevating standards in LTC, including person-centered approaches, technological advancements, interdisciplinary collaboration, and the promotion of HCBS, all aimed at enhancing the overall experience for older adults and fostering sustainable, inclusive environments for aging populations. Additionally, the chapter delves into the pivotal role of the OAA in addressing the evolving needs of aging populations and adapting to changing healthcare contexts, emphasizing its significance in facilitating independence for older adults within their homes and communities. The recent comprehensive update to OAA regulations is introduced as a crucial endeavor to enhance the national aging network, with a focus on improving program implementation and incorporating lessons learned from the challenges posed by the COVID-19 pandemic.

END-OF-CHAPTER RESOURCES

DISCUSSION QUESTIONS

1. How would you introduce a model such as Buurtzorg to your peers, highlighting its distinctive features and suggesting adaptations for the U.S. healthcare system? Additionally, what strategies would you recommend for assessing its effectiveness after implementation?

2. How can interdisciplinary collaboration in LTC improve the quality of care provided to aging adults? What are some potential challenges to achieving effective interdisciplinary care?

3. Successful aging has become a widely discussed topic in recent years. What are some of the key factors that contribute to successful aging? How can we prioritize and promote these factors in the LTC industry?

4. Considering your major or background, how do you envision leveraging your skills and expertise to make a meaningful contribution to LTC, as outlined in Case Study 15.1? Share your thoughts with your peers and discuss potential strategies for utilizing your unique abilities to enhance the quality of care for older adults.

5. How can we ensure the sustainability and scalability of innovative approaches to LTC, as emphasized by the authors? Reflect on recent examples of innovative solutions in the LTC industry that have shown promise. Discuss potential strategies for fostering sustainability and scalability while maintaining effectiveness and quality of care.
6. Health and safety are top priorities in LTC settings. What are some of the biggest challenges to maintaining high standards of quality and safety in LTC, and how can we address these challenges effectively? How can we empower care providers to prioritize quality and safety in their daily work?

SPRINGER PUBLISHING CONNECT™ | A robust set of instructor resources designed to supplement this text is located at http://connect.springerpub.com/content/book/978-0-8261-4935-0. Qualifying instructors may request access by emailing textbook@springerpub.com.

REFERENCES

Administration for Community Living. (2024, February 14). *Older Americans Act regulations: Final rule* [Federal Register, 89 FR 11566]. Department of Health & Human Services. https://www.govinfo.gov/content/pkg/FR-2024-02-14/pdf/2024-01913.pdf

Arku, D., Felix, M., Warholak, T., & Axon, D. R. (2022). Program of all-inclusive care for the elderly (PACE) versus other programs: A scoping review of health outcomes. *Geriatrics*, *7*(2), 31. https://doi.org/10.3390/geriatrics7020031

Black, K., & Oh, P. (2022). Assessing age-friendly community progress: What have we learned? *The Gerontologist*, *62*(1), 6–17. https://doi.org/10.1093/geront/gnab051

Calasanti, T. (2016). Combating ageism: How successful is successful aging? *The Gerontologist*, *56*(6), 1093–1101. https://doi.org/10.1093/geront/gnv076

Chen, C. F., & Fu, T. H. (2020). Policies and transformation of long-term care system in Taiwan. *Annals of Geriatric Medicine and Research*, *24*(3), 187–194. https://doi.org/10.4235/agmr.20.0038

de Boer, B., Hamers, J. P., Zwakhalen, S. M., Tan, F. E., Beerens, H. C., & Verbeek, H. (2017). Green care farms as innovative nursing homes, promoting activities and social interaction for people with dementia. *Journal of the American Medical Directors Association*, *18*(1), 40–46. https://doi.org/10.1016/j.jamda.2016.10.013

Glass, A. P. (2014). Innovative seniors housing and care models: What we can learn from the Netherlands. *Seniors Housing and Care Journal*, *22*(1), 74–81. https://www.oldertenants.org.au/content/innovative-seniors-housing-and-care-models-what-we-can-learn-the-netherlands

Gray, B. H., Sarnak, D. O., & Burgers, J. S. (2015, May 29). *Home care by self-governing nursing teams: The Netherlands' Buurtzorg model*. The Commonwealth Fund. https://www.commonwealthfund.org/publications/case-study/2015/may/home-care-self-governing-nursing-teams-netherlands-buurtzorg-model

The Green House Project. (n.d.). Elders/family members. Retrieved May 2, 2024, from https://thegreenhouseproject.org/elders-family-members

Hirth, V., Baskins, J., & Dever-Bumba, M. (2009). Program of all-inclusive care (PACE): Past, present, and future. *Journal of the American Medical Directors Association*, *10*(3), 155–160. https://doi.org/10.1016/j.jamda.2008.12.002

Hooker, S. P., Seavey, W., Weidmer, C. E., Harvey, D. J., Stewart, A. L., Gillis, D. E., Nicholl, K. L., & King, A. C. (2005). The California active aging community grant program: Translating science into practice to promote physical activity in older adults. *Annals of Behavioral Medicine*, *29*(3), 155–165. https://doi.org/10.1207/s15324796abm2903_1

International Alliance of Carer Organizations. (2020). *Carer Café: Recognising and connecting carers through a grassroots approach*. https://internationalcarers.org/wp-content/uploads/2020/08/IACO-ICP-TAIWAN_web.pdf

Jeste, D. V., Blazer II, D. G., Buckwalter, K. C., Cassidy, K. L. K., Fishman, L., Gwyther, L. P., Levin, S. M., Phillipson, C., Rao, R. R., Schmeding, E., Vega, W. A., Avanzino, J. A., Glorioso, D. K., & Feather, J. (2016). Age-friendly communities initiative: Public health approach to promoting successful aging. *The American Journal of Geriatric Psychiatry, 24*(12), 1158–1170. https://doi.org/10.1016/j.jagp.2016.07.021

Katz, S., & Calasanti, T. (2015). Critical perspectives on successful aging: Does it "appeal more than it illuminates"? *The Gerontologist, 55*(1), 26–33. https://doi.org/10.1093/geront/gnu027

Kotwal, A. A., Holt-Lunstad, J., Newmark, R. L., Cenzer, I., Smith, A. K., Covinsky, K. E., Escueta, D. P., Lee, J. M., & Perissinotto, C. M. (2021). Social isolation and loneliness among San Francisco Bay Area older adults during the COVID-19 shelter-in-place orders. *Journal of the American Geriatrics Society, 69*(1), 20–29. https://doi.org/10.1111/jgs.16865

Kirsnan, L., Kosiol, J., Golenko, X., Radford, K., & Fitzgerald, J. A. (2023). Barriers and enablers for enhancing engagement of older people in intergenerational programs in Australia. *Journal of Intergenerational Relationships, 21*(3), 360–379. https://doi.org/10.1080/15350770.2022.2065400

Krier, D., de Boer, B., Hiligsmann, M., Wittwer, J., & Amieva, H. (2023). Evaluation of dementia-friendly initiatives, small-scale homelike residential care, and dementia village models: A scoping review. *Journal of the American Medical Directors Association, 24*(7), 1020–1027.e1. https://doi.org/10.1016/j.jamda.2023.03.024

Lundy, J., Hayden, D., Pyland, S., Berg-Weger, M., Malmstrom, T. K., & Morley, J. E. (2021). An age-friendly health system. *Journal of the American Geriatrics Society, 69*(3), 806–812. https://doi.org/10.1111/jgs.16959

MacCallum, J., Palmer, D., Wright, P., Cumming-Potvin, W., Brooker, M., & Tero, C. (2010). Australian perspectives: Community building through intergenerational exchange programs. *Journal of Intergenerational Relationships, 8*(2), 113–127. https://doi.org/10.1080/15350771003741899

Martin, P., Kelly, N., Kahana, B., Kahana, E., Willcox, B. J., Willcox, D. C., & Poon, L. W. (2015). Defining successful aging: A tangible or elusive concept? *The Gerontologist, 55*(1), 14–25. https://doi.org/10.1093/geront/gnu044

Martinson, M., & Berridge, C. (2015). Successful aging and its discontents: A systematic review of the social gerontology literature. *The Gerontologist, 55*(1), 58–69. https://doi.org/10.1093/geront/gnu037

National Academies of Sciences, Engineering and Medicine. (2020). *Social isolation and loneliness in older adults: Opportunities for the health care system*. National Academies Press. https://www.ncbi.nlm.nih.gov/books/NBK557974/

Nowak, S. J., Molema, C. C., Baan, C. A., Oosting, S. J., Vaandrager, L., Hop, P., & De Bruin, S. R. (2015). Decentralisation of long-term care in the Netherlands: The case of day care at green care farms for people with dementia. *Ageing & Society, 35*(4), 704–724. https://doi.org/10.1017/S0144686X13000937

O'Brien, K., Liggett, A., Ramirez-Zohfeld, V., Sunkara, P., & Lindquist, L. A. (2020). Voice-controlled intelligent personal assistants to support aging in place. *Journal of the American Geriatrics Society, 68*(1), 176–179. https://doi.org/10.1111/jgs.16217

Papa. (n.d.). *Research*. Retrieved May 10, 2024, from https://www.papa.com/resources/research

Pohnert, A. M., Schiltz, N. K., Pino, L., Ball, S., Duffy, E. G., McCormack, M. E., Oliver, B., Patterson, A., Pelton, L., & Dolansky, M. A. (2023). Achievement of age-friendly health systems committed to care excellence designation in a convenient care health care system. *Health Services Research, 58*(Suppl 1), 89–99. https://doi.org/10.1111/1475-6773.14071

Rogers, E. M. (2003). *Diffusion of innovations* (5th ed.). Simon & Schuster.

Rowe, J. W., & Kahn, R. L. (1987). Human aging: Usual and successful. *Science, 237*(4811), 143–149. https://doi.org/10.1126/science.3299702

Rowe, J. W., & Kahn, R. L. (1997). Successful aging. *The Gerontologist, 37*(4), 433–440. https://doi.org/10.1093/geront/37.4.433

Rowe, J. W., & Kahn, R. L. (2015). Successful Aging 2.0: Conceptual expansions for the 21st century. *Journals of Gerontology Series B: Psychological Sciences and Social Sciences, 70*(4), 593–596. https://doi.org/10.1093/geronb/gbv025

Szanton, S. L., Leff, B., Li, Q., Breysse, J., Spoelstra, S., Kell, J., Purvis, J., Xue, Q. L., Wilson, J., & Gitlin, L. N. (2021). CAPABLE program improves disability in multiple randomized trials. *Journal of the American Geriatrics Society, 69*(12), 3631–3640. https://doi.org/10.1111/jgs.17383

Szanton, S. L., Thorpe, R. J., Boyd, C., Tanner, E. K., Leff, B., Agree, E., Xue, Q. L., Allen, J. K., Seplaki, C. L., Weiss, C. O., Guralnik, J. M., & Gitlin, L. N. (2011). Community aging in place, advancing better living for elders: A bio-behavioral-environmental intervention to improve function and health-related quality of life in disabled older adults. *Journal of the American Geriatrics Society*, *59*(12), 2314–2320. https://doi.org/10.1111/j.1532-5415.2011.03698.x

United Nations. (1982). *Report of the World Assembly on Aging*. https://www.un.org/esa/socdev/ageing/documents/Resources/VIPEE-English.pdf

Walker, A. (2002). A strategy for active ageing. *International Social Security Review*, *55*(1), 121–139. https://doi.org/10.1111/1468-246X.00118

Waters, R. (2021). The big idea behind a new model of small nursing homes. *Health Affairs (Project Hope)*, *40*(3), 378–383. https://doi.org/10.1377/hlthaff.2021.00081

World Health Organization. (2002). *Active ageing: A policy framework*. https://iris.who.int/handle/10665/67215

Index